Endogenous Knowledge: Research Trails

Edited by
Paulin J. Hountondji

CODESRIA BOOK SERIES

Endogenous Knowledge: Research Trails

First published in 1997 by CODESRIA

CODESRIA is the Council for the Development of Social Science Research in Africa, headquartered in Senegal. It is an independent organisation whose principal objectives are facilitating research, promoting research-based publishing and creating multiple fora geared towards the exchange of views and information among African scholars. Its correspondence address is:

B.P. 3304, Dakar, Senegal.

ISBN 2-86978-040-0 (Soft Cover)
2-86978-041-9 (Hard Cover)

Translated by Ayi Kwesi Armah

Cover designed by Ousmane Ndiaye Dago

Typeset by Marie Therese Coron/Diouf, CODESRIA

Printed by Antony Rowe Ltd, Chippenham, Wiltshire

Distributors: ABC, 27 Park End Street, Oxford OX1 1HU

CODESRIA would like to express its gratitude to the Swedish International Development Co-operation Agency (SIDA), the Rockefeller Foundation, the International Development Research Centre (IDRC), the Ford Foundation, the Canergie Corporation, the European Union, the Norwegian Ministry of Foreign Affairs and the Danish Agency for International Development (DANIDA), the Dutch Government and the Government of Senegal for support of its research and publication activities.

Contents

Part III - Medicine and Pharmacology

Part IV - Forms of Transmission

Notes on Authors

Alexis B. A. Adandé: Teaches archaeology at the National University of Benin since 1978. PhD thesis on the History of material cultures (University of Paris I), and has written many articles on archaeology, history, museology and pedagogy. Secretary General of the Benin Committee of the International Council of Museums (ICOM) from 1987 to 1990, and Chair since 1973 of the West African Association of Archaeology. Currently involved in archaeological work in the Mono valley (at the frontier of Benin and Togo), in the Ouéssé region (Central region of Benin) and in Ouidah, the old city of slave trade.

Théodore Comlan Adjido: Doctor of medicine, he graduated from Leningrad University and specialised in Clinical psychiatry and electroencephalography in Paris. Since 1980, teaches at the Faculty of Health Sciences of the National University of Benin. Author of several articles on suicide, migrants, mental health, body language, psychosis, witchcraft in a law abiding state, drug addiction, etc. He is currently head of the National University Hospital of Psychiatry in Cotonou.

Abel Afouda: Moscow trained Hydrotechnical engineer, holds a PhD in Hydrodynamics and a *Doctorat d'Etat* in mechanics from Toulouse University. Author of several articles on hydrology and climatology. Senior lecturer in the Department of Mathematics at the National University of Benin and since 1990.

Gualbert René Ahyi: Psychiatrist from the school of Dakar-Fann (of Professor Henri Collomb) *Agrégé* in Psychiatry in 1980, and author of several articles. Head of the National University Hospital and of the Psychiatric Unit of the Faculty of Health Sciences at the National University of Benin.

Gbénoukpo Dah-Lokonon-Bodehou: PhD holder in ethnopsychiatry and author of several articles. Lectures in psychology, National University of Benin.

Bienvenu Akoha: PhD holder in African linguistics on the *fon-gbe* (University of Paris III, 1980 and 1991). Several articles and works in African languages, pictograms and other non alphabetical types of writing. Lectures at the National University of Benin, and serves as Director of the Benin Centre for Foreign Languages (CEBELAE).

François Comlan Dossou: PhD holder and author of many articles in philosophy and history of sciences. Former Dean of the Faculty of Arts at the National University of Benin.

Victor Houndonougbo: Doctorate degree in number analysis, and author of several articles in algebra and statistics. Lectures algebra at the National University of Benin. And since 1987 Director of the integrated teachers' training college of Parakou.

Paulin J. Hountondji: Alumnus of *Ecole Normale Supérieure de Paris*, and *Agrégé* in Philosophy. PhD Thesis on Husserl and has widely published in scholarly journals including *Dioguène, Présence Africaine, les Cahiers philosophiques africains* (Lubumbashi), *Thought and Practice* (Nairobi), *Quest* (Lusaka), *Genève-Afrique, la Revue sénégalaise de philosophie*, etc. Author of *Sur la "philososphie africaine": critique de l'ethnophilosophie*, translated into English, Serbo-Croat and German. Taught at the University of Besançon (France), at Lovanium University in Kinshasa, at the National University of Zaire, Lubumbashi Campus. Since 1972 lectures at the National University of Benin.

Henry-Valère Kiniffo: *Agrégé* in surgery (1970), and Senior lecturer at the University of Tours. He currently teaches at the National University of Benin and served as Dean of Faculty of Health Sciences from 1981 to 1987. Secretary General from 1988 to 1992 of the African and Malagasy Council for Higher Education (CAMES) in Ouagadougou (Burkina Faso). Associate member of the French Academy of Surgery, and of the International Academy of Francophone Scientists; WHO expert (Geneva and Brazzaville). He is author of several articles in specialized medical journals including *la Revue française de neurologie, le Journal de chirurgie, la Revue du praticien, le Journal de chirurgie plastique et reconstructive, le Bulletin de l'IFAN.*

Pierre Goudjinou Metinhoue: Wrote a PhD thesis on *Le regard des européens sur l'Afrique et les africains aux XV^{é} et XVI^{é} siécles* (University of Paris I-Sorbonne), and other publications on the history of material techniques, namely pottery. Head of the Department of History, National University of Benin from 1984 to 1987 in Cotonou.

Jean-Dominique Penel: Member of the ethnolinguistics research team of the African Studies Unit, University of Paris. Taught for several years at the University of Bangui and at the University of Niamey, Department of Philosophy. Currently teaching psychopedagogy in Djibouti, he has widely written on ethnosciences, epistemology and the philosophy of sciences, including *Anthologie de la Poésie centraficaine,* and a work in two volumes on the literature of Niger, *Rencontre.*

Simone Guiges, épouse de Souza: Doctor in natural sciences, post-doctorate work in Botany (Paris 1979). Author of *Flore du Bénin* in three volumes, *La famille de Souza au Bénin-Togo* (Cotonou 1992). Author of articles in botany in several specialised journals, also Senior lecturer at the National University of Benin, and since 1993 lectures at the Aix-Marseille University (France) .

Toussaint Yaovi Tchitchi: Doctoral Thesis on *la systématique de l'ajagbe* (University of Paris III-Sorbonne nouvelle, 1984) and several articles and studies on African linguistics. Teaches at the National University of Benin and proceeds with his works at the National Centre for Applied Linguistics (CENALA).

Introduction: Recentring Africa

Paulin J. Hountondji

The Logic of Extroversion

The fact bears repeating: in the fields of science and technology, Third World countries, especially those in Black Africa, are tied hand and foot to the apron strings of the West.[1] Of the degree of this dependence we are sometimes only hazily aware. African researchers, as long as they narrow their vision to take in only individual performance and careers, see little wrong with the present situation. Some see nothing wrong at all. The most critical may deplore shortages of funds, equipment and other material resources. But they might not see this lack of resources, taken in isolation, as necessarily catastrophic. It could be simply symptomatic of the fact that science in Africa is in its teething period, that compared to the scientific establishments of the great industrial centres it is a latecomer, and that given time, the continent might naturally make up its handicap, as the urge to scientific excellence takes hold in Africa, nurtured by our existing institutions, within the framework of intellectual production relationships as they exist today.

A closer look reveals that this sanguine scenario is much too simple. We need to look beyond merely quantitative comparisons. We need to go beyond appraisals of the work of isolated individual scientists, beyond assessments of the output of particular research teams. We need to look farther than evaluations of the competitive acumen of unique, outstanding research centres and scientific laboratories, probing until we hit the root of the problem. Where, for instance, does all the equipment used for research come from? How are research topics selected? On what social needs or other practical requirements are they based, directly or indirectly? Where on earth are these needs felt? Who in reality are the intended beneficiaries of this research? Where will its findings end up?

Where and how are the data produced dispatched, stored, capitalized? How do they get translated into practical applications? What complex ties link our research establishments to industry in particular and the business world in general? In addressing these questions, we shall need at every step to ask: What is the purpose of this research? Who benefits from it? How does it fit into the society producing it? And to what extent is this society able to take charge of its findings?

Once we approach the issue from this standpoint, it becomes clear that the difference between scientific work in Africa and in the industrialized metropoles is not only quantitative but also qualitative; not merely a matter of degree or of levels of development, but also a question of fundamental attitudes and operational modes. For here, research is an activity oriented outwards, focused on the external world, ordered by and subordinate to external needs. Its focus is not inward. Its primary purpose is not, as it should be, to address issues raised, directly or indirectly, by African society itself.[2]

Ultimately, then, the Third World is scientifically dependent in the same way as it is economically dependent. Situated in the context of its historical origins, this ideational dependence is one more manifestation of the steady integration of the Third World into the world-wide process of intellectual production managed and controlled by the Northern countries.[3]

As everybody knows, in colonial days, conquered territories served as economic reservoirs from which metropolitan factories drew the resources they needed. What is less well known is the fact that the economic linkage had a scientific counterpart, and that metropolitan scientific establishments also tapped raw materials from the colonies. For colonies were no less than immense strove of new information, gathered as raw data for transmission to metropolitan laboratories and research centres, the only establishments empowered and equipped to process them, interpret them, spin them out into hypotheses and theories, before integrating them into the ordered, comprehensive system of scientifically recognised and acknowledged data.

In other words, a standard feature of economic activity in colonial territories was the practical absence of industry. An equally standard feature of scientific activity was a howling absence of theoretical work.

Just as there were no colonial factories, there were no colonial laboratories or think tanks. Now generally speaking, advances in all branches of knowledge, whether they belong to the natural sciences, the social sciences or the humanities, necessarily begin in laboratories, broadly defined as venues for the systematic processing of intellectual and scientific knowledge.[4]

Colonies, the powers that be supposed, could have no earthly use for places specially equipped and outfitted for conceptual work. Quality libraries would be out of place there. As for the technical apparatus necessary for scientific experimentation — the transformation of crude data into tested knowledge — it was too complicated for the colonies. Meanwhile metropolitan laboratories fetched precious new information from the colonies, exploiting priceless opportunities to enrich their stores of knowledge, to advance their research work, to rise to encyclopaedic, universal heights in their quest for knowledge, and to enhance their practical mastery over the human environment.

Apart from providing raw materials, colonies also served as outlets for industrial and other products from the metropolitan countries. That much is well known. But here again a parallel fact has escaped notice: colonies also served as outlets for the output of metropolitan scientific research establishments. In the colonial past hawkers in Dahomean markets sold Palmolive soap made in France from Dahomean palm oil; they still do today.[5] Similarly, in colonial times, teachers in Dahomean schools used textbooks on tropical geography (or even on the geography of Dahomey) produced in France using information gathered in Dahomey or in other tropical countries, and processed in the workshops of the French National Cartographic Institute in Paris. Dahomey is now Benin, but geography teachers still use textbooks and atlases made in France to teach students about their own country.

Another aspect of the same process was and is the importation of rolling stock, cars and various types of equipment and machinery, the product of the technological application and industrial use of knowledge accumulated in the metropolitan countries. Colonies specialized in the consumption of scientific knowledge and products, in much the same way that they specialized in the consumption of finished industrial goods. In both cases the commodities were imported. The local population, while perfectly aware that they came from abroad, knew little about the places where they were produced, or how they were manufactured. Little wonder, then, that they saw them as surreal artefacts beyond their understanding, magically dumped into their daily lives.

It would be worthwhile to make a detailed study of the resulting culture of scientific consumerism in the peripheral countries, to measure its scope and to make statistical assessments of the discrepancy between the volume of imported information and the more or less embryonic output of the local scientific establishment. Such a study could provide precise indications of the degree of scientific and technological dependence in various countries, or in various sectors within the same country. It would be equally enlightening to analyze the nature and relative importance of raw data exported from the colonies to the research centres of the metropolitan countries, and to compare this flow of unprocessed intellectual resources with the flow of raw material resources exported from these same countries to the factories of the metropolitan countries. That done, the next step would be to establish a set of handy evaluative criteria for distinguishing between the two categories of 'primary resources'. This would be a complicated task. After all, even industrial raw materials are sometimes given a preliminary 'scientific' going-over before they undergo actual processing in the factories.

Lastly, from a historical and epistemological viewpoint, it would be intriguing to assess the debt European science owes to the Third World, the nature and scope of knowledge resulting from the theoretical processing of the voluminous quantities of fresh data extracted from there, the real function of the new disciplines based on that knowledge (tropical geography, tropical agriculture, African sociology, anthropology, etc.), and the shifts and shake-outs caused in old disciplines by these new discoveries.

The problems touched on here are complex and we cannot here presume to solve them. What we intend is to note, as a starting move, the practical parallelism between the complementary roles of colonial and metropolitan economies, on the one hand, and the complementary functions of colonial and metropolitan science and scholarship, on the other. In both cases the analogy of extraction is apt. In the first instance, there is the extraction of material resources from colonial mines and plantations at the periphery to supply metropolitan factories. In the second, there is the siphoning of information from the Third World to feed metropolitan universities and research centres.

Apt though it is, the analogy is no doubt imperfect. For one thing, the export of information does not in itself make the source country any poorer. The export of gold, ivory, palm oil or groundnuts certainly does. Still, given our central focus, this difference is of minor importance. As a matter of fact, what is involved here is much more significant than this secondary difference. Beyond the aptness of the analogy, there is also the fact that two forms of extraction — material and intellectual — which are in a more profound sense not discrete realities but two sides of the same coin. The name of that coin is accumulation on a world scale.

For scientific activity can be conceptualized as a specific mode of economic activity. It is one more productive activity, and the fact that the artefacts produced are intellectual concepts instead of material commodities does nothing to invalidate the point. It was altogether natural, given such a perspective, for the physical, geographical annexation of the Third World and its integration into the world capitalist system through the slave trade and colonialism to go hand in hand with its intellectual annexation and integration. It was altogether logical for the pillage of material resources to go arm in arm with intellectual and scientific exploitation, the extortion of esoteric and other useful information, and the purloining of artistic treasure to stuff metropolitan museums.[6]

But let us warn against an easy mistake. We shall have missed our aim completely if all we achieve with this historical note were to swell the flood of facile, belly-aching rhetoric that has become such a fixture of intellectual discourse in Africa, that copious rhetoric which enables us to blame others for all our ailments. Yesterday, the blame-bearers were imperialism, colonialism and neo-colonialism. Today they are called the World Bank and the International Monetary Fund. Tomorrow, no doubt, the same devil will sport new names. For our part, we think the point is not so much to cast blame as to understand the mechanism involved, and then to share our understanding. The mechanisms are operative to this day and they will continue into the future shrouded in mist unless we take pains to elucidate them within a historical perspective. We hold that there is no such thing as innate underdevelopment. Underdevelopment is always the outcome of historical processes. Likewise, scientific activity in Third World countries, admittedly obeys the same historical rules, and is inseparably linked to economic life. Still, it is also historically true that human beings invariably bear some responsibility for what happens to them. Often, the accuser's rhetoric merely camouflages an inadequate response, a subtle acquiescence in mediocrity.

What we need to do is to observe reality with clear sight and analyze it with clear logic, while staying detached from the fashionable rhetoric of the day, the we-are-the-world verbiage which, not content to acknowledge integration into the world market as a fact of current life, presents it as the only salutary path open to the Third World. We keep our distance, equally, from the lazy, perennially whining romanticism of the left. For in our opinion, what we need to do is simply have the courage to face reality with open eyes, a minimum of prejudice and preconceived ideas, and a firm determination to understand.

We have by all means left behind the heyday of the colonial pact, when economic life in our countries was totally devoid of industry. By the same token, scientific activity in our countries is no longer marked by an absolute lack of theoretical facilities and endeavour. In countries that were formerly colonies, there are now factories, universities, research laboratories and institutes. Some are admirably equipped. The problem remains, however, that the increase of factories has not resulted in any genuine development. In the best cases it has merely led to 'growth without development', to use Samir Amin's cogent phrase. The installation of vehicle assembly plants and similar industrial units has done nothing to change old extroverted economic patterns. In the main, neo-colonial industry is tied to the needs of peripheral bourgeoisies. Such needs are, fundamentally, no different from those of metropolitan bourgeoisies. The vocation of neo-colonial industry is to turn out luxury consumer items for privileged minorities. It does not care about producing consumer goods for the masses. It is therefore incapable of serving the social advancement of the majority of the population. Yet that service is the core process of real development.

Mutatis mutandis, the multiplication of facilities for intellectual and scientific production in the peripheral countries (universities, research centres, libraries, etc.) has so far mainly served to facilitate the export of information. It has thus intensified data outflow, accelerated the revelation of esoteric lore, pushed 'traditional' knowledge to the fringes of respectability, and enhanced the slow but inexorable integration of the entire proto-scientific and scientific legacy of the South, along with any other useful information, into a process of intellectual production on a world scale managed and controlled by the North. In plain words, the scientific facilities of the Third World, like vehicle assembly plants, also operate in the manner of import-substitution structures. They do nothing to end the outward orientation of Third World countries. Instead, they reinforce it, deepening the dependence of the periphery on the centre.

Let us look at selected indices of this extroversion:

1. In our countries, scientific work depends largely on the use of apparatus imported from the centre. We have never produced a microscope, to say nothing of the increasingly sophisticated equipment needed for leading-edge research today. Thus we see the first link in the intellectual chain — the manufacture of research apparatus, the production of the means of scientific production — slip through our fingers from the word go.[7]
2. Our intellectual work is to a large extent dependent on journals, libraries, archives, publishing houses and other support facilities in the North. In a more general sense, it is dependent on structures designed for the storage, preservation and dissemination of research findings. These are the facilities where the memory of humanity is physically stored. Most are concentrated in the North. Admittedly, over the last few decades, countries in the South have made tremendous progress. Credit must be given to those who have worked to create university annals, scholarly journals and various other publications, along with increasingly business-like publishing houses. Still, these advances are far from adequate to reverse old extroverted trends. Witness the fact that scholarly publications in the South still have their most numerous and reliable readership in the North. There is no point bewailing the fact. It needs to be observed, analyzed, and understood.
3. Here we come to the issue of theoretical extroversion, strictly defined. What it means is that the work of our scholars and intellectuals is always much better known and read in the North than in the South. Now this could be considered a purely external reality. What makes the situation worse is that our own intellectuals invariably internalize

it, going so far as to modify the content and even the orientation of their work, choosing research topics and design models in accordance with external norms. In this way, Third World researchers tend to let themselves be guided in their scholarly work by European expectations and concerns, since their readership is to all intents European.

4. One consequence of this theoretical extroversion is that research in the peripheral countries is most often focused on the immediate environment. Tied to the local scene, it is trapped in particularistic details, unable and unambitious to break through to the level of universals. At first glance, it might appear odd that we present this local focus as an index of intellectual extroversion. After all, it would seem instead to indicate the independence of researchers in the South from the main topics of research in the North. In other words, it would seem to signify that researchers in the South are more interested in addressing issues of direct consequences to their own societies. The truth is sadder. For when we look at the general sweep of intellectual and scientific history, we see that specialist territorial disciplines are so many more European products, and that at their inception they were tailored to the satisfaction of Europe's practical and theoretical needs. African Studies, for instance, in all its professional and ideological ramifications, truth to tell, belongs to the roster of European inventions. African researchers, content to say within the confines of that discipline by that token accept the role of well-educated informants serving European scientists and intellectuals in subaltern positions. It is perfectly legitimate for Southern researchers to focus primarily on their own societies. But when that focus becomes crudely exclusive, it may lead researchers into fearsome pitfalls. For then they may become obsessed with immediate realities, afraid to take wing and fly into challenging intellectual realms. Then they become intellectually ingrown, and thus miss an indispensable phase in the well-rounded intellectual itinerary: the independent creation of theoretical models, the making of comprehensive conceptual designs which later facilitate the accurate understanding of particular details as such.[8]

5. Scientific extroversion may also originate from more down-to-earth considerations, and have a more practical impact. It is quite possible

to find situations in which choices of research focus are not just indirectly conditioned by the concerns of a European readership, but are directly imposed, with no ifs, buts or nuances, by the imperatives of a frankly extroverted economy. Not so long ago, agronomic research in Africa was a glaring case in point. For the work done by most agronomic research institutes was principally concerned with improving the cultivation of such export crops as oil palm, coffee, cocoa, groundnuts and cotton. These were the crops that went to feed the factories of the North, or the few 'import-substitution' factories scattered here and there in the South. Food crops, the staples of the vast majority, on the other hand, were given short shrift. Some progress has been made since then, but still the basic trend is the same, and agronomic research is still overwhelmingly geared to the trading economy.

6. From this perspective, the much-discussed brain drain that takes Southern intellectuals on a Northward trip reveals a novel aspect. It is an existential expression of the general extroversion of our economic life, and a specific expression of the extroversion of our intellectual life. It would be senseless to treat it as if it were some unique problem. It is, instead, the visible tip of a gigantic iceberg. Our task is not to treat it as an evil in itself but to examine it carefully, to understand it, and then to find ways of lifting it outright, if we can. The fact is that those who pack up and take off for the North are not the only African intellectuals caught in the fever of extroversion. Those who remain at home suffer from the same disease, if only indirectly. For the truth is that all Third World intellectuals, whatever their disciplines ad specializations, are driven in one way or the other by the potent impetus of international scientific endeavour as organized today, towards the centre of the system. A few 'settle' out there in the North. Others shuttle eternally between centre and periphery. The remainder, unable to make the passage, survive as best they can on the periphery, waging sisyphean battles against cynicism and despair while keeping a sharp eye out for openings through which they too might wriggle into Northward brain drain. Meanwhile, it is from the North that most of their research instruments, traditions, publications, methodological techniques and theoretical models, with all the attendant values and idiosyncrasies, come.[9]

7. There is a minor form of the brain drain that has so far drawn little notice. This is the intellectual tourist circuit linking North and South. In the normal career of Third World researchers, the outward trip has become an indispensable component. Third World researchers invariably have to make the physical trip to the great industrial metropoles. Some go to take advanced courses near the end of their academic training. Some go to leverage their ongoing research careers beyond ceilings already reached back home. The point is not to determine whether such trips are fun. Many obviously find them delightful, especially as they embark on new careers. Others find them weirdly repetitive, and there are those who find them particularly unsettling. But considerations of personal enjoyment or bewilderment are beside the point, because they leave the kernel of the problem untouched. That kernel is that such intellectual tourist trips have become structurally necessary, because there are real life constraints making them inevitable, and all intellectual pursuits in the Third World now bear the stamp of these constraints.

Our observations here are not meant to gainsay the tremendous scientific profit afforded by such trips. But what we wish to focus on is the fact that those trips remain, under current circumstances, the *sine qua non* condition for such a profit. It would thus be absurd, for instance, under such circumstances, all other things being equal, for anyone to seek through various coercive means to halt the North-South scientific 'tourism' insofar as it is demonstrated that strictly speaking, it is no tourism at all. The real issue is altogether different. What we have to do is to make profound changes in existing relations governing scientific productive work. What we have to do is to promote the growth, in countries now on the periphery of the world system, of a process of inner-directed scientific productivity and creativity.

It might be objected that even at the centre of the world system today, researchers cannot stay put, that they have to be mobile on pain of heading towards a slow death. It might further be pointed out that even within the centre there is a core, the absolute hub that is the United States of America, the country that increasingly attracts the cream of international-calibre researchers to the detriment of Northern Europe and Japan. To this there is a ready rebuttal that the scientific tourism then does not have the same meaning. The flow of researchers from one Northern country to the other is not the result of any internal imbalance in the process of scientific research as conducted in second-rank capitalist countries. Each of those countries has a viable, autonomous and inner-directed scientific tradition. If push came to shove, they could survive independently as intellectual centres. So when European scientists and researchers travel to the United States or, in the case of selected disciplines, to Japan as a matter of course, they look for a leading edge, an extra quality. Compared to the objectives behind the South-North intellectual exodus, those motivating the North-North process have more to do with luxury than with vital needs.

8. There would be a need to consider, for the sake of thoroughness, another form of scientific 'tourism', i.e. the North/South movement, whereby a researcher from an industrialized country goes to a country on the periphery and which never has the same function as the reverse itinerary. European or American scientists go to Zaire or the Sahara in search not of knowledge but only of materials that lead to knowledge and, if need be, to a testing ground for their findings. They do not go searching for paradigms or methodological and theoretical models; rather, they go hunting for information and new facts that are likely to enrich their paradigms on the one hand, just as on the other hand, they prefer distant territories where with the least possible ill-effects on their own environments, they can conduct nuclear tests or other types of experiments that are dangerous in various degrees.

Whole layers of contemporary knowledge have emerged from such scientific investment in the South by the North which brought forth new fields such as social and cultural anthropology and various specialised subjects within previous fields of intellectual endeavour. As a result, knowledge thus acquired on Africa and the Third World escapes entirely from Africa and the Third World altogether, only to be ploughed systematically back toward Europe, repatriated, capitalized and accumulated at the centre of the system. There is no extroversion, therefore, in the North / South movement, but a mere tactical detour in the service of a reinforced self-sufficiency and technological know-how.

9. Scientific extroversion manifests itself also through the use of Western languages alone seen as scientifically sound languages, and the obligation for the researcher from the Third World to accept to put on the straight jacket of those foreign languages in order to have access

> to knowledge and, more so, to reproduce and extend such knowledge. Undoubtedly one must guard against exaggerating inconveniences resulting from such a situation, or against falling into the excesses of a linguistic romanticism whereby every language, in itself and by itself, appears as the expression of a given world view, and a mother tongue, therefore is the only one medium that can express each and everybody's true identity.[10] Certainly there is a need to bring language back to its role as an instrument and to allow for the modern demands for broad communication, in a world where no one can any longer, on pain of suffocation, withdraw entirely within him or herself. One must just as well acknowledge the abnormal nature of the actual assessment that is made nowadays in some Third World countries, and particularly in Africa, regarding local languages and imported languages, the *de facto* marginalization of the former for the exclusive benefit of the latter, their down-grading to second-class languages, or worse still, 'dialects' or 'patois', only good enough to express everyday life platitudes. Lastly there is a need to consider the lack of a daring project aimed at eradicating illiteracy on a large scale and using those languages as vehicles for teaching and research at the highest level, for purposes of true democratization of knowledge.[11]

So, from yesterday till today, the same scientific dependence has kept on showing itself in new shapes that are however always easy to recognize. So, in all spheres of human activity, scientific, economic or otherwise, that same logic of extroversion goes on, whereby we expect motivations, initiatives and starting signals for our deeds to originate from places other than our own societies. To break that logic at last, to recover individual and collective initiative, to become ourselves again is one of the major tasks prescribed by History. That task, within the specific field of knowledge, amounts to taking an informed enough view of current practices in order to work out other possible modalities of producing knowledge, other possible forms of technological and scientific production relationships, first between the South and the North, but also in the South itself and inside each and every country.

Status of the 'Traditional'

It is in such a context that thoughts on 'traditional' knowledge must be placed. Nobody can nowadays deny that there exist, in our oral cultures, corpuses of knowledge sometimes very elaborate, faithfully transmitted from one generation to another and often gaining quality substance in the process of such transmission. Then, in the context of the massive extroversion of our societies, one may wonder, what becomes of such corpuses? What of their relations with assumedly modern science, that is, the progressive, conquering heuristic activity now developing in our universities and other centres of intellectual production, the institutional research which eats deep into credit funds but which otherwise depends structurally on the West, as we have just shown? What one realises is that instead of developing and gaining in accuracy and strictness as a result of contact with exogenous science and technique, this ancestral knowledge of plants, animals, health and illnesses as well as the age-old handicraft and agricultural know-how rather tend to fall back upon themselves.

Instead of fitting into the dynamics of contemporary research through a neat articulation with imported knowledge, with a view to leading to a living and original synthesis, 'traditional' knowledge is seen, in best cases, *side by side* with the new one, in a relationship of simple juxtaposition, exclusive of all true processes of exchange and of all manners of reciprocal valorisation. In the worst cases, such knowledge even ends up fizzling out of the collective memory.

So, the integration of the Third World into the world process of knowledge production entails, among other palpable effects, a marginalization of old elements of knowledge and know-how, along with their steady withering and impoverishment, and in worst cases, their sheer disappearing and vanishing out of people's conscious memory. In sum, the logic of extroversion which commands the so-called modern scientific activity in the Third World and singularly in Africa, has a binding corollary, a logic of marginalization. Peripheral to science in the metropolis, institutionalised research in Africa entails in its turn a further push of endogenous elements of knowledge to the periphery, thus relegating these to the periphery of the periphery, as mere survivals, intellectual and technological curiosities and lifeless, inert cultural objects, only fit for exhibition in museums for the titillation of antiquaries and other lovers of exorcism.

Unfortunately for the institution, such logic of marginalization never reaches its aim fully. There is an impressive record of repeated failure of hospital medicine, a howling inadequacy of officially sanctioned knowledge; and this has brought about a steadily stronger turn towards a so-called traditional medicine, and more generally towards those millennial stores of learning hastily dismissed out of mind, in order to find therein effective or tentative solutions to problems which are considered intractable today. The process of Westernization has thus turned out to be self-limiting. The backfires of the system have forcibly led to the emergence and valorisation of counter-systems, of the vast domain of the informed sector, or more accurately in this instance, of the teeming complex world of 'yet unstructured doctrines', as per Georges Canguilhem's apt expression (Canguilhem 1972).

The core question, however, is this: at this juncture, are these isolated sorties off the beaten paths of official science sufficient? Is it sensible to continue treating the counter-systems, the ancestral knowledge and know-how as sporadic seasoning, used only occasionally to camouflage failures or shortcomings, seen in turn as accidental mishaps in the dominant system? Shall we keep passing now and then from within the dominant system to counter-systems, and then back again, never wondering if the two realms are compatible or 'compossible', to use a concept suggested by Leibnitz? Should we not explore the possibility of harmonizing them in a more viable composite, bringing them into a logical union, and thus finding out if they can in theory and practice yield coherent concepts and technical procedures that might at the very least prove minimally meaningful? Can we nowadays be satisfied with seeing formally trained nurses, doctors and top-level specialists in surgery or paediatrics, when they fail to treat some complicated disease, counselling their patients to 'go back to the village', to consult traditional healers or even quacks, with no rational explanation to back up their advice, with no attempt to understand why they themselves have failed, or why their traditional counterparts do or might succeed? How far is it acceptable for our degree-burdened scientists, once they leave their laboratories, to go seeking out local weather specialists to find out the best times for holding family celebrations with the least risk of their getting rained on, without taking the trouble to understand the mechanism and mode of operation, the scope and limits of the know-how possessed by these local specialists? How much longer shall we continue agreeing with this watertight compartmentalization of thought and deed, this self-devastating duplicity, this ill-disguised schizophrenia?

This work would not have seen the light of day, were it not for the conscious determination of its authors to move beyond the present impasse. For we have to go further and, beyond the mute coexistence of discourses, to examine each and every mode of thought within their specific frames, then if possible, to bring them face to face within the unifying context of the kind of rigorous thinking that is careful to ensure its own coherence as well as the intelligibility of its practical procedure. We have to develop in ourselves the ability to shift from one mode of thought and one logical universe to another, not in a blind leap, and certainly not in the kind of reckless jump that has somehow become our daily bread — but in a conscious, intelligible movement, step by clearly identifiable step.

Such option for a rational approach requires an attitude, a relationship to 'traditional knowledge' entirely different from those prevailing today. The new approach calls for the working out of new methodologies in the various subject areas designed to help examine and evaluate and in total, in various proportions, to discard or to validate 'traditional' knowledge, thus integrating it critically and utterly carefully into the trend of current, living research work. The critical validation of the traditional element with a view to facilitating its active reappropriation, is likely to cause within the body of existing knowledge, shifts and shake-ups of which we at the moment have no way of predicting either the scope or the impact. The main thing, however, is to create bridges, to re-create the unity of knowledge, or in simpler, deeper terms, the unity of the human being.

The bulk of this work is made up of a revised and extended series of papers presented at a research seminar organized for Masters degree students in Philosophy and Sociology at the Université Nationale du Bénin, Cotonou, in 1987. The seminar was ordinarily open to registered students only. But other students, interested faculty and researchers in various fields were invited to a series of 'open sessions'. This introduction by the seminar director and eleven out of the thirteen following chapters are the outcome of the 'open sessions'. To those, we added a paper by

Jean-Dominique Pénel, who was invited but unfortunately could not attend. We also included a separate chapter by Abel Afouda, a hydrologist, which is a contribution to the discussion on 'rain makers'.

Right at the first seminar session there arose a terminology problem. The initial title was in fact 'traditional knowledge'; and the quotation marks between which the word *traditional* was put were already an indication of some lack of satisfaction as well as the awareness that, in such a phrase currently used, and doubtless effective with regard to empirical identification — in as much as everybody knows or believes he or she knows what 'traditional knowledge' refers to — the adjective *traditional* is innocent only in appearance. Spontaneously used in contrast to 'modern', that adjective connotes the obscure idea of a radical cut of the old from the new. It thus conveys of the old a shallow, uneventful, uniform, static picture in which all points appear as rigorously contemporary, keeping for the new order the prestige — or misfortune — of movement, of change, in short, of historicity.

We had already in other circumstances observed the mirage effect produced by passage from the noun *tradition* to the adjective *traditional*; we therefore proposed as a corrective the return to the noun system.[12] Behind the caption 'African traditional thought' pinned down and petrified as it were by a long ethnological practice, there was an invitation to a re-discovery of African *traditions* of thought, in their own dialectics and their eventful history; and beyond the hint at 'traditional' religions, supposedly static, cold and ageless, there was a reference to manifold, living religious *traditions*, inseparable from social groups supporting them and from functions which they fulfil in different political, economic and cultural contexts and which are marked by their convergences and divergences, including, as the case may be, wars and other categories of conflict which they instigated in the past, directly or indirectly. Likewise, behind 'traditional' knowledge held as definitive and foreign to history, one could hereby wish to seek out manifold, living knowledge traditions, corpuses of knowledge endowed with variable coherence, forming a system in varying degrees or resistant to every abstract systematization, coexisting in a relationship of simple juxtaposition or logical articulation, moving as a group or separately and inducing at each stage, variably efficient techniques and other practices.

The quotation marks meant all that at a time, i. e., those legitimate reservations, that criticism of a reductionist perception of non-Western cultures, that refusal of ignorance or *a priori* evacuation of the history, the internal movement as well as the change inherent in precolonial social formations and their spiritual productions. Putting the word 'traditional' in inverted commas in the seminar title itself, was an implicit acknowledgement that the adjective was improper and that as much as possible, beyond the empirical identification which was allowed and maybe favoured by such a usual term, there was a need to undertake the enormous work of ideological deconstruction necessary to re-establish the facts.

But then, quotations marks are written signs, not sounds likely to be heard. The graphic precaution appeared insufficient, right from the first session of the seminar. A satisfactory designation was required both for the ear and the eye. Was it necessary for such a purpose, to evoke 'so-called traditional' or better still 'assumedly traditional' knowledge, in order to express the acknowledged impropriety of the usual qualifier? The group concluded to the inadequacy of that very oratorical precaution which, as it rendered the research programme title rather clumsy, could only confirm the impropriety which it set out to denounce.

The group therefore preferred to find another phrasing. 'Endogenous knowledge' appeared to be a better choice. The term evokes the origin of the kind of knowledge in question by identifying it as an internal product drawn from a given cultural background, as opposed to another category of knowledge which would be imported from elsewhere. Certainly one will object that such distinction itself is relative altogether and is valid only in a first approximation, since what today appears endogenous may have been imported at a distant time in the past, prior to its later assimilation and its perfect integration in the society, to the extent of obliterating its foreign origins. Certainly one can quote instances of the case in point; for example, maize in the eyes of any tropical African farmer appears as an autochtonous crop, whereas it originates actually from the American continent and in Africa does not date further back than the 17th century.[13]

But, rightly, here lies the crux of the matter. That a cultural borrowing is assimilated to the point of being at one with the collective heritage thereafter, means that such borrowing is fully mastered and integrated into the initial culture itself.[14] Endogeny therefore is not necessarily static, it can be dynamic. Maybe there is, after all, no absolute interiority, nor an absolutely first origin. Maybe one is rather a witness to a never ending movement of interiorisation and appropriation of values derived from elsewhere. Far from forbidding however that a distinction be made between the endogenous and the exogenous, the above realisation, on the contrary, compels one to maintain it in its principle, while shifting the dividing line according to periods and stages in the history of a given culture.

One will therefore describe as endogenous, in a given cultural set-up, such knowledge as is experienced by society as an integral part of its heritage, in contrast to exogenous knowledge which is perceived, at this stage at least, as an element of another value system.

Just as the endogenous does not refer to absolute interiority, so it cannot be taken as a synonym of indigenous. In fact the indigenous is what appears to the foreign observer — explorer or missionary — as a purely local curiosity that has no effectiveness outside its particular context. The term always has a derogatory connotation. It refers to a specific, historical experience, precisely one of integration of autochtonous cultures into a world-wide 'market' in which these perforce are pushed down to inferior positions. The endogenous becomes 'indigenous' in and through such a world-widening process. What is proper thereby becomes improper, and sameness turns out as difference. Viewed from the outside, and perceived as an object, as a thing, the autochtonous person sees him or herself endowed with a new function, that of a 'primitive', a privileged witness of humanity's imaginary beginnings. Worse still, if that person does not take care, he or she can very quickly interiorise the new values and, looking at him or herself henceforth with other people's eyes, perceive him or herself as an 'indigenous' being. Such is truly, as occurs in every historic encounter, only the first moment of a dialectic, which may suddenly bring in a reverse movement. The autochtonous person therefore by reaction and through revolt, happens to claim his (or her) 'indigenousness' just as the Negro, more especially, does his (her) 'negritude'. One knows which literary movements, which political and ideological trends were born of such a reaction, and how such movements and trends, after forcefully expressing the awareness of a collective identity, in some cases contributed to keeping up an utterly stale conservatism and building a resistance to progress, a real obstacle to self-abnegation.

But there will be no emphasis here on that dialectic. The important thing is seeing how the world-widening process affects all fields of human activity, how it entails the belittling not only of the existing knowledge, but of cultures in general, not only of cognitive values, but of practical and aesthetic values, how it entails the marginalization of the whole economy, that is to say, the whole productive activity, which is henceforth ordinate and subordinate to an external demand, and totally deprived of autonomy and self-regulating power.

Endogenous Technologies

The following chapters fall into four sections: Endogenous Technologies; Conceptual Structures; Medicine and Pharmacology; Transmission Methods.

The chapter by Pierre G. Mêtinhoué, 'The study of "traditional" techniques and know-how: methodological issues' deals first and foremost with the issue of the current terms of reference of History in Africa. As it highlighted conflicts such as wars and other heroic deeds, furthermore as it affirmed the primacy of the written word, the traditional approach of that discipline narrowed considerably the scope of possible investigations in Africa. In order to uncover the African historian's mind's eye and open up new perspectives, there was a need therefore to start rehabilitating oral traditions as materials conducive to proper knowledge of the past, and with regard to conflicts such as wars, to highlight the study of civilisation facts, in particular material cultures. The new approach to history thus offers a vast field to the researcher: that of endogenous techniques. All has not been said, the African historian does not lack a purpose, innovation remains possible, just as there is hope for an increased contribution to collective repossession of self and the world.

To illustrate his views, Mêtinhoué lists up to forty-three (43) research studies conducted between 1985 and 1988 by material culture history and archaeology students at the National University of Benin. These students, somehow, showed the way forward, but their topics obviously are only a few pointers among hundreds or even thousands of others.

The history of material cultures, of which the relevance is thus pinpointed, however offers an 'unprecedented methodological challenge' to the researcher. Grounding his argument on authors like Jean Devisse and André Leroi-Gourhan, Mêtinhoué shows how the solution to the challenge presupposes, not only streamlining oral source study critical methods, but also resorting systematically in a spirit of interdisciplinary approach, to data from other subject areas like archaeology in the first place, but also palaeography, palaeobotany and 'little by little, the whole modern knowledge and technology'. The chapter closes with a case study, consisting of a description of the making of distilled palm wine, which the author presents here as an illustration of how the history of endogenous techniques readily blows up what Joseph Ki-Zerbo termed the myth of the historical passivity of African peoples.

The chapter by Alexis Adandé, 'Traditional Iron metallurgy in West Africa' is basically an answer to the same preoccupation: to re-establish the historical truth, beyond all the shrewdly kept up complexes whereby Africans were made to believe that they had never invented anything through their own means.

Secondary metallurgy is a well-known activity in black Africa, and the business of blacksmiths has been studied thoroughly by ethnographers and historians. What is less known however, is the existence of a primary, very ancient metallurgy in Africa. Recent archaeological research enables one to locate in West Africa today, namely in Ghana, Nigeria, Burkina Faso, Mali, Senegal, Mauritania, Togo and Benin — many sites where blast furnaces in olden times were used for separating iron from its ore through the 'direct method', that is to say, without going through the intermediary cast iron stage.

Given that obvious reality, the great controversy among specialists would not deal with the existence, but with the origin of that technology. While researchers at the beginning of this century admitted easily that iron metallurgy was born in black Africa prior to its dissemination towards Europe, directly or through the Near East, another group of colonial researchers, from the years 1930, finding it hard to imagine that Africa itself could ever invent such a technology, thought it clever to suppose that the technology came from the Near East or India: a quaint interpretation of the diffusionist school of thought strongly contradicted however by more recent research work that leads to placing in Africa itself the origin of iron extractive metallurgy.

The study by Alexis Adandé starts with a few definitions and conceptual preliminaries; then it draws a balance-sheet of current knowledge on ancient iron metallurgy and shows the relevance of such a research field.

Divided by some archaeologists into three periods, the iron age in Africa would therefore comprise an early period extending up to year 650 in our era, a subsequent period going from VIIth to XVIth century and a recent period stretching from XVIIth to early XXth century. Up to this day, three large areas relating to the early period have been identified, that is the Nok culture complex in Central Nigeria, the Aïr region in Northern Niger and Daboya in Northern Ghana; but the main thing is that the dating data obtained through the most rigorous methods no longer today allow for the least doubt about the ancient origin of iron technology which in Africa goes perhaps back to the beginning of the first millennium before Jesus-Christ.

The major question then is how these metallurgical traditions ended up vanishing, and why the vast historical regression at the term of which those iron-ore processing operations which were once conducted on a large industrial scale, are carried on nowadays only in a few isolated places, seen as 'the ultimate traces of a once widely practised activity'. Alexis Adandé mentions two causes here: the impact of slave trade, of which one has good reasons for thinking that it drained an important group of African foundry-workers and blacksmiths to the Americas, where the natives until then knew only gold, copper and bronze metallurgy; the other cause mentioned by Adandé is the brutality of a colonial administration which deemed it expedient to protect the market of imported iron items by suppressing local metallurgical practices. In addition to that historical regression problem, other issues arise, regarding namely the metallurgist's and blacksmith's social status, and more generally forms of iron production social organisation which vary considerably from one region to another, or regarding the influence of that production on the economy and politics, on relationships between social formations, development of religion and magic, and ecology.

With the paper by Gbênoukpo Dah-Lokonon-Bodehou and the lively debate that follows, we are at the heart of an essential problem and of a difficulty. The question which the speaker was asked to answer was clear: how much myth and science is there in the practice of 'rain makers'? How can the core of proven techniques be identified as opposed to mystification and sheer magical/religious delirium? We would not have raised such questions if we knew the answers, or if we were sure that, in the local weather specialist's claim to atmospheric management, all is mere myth and illusion. Besides, Dah-Lokonon's paper, beyond its obvious informative richness, will certainly amaze its readers owing to its deliberately apologetic character, its unmitigated valorisation of something which precisely is at stake, and therefore its tendency to suppress questioning, as several speakers remarked during question time. This is a proof of the extreme difficulty of having to sit on the fence, of knowing from the inside technical and magical practices inherited through a tradition dating back to time immemorial, and of keeping towards the discourse supporting or expressing such practices — the critical distance necessary for a fully rational assessment.

But there lies, precisely, the relevance of the paper the author of which should be given due credit, first for managing to support the views of those he deferentially calls the 'wise ones' in our countryside, then for agreeing to take on questions and observations from speakers who, in their large majority, were rather sceptical, in order to attempt building with these a common knowledge in a dynamic manner. In that dialogue which occasionally resembles a proper disputation, rationality can be seen at work inside or starting from a discourse which still remains, thoroughly, the speech of the ancestors: *mythos* in its literal sense.

From Dah-Lokonon to Abel Afouda, there is a need for a giant's step. The hydrologist right away betted on rationality, that is to say integral intelligibility; a firm position backed up with utterly strong heuristic principles with which he questions pre- or proto-scientific practices still partially caught up in myth, and of which he aims to work out the meaning and limitations. He also wishes to confer a new value on endogenous knowledge, but through a recuperation process subsequent to a preliminary rupture, instituted precisely by 'fundamental principles of modern science'.

It is therefore in the light of a positive knowledge of the usual mechanism of atmospheric precipitations that Abel Afouda wishes to interpret 'the experimental device of a rain maker', as observed by himself in August 1978. That the experiment held as a reference should have ended as a failure is only a minor detail to the hydrologist, whereas such a failure would have been sufficient to make the experiment irrelevant in the eyes of the apologist or ideologist. The whole trick is explained thus:

> The big wood fire acted as a generator of a smoke panache containing fine particles necessary for nucleation. The necessary hygroscopic properties would be conferred on the panache by the fine particles obtained from the burning of salt or herbs and leaves used as ingredients for the experiment, etc.

And that is not all; there exists on the issue a plentiful scientific literature which gives a minute account of various artificial precipitation experiments. Important elements of knowledge have been accumulated on the issue and have sometimes given rise to industrial implementations in the United States, the former Soviet Union, Israel, France, Chile, India and Africa.

In the light of such experiments, one cannot help thinking that mental sinking in the mythical discourse comes from a regrettable lack of information; although there is a need to guard against nullifying endogenous practices. Indeed, if the artificial causation of rain is not a phenomenon peculiar to Africa, nevertheless, the fact remains that 'African methods can have their particularities'. In that regard, Abel Afouda opens up paths of research that hold out promises of fecundity, aimed at an active reappropriation of traditional know-how.

Conceptual Structures

Under the title 'Conceptual Structures', part two of the book covers a series of thoughts on the African numerical system, then another on the mathematical foundation of geomancy, and a third on zoological taxonomy in Hausa.

How to count up to one thousand, up to one million and one billion in African languages? What is the mechanism of numerical systems in those languages and which transformations and new abstractive processes should be introduced to make them more manageable and more able to express and enrich modern arithmetic thinking?

These questions received answers from Toussaint Y. Tchitchi, on the basis of a Beninese language, *Ajagbè*.

After describing the real functioning of the *Aja* numerical system and examining successively in that framework, the formation of cardinal and ordinal numbers, and of what he calls iterative numbers, the expression of currency, and lastly terms of connection enabling the expression of the basic arithmetic operations (addition, multiplication, subtraction, division) — the author raises the issue of the transformations necessary for adapting the *Aja* language to the pressing needs of modern arithmetic thinking. Hence the question of decimalization, an essential issue of which Tchitchi's laconic presentation indicates however clearly the intractability just as it proposes a solution, as follows:

The *aja* traditional system of numeration uses two 'basic numbers': 10 and 40. Eighty, one hundred and twenty and one hundred and sixty are 'twice forty', 'three times forty', 'four times forty', and so on. So that beyond forty, 'whole powers of forty served ... as connecting modes in the system'. Hence the difficulty in expressing very large numbers, and the high propensity of the system to numerical saturation.

A team of reformers, bent on simplifying the system through decimalization, at the end of a series of careful field enquiries and after consulting with elders in the community — had to propose new terms for saying ten, one hundred, thousand, million and billion. Thus, instead of saying the number ninety, the way it is naturally done in the language, that is *kave ho wo*, literally: two ropes plus ten (one rope standing for the simple unit 'forty'), one will say in the new terminology: *ta-shidekè*, literally: nine 'heads', or more accurately (even though Tchitchi does not specify it) nine heaps, a heap standing henceforth for the simple unit 'ten'.

Finally, asking himself the relevance of the reform, the author observes that if it does not lead necessarily to shorter numeric terms and does not therefore entail an economy in the enunciation, nevertheless it eases management of large numbers and figures. The testing of the new system by farmers in the Mono Region — within the programmes of the

Centre for rural development regional action (CARDER) — invites one to assert the efficiency of the new system, the author concludes.

The message of Victor Houndonougbo has a different orientation in as much as the author aims not to transform but to elucidate, not to adapt existing resources for the sake of a more secure production of the rational, but to lay bare the concealed rationality of a seemingly mystical practice. Behind the geomancy of Ifa, already abundantly described through a whole ethnographic literature, behind the complex signs interpreted by the diviner by means of schemes and a whole set of symbols which emerged as a result of the force of tradition, Houndonougbo discovers a few simple rules, a few combinatorial elements that refer to familiar mathematical theorems.

Calculation of probability therefore allows a rational interpretation of the three modes of divination, which include both the most simple and the most complex, i. e. divination by a throw of kola-nuts, cowries, or use of beads. Houndonougbo's approach consists in construing mathematically, from a given divinatory material (four lobes of kola-nuts in the first instance, sixteen cowries in the second case, a string of eight bead items in the third case) — the different possible arrangements of such materials; the author also calculates the probability for each arrangement of such materials. The result of the exercise can be formulated by means of a theorem whereby the aleatory variable (number of lobes facing down in the first instance, number of cowries facing up in the second case) is distributed according to well-known probability calculation laws.

No matter who can understand formulae and graphic representations, as well as mathematical concepts whereby the author accounts for those phenomena: Bernoulli's binominal law, associated probability space, arborescent exploration with unicolumn matrix notation, factorial tree, Pascal's triangle, Gauss' bell, application of a set of x elements, equiprobability, quantity of information equal to logarithm of n, with 2 as the base ($q = \log_2 n$), etc.. The essential thing for the common reader basically is the process itself: the laying bare of a concealed rationality, the endeavour to formalise a practice perceived by all and perceiving itself as mystical, the 'mathematisation of an unstructured doctrine', to use Georges Canguilhem's phrase (Canguilhem 1972).

However, one will note, in passing, the following implication: betting on rationality presupposes a complete evacuation, a blowing up of the mystical horizon which thus far encompassed divinatory practices. Houndonougbo comes back to it three times at least: no esoteric or psychic influence, no mystical entity directs the kola lobes or orients the cowries, just as no mysterious power influences the lay-out of the beads thrown many times in succession. Such definitely is not the opinion of the diviners themselves, who on the contrary assert strongly that each lay-out of beads is guided by a divinity whose message it transmits faithfully. The mathematical approach proceeds therefore from taking the sacredness away from the real world. The mathematical approach is god-killing. Such is the splendid assassination which Victor Houndonougbo performs without saying it, or rather saying it in his own way, with the quiet assuredness of the scientist.

We are back to the language issue with J. D. Pénel's paper entitled 'Epistemological reflections on animals' names in Hausa. As in Tchitchi's text on traditional enumeration systems, the object consists in questioning the functioning of an African language chosen as an example, with regard to a given knowledge field.

Pénel's intention is to compare the mode of classification of animals in Hausa and that of modern zoology, as was established in the main, by Linné in the 18th century.

While Linné's classification goes according to hierarchy and 'interlocking' of categories, names of animals with the Hausa people are primarily in keeping with features likely to be observed directly by the five senses as for that matter, they themselves supply valuable information on morphology and behaviour, natural places, seasons and other times of appearance of such various animals. Designations thus constitute in themselves 'a contribution to knowledge which zoology can utilise and integrate'.

Pénel pinpoints also in the process of naming some animals a 'projection of the social world on the animal world', but the author soon realises that such anthropomorphism which has a massive presence in Hausa zoological lexicon, is not wholly absent either from a so-called scientific terminology.

The most important point, however, is the examination of classification processes used in compound names. Indeed, the naming approach which consists in taking a basic name and adjoining to it one or several attributes — 'operates as the root or ancestor to Linné's procedure', which itself surely as well started with an external but rigorous observation of some parts of the bodies of animals and plants, prior to rising to distinction between gender and species and to the whole theory that carries it. Then all of a sudden one sees clearly the relevance of Hausa taxonomy and its limitations, its richness, but also the unreliable nature of analogies grounded on external description alone, with no reference to anatomy and physiology, that is, to structure analysis and to study of functions. That is a valuable pointer to what remains to be done, provided that one wants to go beyond the limits of the present for a self-projection into the future. And that is a task all the more important since all in all, zoological vocabulary itself is far from reaching, today, a measure of strictness comparable to that of the concepts of physics or chemistry. 'Latin does not in itself create science and ... is only a convenient convention for avoiding friction of national feelings among scientists'. In summary, zoology is still in the making, that is, in a state of incompleteness which gives additional sense and justification to a research process that would endeavour to take into account the contribution of local knowledge by inserting it into a new theoretical environment.

Medicine and Pharmacology

The Third part of the book deals with medicine and pharmacology. In her presentation of some of the most famous medicinal products in Benin pharmacology, including fourteen (14) fruits, eight (8) seeds, three (3) bulbs and rhizomes, one (1) shell and nine (9) mineral items — Simone de Souza ensured that she indicated for each of them, not only local names as well as the scientific, that is to say, Latin corresponding words, but also and above all, proven, objectively experienced medical, effects, then supposedly magical effects, and lastly both medical and magical effects.

The value of the paper does not derive from its information content alone. Between the lines of such a brief, unassuming itemized list, two issues at least can be seen, looming up at first, then becoming truly unavoidable — as discussions showed. First, how can one discriminate between medicine and magic? Why are they so closely tied up in so-called traditional therapeutic practices ? In substance, the same question arises with regard to rain-makers whose procedures already called for thoughts on the dividing line between myth and reality, positive technique and wild ritual.

Then and above all, grounded on that first question, there is a concern which amounts to the very one lying at the heart of this book, in terms of how, by which methods, by which ways and means one can recuperate and put to the service of our societies today, what is most valid in local pharmacology ? The reader will be left to make his (or her) own assessment of the author's answers to these two questions, and to carry on by him or herself the thinking thus started, possibly through a translation into an action programme.

Questioning traditional etiological models, from the case of Benin republic, Gualbert Ahyi observes that mental illness is linked to two causes: it is the work of a human being or of a spirit. In the former case, it results from a direct or indirect aggression; direct when somebody attacks somebody else without an intermediary, by virtue of a genuine power which is witchcraft. The aggression is indirect when somebody attacks somebody else through a third person, perceived as an initiate, a magician or a 'marabout'. In the latter case, on the contrary, the aggression comes from a spirit that partakes of ancestral religions or imported religions.

The consequence of such aetiology is that in his or her diagnosis, the healer will concentrate not so much on visible symptoms of the illness as on signs which can allow him (or her) to identify the aggressor. And such signs he will find above all in what the patient or the family says and the quality of the relationships linking the individual to the group; which definitely puts the psychiatric fact outside the field of mental illness, strictly speaking: 'The trouble is neither in the body, nor in the sick person, but in the aggression'.

What is the therapeutic virtue of such models? Ahyi then asks himself. Both models refer to conflictual situations. Aggression by witchcraft refers to a basic conflict within interpersonal relationships, and finally, to an original relationship with the mother. The witch who 'eats' a victim is only an avatar of the devouring mother. As for the healer, he or she is also necessarily an adept of witchcraft, that is, the one which does not eat, nor kills, nor uses its power to cause harm but which on the contrary is meant to prevent others from eating, killing and harming potential victims.

Aggression by spirits refers not at all to a dual relationship, but to a relationship with the law of ancestors, tradition, taboos. Illness is then a sign indicating that a taboo or a rule has been violated or forgotten. It is a call to order, a message signalling that something abnormal has happened in the dynamics of the family or social group, that there has occurred a rupture which can be overcome only through special rituals which the healer, a priest of a kind, will as a duty prescribe.

Regarding such traditional models, the author recommends the minimal humility which is required for taking seriously a type of discourse wholly nonsensical at first. He even goes further. The African aetiology, he acknowledges, is very much like 'a big joke' ... However, it is an efficient joke, 'a lie that works somehow'. The most original contribution of the paper lies probably in the theory of the efficient lie! 'Thus, the Black man would have understood things which he cannot name, because naming them would serve no purpose, except for breaking families'.

A child who killed his (or her) mother could not have done it on his (or her) own; he (or she) must have been disturbed by a spirit, because of the family's failure to perform such or such a sacrifice. As a result, the culprit is perceived as a victim and in this capacity, is taken charge of by the group. What purpose would it have served to spell out the crude fact of the crime? A crude denomination, a positive designation of reality can lead to a deadlock, whereas a symbolical clothing could conversely allow preservation of social cohesion. Gualbert Ahyi sees therefore in such African therapeutic practices a 'recovering' technique: 'It is perhaps because truths are not spoken but thrown away elsewhere that the system operates. For if the truth was unveiled, one would from a certain moment be forced with a truth upon which one could perhaps no longer work'.

Do 'mystical shootings' exist really or not? Any little child in Benin would find such a question as preposterous as when one wonders if the earth and trees do exist. Belief in '*tshakatu*' (mystical shooting) and belief more generally in occult forces — are here a matter of course. But then is this mere belief, sheer fantasy, and the outcome of an 'animist' vision of the universe (according to Tylor) or of a 'primitive' mentality (according to Lévy-Bruhl)?[15] It is as a surgeon, that is to say a practitioner of one of the most positive or materialistic branches of medicine that Henry-Valère Kiniffo answers the question. As a matter of fact, his answer, one must say it plainly, is quite disturbing.

That a child should have the broken tip of a pencil fall into his or her ear, swallow a button snatched off a shirt, or breathe a tiny ball into his or her nose, that a stray bullet should hit deep into somebody's backbone or that a clumsy or careless surgeon should leave a blade unnoticed in a patient's body — such are cases where a foreign object being found out in a human body, far from appearing as a surprise, is seen by all as resulting from a material, causal process which can be observed empirically. The author starts by presenting a typology of such parasitic objects according to their mode of introduction into the human body, then he indicates in each case, the most effective techniques of extraction.

There are however cases where the presence of a foreign object could not be explained in such an 'obvious' manner and does not refer to any causal, observable process. Tapping his own rich medical experience, Kiniffo cites specific examples. In two such cases which remained famous, the renowned surgeon patiently managed to extract sewing needles stuck deep in various parts of a catechist's fore-arm, and also a bundle of black and red hair plaiting thread nestled quaintly in a young girl's stomach. There is no denying the facts, hard and properly established as they were. However, one will seek first to explain them positively by casting onto their background an empirically intelligible, causal reasoning. But then things get complicated: the catechist did definitely *not* fall unto a bag of needles, nor did little Agathe swallow plaiting threads. The 'mystical' explanation appears therefore to be more simple, in this instance, that is, more economical: 'The matter has to do not with swallowed threads but with a thing sent out' (*sic*), which is a literal translation of a stock phrase in local languages. The author seeks no further explanation. At most, he adds, in his capacity as a therapist, that what he himself achieved by dint of patience and owing to what one is inclined to see as a piece of surgical success story, the traditional healer performs otherwise, that is, through magnetic charm. The ultimate nature of such therapeutic process will however not be questioned, nor was that of the mystical projection of which the process is considered as the antidote.

What a pity (that) the recording of the long discussion which then followed got lost! Questions were full of passion, one guesses easily, just as the clash of arguments was stimulating. One sees what the case in point could be: value and limitations of rationalism in general, or at least, of that common rationalism which some describe, wrongly or rightly, as pertaining to Descartes, and which appears to many as a very narrow approach which singularly reduces and impoverishes reality.

The paper by Comlan Théodore Adjido relates directly to that debate. Let us not jump to conclusions too quickly, the author warns, and let us not give up understanding. One must get out of the closed world of witchcraft to be able to deal thematically with witchcraft itself, that is, to take it as a theme, as a topic for study. For 'witchcraft is one of such phenomena as descend suddenly upon the people; and by definition, epidemiology is one of such sciences as deal essentially with phenomena that descend suddenly on peoples'.

In other words, the real issue is not witchcraft itself, but *belief* in witchcraft. And that belief which pervades our reference societies, has all the features of a scourge, such as small pox or cholera epidemic.[16] For Theodore Adjido, psychosomatic medicine, such as it develops nowadays, offers altogether if not complete explanations, at least a satisfactory model of explanation of witchcraft phenomena which usually appear to us so mysterious and which we consider wrongly as specific to Africa. What is being questioned therefore, on careful examination, is not rationalism in general, but at most a narrow rationalism which would take into account, in terms of etiological explanation, only a series of causes exclusive of all others, and which, in like manner, would ignore the complex relationship between the body and the mind. It is to a better knowledge of processes whereby the human body responds to environment, that the author invites us. The reader will certainly be frustrated for finding in the first chapter on 'synopsis of psychosomatic medicine' only a brief overview on authors, works and concepts which would probably deserve a major emphasis. But one will understand easily that one cannot do better in a presentation aiming only at showing a possible way for research. Maybe it will be regretted also that the author does not show further, relying on his experience as a psychiatrist the practical implications of his approach. Such however was not his aim either, and in that general discussion on etiological models, the only clinical case which was cited could be more than enough.

Me we no di bo bo no di: evil strikes only somebody who is ready for it. The above saying quoted from the *Fon* language by Adjido, sums up the content of his paper and shows also that, even inside a culture where belief in witchcraft remains not only omnipresent but basic structurally, there exist discordant voices, non-conformist voices which express scepticism and proclaim its legitimacy, thus showing to all and sundry the way to a possible psychological liberation.

Transmission Methods

At the end of this intellectual journey, while it is no longer possible to doubt the existence of endogenous knowledge and of the complex problems related to its identification and actualisation, one is forced to raise questions on the mode of transmission of such knowledge in the past, and in particular on the respective roles, scopes and limitations of written and oral means of communication. Such is the object of the fourth part of this book.

As a true argument in favour of orality, and keen on rehabilitating a form of communication which it deems unfairly despised by the intellectuals, those who in Benin go by the name of *akowe* — a yoruba word meaning literally scribes — the text by François Dossou starts by asking a definite question, which relates to the intrinsic efficiency of orality, that is to say, specific means at the disposal of a given culture for selecting, stocking and transmitting from one generation to another such knowledge as it deems useful, without resorting to writing. Once the question is thus put, the author proposes a few definitions which he sees as just as many 'warnings'.

So he vigorously denounces the semantic shift which makes the illiterate appear, no longer as simply somebody ignorant of the alphabet, but as an absolute ignorant; likewise, orality is conceived of, restrictively as mere absence of writing, whereas very positively, in the same capacity as scripturality of which it is the alternative, orality is seen as a particular form of communication and transmission, of which the functioning deserves a close examination. Finally François Dossou points out that writing was invented in the beginning in response to practical and not literary or scientific needs and that it served the exclusive interests of social classes the members of which were then in positions of power. Next comes the examination of what the author calls 'verbophilia' and 'scriptophilia', that is to say, an exclusive cult of speech or writing, as illustrated respectively by Rousseau, Lévi-Strauss and Saussure on the one hand, and on the other — mind you! — by Jacques Derrida and ... Paulin J. Hountondji. One first expectation is that the author should brush aside both antagonistic attitudes and instead propose a global, more balanced approach whereby the respective and complementary functions of speech and writing would receive their fair share of appraisal. But it appears very quickly that for the author, the absolute evil is 'scriptophilia' — which shows up as a theoretical peroration of oral civilisation and which tends to consider as savage and primitive, peoples with no known writing traditions.

Little wonder therefore that a third and last paragraph serves as a special renewed contribution to such criticism under the title: 'Mystification of the written word'. François Dossou, as always, warns against 'fetishism of the Alphabet', which considers orality as incapable of conveying knowledge, leading us to 'kneel down in front of the written word', to believe at the limit that 'what is not written is thoughtless', and to look at orality 'as ... a weakness, ... a synonym of illiteracy, of ignorance, and at the limit, of primitivism'. The author analyses the reasons for such a mountain of prejudices and invites the reader to give back to orality all its value by going beyond the notions of individual authorship, individual merit and copyright, which are bound up with our bourgeois world as well as transcending reflexes linked up with the triumph of modern bureaucracy and of 'paper civilisation' in societies which had till then managed to do without them.

One will not be surprised at the direct and fairly lively nature of the discussion of which there is a deliberate faithful transcription here, along with its occasionally intra-Beninese polemical heights. For science is all that as well, that is to say, the outcome of misunderstandings which sometimes are dissipated and otherwise persist in spite of clarifying efforts, ingenuous or ill-intentioned questions, which sometimes resemble disputations and are not always innocent of charges of bad faith while finally and in their own ways, they contribute to progress of knowledge.

With the paper by Bienvenu Akoha, beyond the ideological and impassioned debate, one comes back to a question of fact: the actual history of writing.

To put writing systems at their proper places in precolonial Africa, the author starts with a general reminder of the different stages of the writing process: that of the very first form of writing, where the signifying function is attributed to various objects chosen as symbols or, at a later stage, to the graphic representation of such objects; next, there is the stage of pictography, where a sign or group of written signs aims to suggest a whole sentence, a trend of which the *Fon* culture in Benin, offers numerous illustrations; then comes a third stage deeply innovative regarding the preceding ones, namely the ideography stage, where the written sign no longer calls to mind a sentence, but a word; lastly, we have the phonetic system of writing, where the graphic sign represents either a syllable (hence the writing system is said to be syllabic), or a sound or phoneme (hence the writing system is said to be alphabetical).

It is in the light of such concepts as are presented above, and convinced, like all linguists, of the superiority of the alphabetical system of writing, deemed to be more economical and therefore more efficient, that Bienvenu Akoha examines what could correspond, in Africa, to those different stages of the writing process.

In such a way, evidence is given on our continent, first, of 'forerunners of the written word', as are largely illustrated in the author's reference culture — the *Fon* culture — through the famous 'récades' — wooden and iron emblems in honour of Kings of Abomey, through maps serving as tapestry drawn by spies to help identify strategic points in towns to be conquered, bas-relief showing war scenes, Ifa symbols as interpreted by diviners, as already discussed above. Evidence is also given, in precolonial Africa, of more elaborate forms of non phonetic writing system, such as pictography, of which the author cites numerous examples borrowed from *Ashanti*, *Ewe* and *Fon* cultures, and ideography or word-based writing system, of which Egyptian hieroglyphics offer shiny examples. Finally, evidence is given of more or less elaborate phonetic writing systems, such as Vai, Mende, Somalian, Ethiopian and Arabic.

Once facts are thus reconstituted, comes the inevitable question: how can one account for the stagnation and decline of African writing systems? Why did Africa, unlike the West, never put a premium on writing as a means of communication? Given that question, Akoha discards formally a bad answer which would consist in seeking the cause of such stagnation in the writing systems themselves. One should rather question history and sociology — he cautions — just as one should examine closely the mode of collective use and appropriation of writing systems in African societies and the relations of such societies with the others. The author's assumption is a strong one: it sees in the scientific and cultural marginalization of Africa the combined effect of two phenomena which are distinct but complementary with regard to Negro Slave Trade which, from XVIth to XIXth century, compelled societies on the Black continent to live on the defensive by withdrawing within themselves, at the very time when the invention of printing in 1434, made intensification of intellectual exchange possible in the rest of the world.

No doubt it will be objected that such assumption is valid only for a very thin layer of African and international history, as re-placed in the long perspective. One could however not deny the relevance and richness of the assumption at least with regard to recent history, nor could one ignore the strategic importance of the period in relation to the history of writing in the world. There is therefore a need to take the reading of facts seriously, as proposed by Akoha, who sees in the history of writing in Africa the story of a lost opportunity, the missing of a decisive turning-point in the evolution of mankind.

Such is broadly the problem posed in this book, which raises issues some of which are essential; but while there is no claim to giving final answers to those questions, the intention is simply to open up paths and to show possible ways for thought and action. Forms of knowledge exist; the point is how to learn to find them out, to recognize their inner truth and coherence by re-placing them in their original contexts, in the dynamics that carries them and likewise spells out their specific limitations. There is a further need to learn to *scrutinize* them in order to extract the essential kernel, to *purify* them by separating the myth in which they are wrapped up, just as right here in Africa, metals used to be separated from mineral ores. Finally, one must learn to re-integrate such forms of knowledge thus reclaimed into the movement of living science, into the new dynamics that carries us nowadays forward, us and our societies.

In the following pages, one will find very little erudition: few quotations, few references to existing science literature; rather, one will find the direct expression of context-bound preoccupations, a theory-building approach obviously marked by the limits of scientific information on this periphery of the world market of concepts, polemics which one will perhaps deem naive in some cases and which would make one smile if one were not aware that science can also be done in a hole and that everybody's task today is precisely to ensure that there should be no such holes any more, by creating conditions for a more equitable sharing of information.

To demarginalize Africa and the Third World with regard to knowledge as well as in all other respects, to ensure that on this periphery of the world capitalist market, the common heritage be appropriated as the fruit of the work of all and sundry and that the margin be no longer margin but part and parcel of a multifaceted whole, a centre of decision among other centres of decision, an autonomous centre of production among others, such is today a major task. But such appropriation by the periphery of all the useful knowledge supposes further, a conscious effort towards a critical but resolute reappropriation of one's own practical and cognitive heritage, a negation of the marginality of one's endogenous knowledge and know-how, and a re-insertion of the 'traditional' into a living tradition that looks out to the future.

The question of questions, one can see, is still and always the same: what next? The issues raised in this book refer to problems of science policy and of politics, pure and simple. They are born of practical preoccupations and must lead, beyond the nexus of theoretical analyses, to answers to such preoccupations.

Notes

1. In this first paragraph, I have incorporated the substance of texts already published (Hountondji 1984, 1986, 1987, 1990a, 1990b, 1992).
2. In this regard, I recommend the reading of a special issue on 'Scientific research' of *Recherche, Pédagogie et Culture* (Paris) No. 38, nov. — dec. 1978; as well as Rossi 1973, Moravcsik 1976, Latour 1982, 1983.

3. Underdevelopment as *an end product,* that is to say the contrary of a native property or of an atavism: it is worth emphasizing the relevance of the approach which, better than the evolutionist theories which were dominant up to the end of the nineteen sixties (Parsons 1951, 1964; Leibenstein 1957; Rostow 1960; Hoselitz 1960; Szentes 1971) enables the understanding of the phenomenon of underdevelopment by putting it in historical perspective. Hence, the admitted opinion nowadays that no country is in itself underdeveloped, but that all can become underdeveloped in proportion with their annexation by the world capitalist market (Frank 1967, 1972; Amin 1970, 1973; Rodney 1972; Wallerstein 1974). We shall endeavour, in this introductory part, to apply that pattern of explanation to one particular, all too often neglected aspect of the same phenomenon, which is *scientific* underdevelopment.
4. Bruno Latour in *La vie de laboratoire,* makes a thorough description of the daily functioning of a small-sized experimental research unit, thus giving an excellent example of what science anthropology can be (Latour 1988). What is proposed here is a generalisation of that notion of laboratory in a perspective which is not anthropological but epistemological. So, authors such as Alain Badiou, Pierre Raymond, Xavier Renou propose to consider mathematics itself, not as a purely ideal or *a priori* science, but as an experimental science whereby thought moves forward only owing to physical actions being brought to bear on a material device: the written formula being an exact equivalent of the microscope or of other more or less sophisticated material equipment items (Badiou 1969; Raymond 1973; Renou 1978). In that context, and in the light of that experimentalist vision of science, it is proposed here that the term laboratory, in its broad sense, should be used to designate any organised space containing equipment items and other material devices that are meant to enable transformation of information into knowledge.
5. Statistics show a considerable downfall of that production from 44,000 tons in 1971 to less than 13,000 tons per year from 1979 till this day. This is however only a minor point with regard to our problem.
6. If reference to the colonial system is a particularly eloquent illustration of the functioning of underdeveloped economies, the fact remains that integration into the world market is older and goes back to the Slave trade, as far as Black Africa is concerned.
7. Léopold Gnininvi, while director for scientific research in Togo, during a round-table meeting, talked jokingly about such embarrassment as can arise from a microscope breakdown, or from the dysfunctioning of some other apparatus in an African laboratory: the only alternative is to wait for the maker to choose to send the spare parts from Europe or elsewhere.

For serious breakdowns, there was a need to send back to the maker the apparatus themselves for repairs (*Recherche, Pédagogie et Culture*, 1978).

8. Ethnophilosophy is a good example of such scientific closing-in. One understands therefore that criticism of ethnophilosophy should always go hand-in-hand with criticism of Africanism or, at the least, of extreme forms of Africanism, and with a claim to what could be called the right to universality (see Hountondji 1977, 1983; Towa 1971; Njoh-Mouellé 1975; Mudimbe 1988). One remembers Aimé Césaire's warning that 'there are two ways to losing oneself: through walled segregation in the particular, and through dilution in the universal' Césaire 1956). Scientific closing-in relates to the former way to perdition. The latter form, on the contrary, would be that abstract universalism which, taking a pretext out of the universal validity of science, would hold as superfluous every question concerning the relationship to science, the historical modes of appropriation of knowledge, the relationships of scientific and technological production world-wide.
9. Here, an attempt is made by various authors to do justice to a well described phenomenon. But the method used is more narrative than analytical, as in this remarkable testimony by Jacques de Certaines: *In the African Universities where I trained, a highly valid scientific teaching was provided with respect to the subjects I studied, but... all this 'good' teaching only led to a feeling of subordination to the sites where science was really being undertaken. I was somewhat told: here, we work at the periphery of science, but if you really want to go to the heart, then you must go. All my school mates continued their studies in biology, a number of them engaged in secondary school teaching, but those who engaged in research left. Can our educational system which is in such a state of dependence, lead to a genuine development?* (Collectif 1978b:41).
10. For an African version of that linguistic romanticism, one will refer, for example, to the famous book by Alexis Kagame (Kagame 1956). Such treatment of language, one knows, however goes back to the XVIIIth century as illustrated particularly by Herder (Herder 1766) prior to being taken up and developed in the following century by Wilhelm von Humboldt (Humboldt 1835, 1974). In order to appreciate that form of romanticism and relativist theses which derived from it, we recommend the reading of our article on the issue (Hountondji 1982).
11. For easily understandable historical reasons, linked namely to prevalence of the assimilationist ideal in the French colonial doctrine, linguistic extroversion as described here, is more marked in francophone Black Africa than in the rest of sub-Saharan Africa. The phenomenon is none the less general, and it is little wonder if occasionally it causes violent

rejection reactions on the part of both anglophones and francophones, and oddly enough with those among them who master the colonizer's language best. Witness the pathetic 'farewell to the English language' which opens the last book published in English by the Kenyan writer Ngugi wa Thiongo, entitled *Decolonising the mind* (Ngugi 1986).

12. See Paulin J. Hountondji: 'Evidence of such evacuation of history is the use of the adjective 'traditional' which has become habitual ... Replacement of the word 'precolonial', which implies simply a conventional periodisation of History with no relation to the internal characters of the object — by the qualifier 'traditional', which appears to express an internal characterisation, does translate the will to simplify the cultural History of Africa, to reduce it to a convenient, handy pattern, to empty it of its tensions, its enigmas, its equivocations, and finally to close it [...]. Rather than speak of 'traditional Africa', better speak of African tradition, or better still, African traditions. For nothing such as 'traditional Africa' can be found out in the sense that the adjective would qualify invariants remaining identical with themselves throughout the millenniums of a supposedly repetitive History. But there exists an African tradition, or more accurately African traditions. For nothing such as 'traditional Africa' can be found out in the sense of complex heritages which are plurivocal, contradictory, and transmitted from generation to generation through the waverings and somersaults of an eventful History (extract from an unpublished paper written for UNESCO in 1974).
13. In that regard, read the beautiful paper by Alexandre Adandé, Le maïs et ses usages au Bénin méridional (Adandé, Alexandre, 1984).
14. On the exact meaning of those terms as used by Tylor and Lévy-Bruhl, read namely by the former author the very great classic, entitled Primitive Culture, and by the latter, Les fonctions mentales dans les sociétés inférieures, as well as La mentalité primitive (Tylor 1871; Lévy-Bruhl 1910, 1922).
15. Marc Augé very accurately posits the issue in a remarkable text on 'Witchcraft beliefs'. By the same author, we recommend the reading of Théorie des pouvoirs et idéologie (Augé 1974, 1975).
16. We are all the more grateful to CODESRIA's research teams who kindly joined in the work by proposing to us additional bibliographies, particularly useful for pushing the analysis further. We are pleased most specially to thank Valentin-Yves Mudimbe, from Duke University (USA) whose friendly support is appreciated once again, subsequent upon many other such occasions.

Part One

Endogenous Technologies

1

Methodological Issues in the Study of 'Traditional Techniques' and Know-How

Goudjinou P. Metinhoue

What possible contribution might history make to the development of Black Africa? A serious, pertinent question addressed to all disciplines, it is especially relevant to the study of history. An examination of traditional techniques and know-how is a direct response to this question. This chapter focuses on three issues: a) the vast field of traditional techniques; b) the issue of methodology; and c) a case study of the production of sodabi, a local brand of alcohol distilled from palm wine.

The Vast Field of 'Traditional' Techniques

Until recently, historians had little time for the study of know-how. African know-how, in particular, got even shorter shrift. Textbooks on African history rarely discussed ways in which past generations of Africans coped with the practical problems of daily life. History, according to the prevalent approach in those days, was a top-down process. The approach, fortunately, has changed, and historiographic practice has been transformed.

The time is past when historical research could stay blinkered behind supposedly orthodox, universal approaches and topics. In Black Africa the need to move towards innovative approaches has been particularly keen. Our interest in endogenous techniques is part of the move to broaden the scope of historical scholarship. Hountondji (1987a) calls research on traditional technological knowledge and practices ethnotechnology, a pursuit he justly places within the general context of ethno-science, along with such counterparts as:

> ethno-zoology, the study of traditional zoological knowledge; ethno-botany, the study of traditional botanical concepts; ethno-mineralogy, the study of traditional knowledge of mineral resources.... We define ethno-science generally as the study of a corpus of knowledge, information and know-how handed down from generation to generation.[1]

Hountondji (1987) has called the survey conducted by Alexis Adande and myself on local techniques an ethnotechnological study. His point is well taken. Hountondji raises a further, and, in his judgement, crucial question concerning this type of work: the question of the 'field of knowledge'. His argument is as follows:

> When anthropologists survey traditional knowledge in a given field, are we to assume that the knowledge thus identified makes up a complete, self-contained system within the culture under study? Or should we suppose that it develops or gets a new lease on life through the scholarly presentation of the anthropologist?

Hountondji (1987a) illustrates his query by wondering whether scholars studying a craft such as basket-weaving or pottery simply describe forms of knowledge already systematically organized in the background culture itself, or themselves impose that systematic organization in the course of their scholarly investigations.

It is our responsibility to answer the query as honestly and objectively as possible. The findings of researchers reflect the way they approach and assess African knowledge and know-how. It is important, in my opinion, to distinguish between a general corpus of knowledge and particular techniques. The former are more theoretical. Their assessment is therefore more complicated and delicate. As a rule, African cultures operate in a non-literate mode. It is therefore tempting to reduce African knowledge to a series of material cultures with no foundation in scientific philosophies capable of theoretical insights and abstract formulations. That temptation should be resisted. For a close study of all factors that might and should interest historians of material culture indicates that technological achievements are invariably based on theoretical premises. That is altogether natural and logical.

To quote Hountondji again (1987a, see also 1987b):

> There is a whole range of knowledge about plants and animals. Our plant and animal names are informed with tacit systems of zoological

> classification and botanical taxonomy. When these classificatory systems are reconstituted and compared with accepted modern zoological and botanical systems, it becomes clear that matters are far from simple, and questions arise as to the way the traditional classificatory systems actually operated in African society, as distinct from the way modern researchers perceive, reconstitute or reconstruct them.

It is possible that the reason we now wonder about the existence and *modus operandi* of the science in question is that Africa's learned practitioners did not and do not have the competitive attitudes of their Western counterparts. Experience shows that Africa has a corpus of theoretical science, with its share of limitations, but that it is esoteric, becoming clear only to those who seek to understand it.

A study I conducted on the *hungan* (literally, the big drum) at Sè, in the Mono area of south-west Benin sheds some light on this issue. It provides evidence that it is not always the researcher who imposes a systematic structure on African knowledge in the act of presenting it to readers. *Hungan*-playing follows precise rules, and it is accomplished under clearly defined conditions, its purpose being the transmission of messages. The drum language involved uses a specific vocabulary referring to inanimate objects and living beings, and known to selected initiates. The choice of objects and beings thus named is also determined by set rules, and it is necessary to identify and clarify them.

'Traditional' techniques cover a vast field. There is an urgent need for specialists from various disciplines to put their heads together, map out that field and begin to explore it. The time has come, in other words, to conduct a responsible identification of 'African values'. It is such values that would constitute the ground frame for all development projects aspiring to be endogenous.

Pioneering work for a research programme on endogenous technologies has already been done at the National University of Benin. Within the framework of a research seminar entitled 'Archaeology and History of Material Cultures, organised by F. de Medeiros, Alexis Adande and myself, the departments of history and archaeology have been conducting a series of studies since the 1985-86 academic year. This seminar has persuaded me that historians can render an invaluable service to Africans by helping them find their technological and scientific roots, and by urging them to plan for the future in full awareness of the whole extent of their ancestral heritage.

From October 1985 to July 1988, forty-three (43) topics covering every aspect of life were examined by three (3) classes of fourth-year history students led by the seminar organizers. In terms of quality the work presented differed from student to student, but in doing it all students came to discover an area of history practically untouched by prior research. The excitement of our young students was palpable as they found out how pottery was manufactured, how palm oil was made, how *sodabi* was distilled from palm wine, etc., in various regions of Benin. This is the fresh approach to history Devisse (1984) refers to when he writes: 'Students nowadays are much keener to understand a history without heroes, an extensive, profound history grounded in material culture, than to hear ludicrous accounts of battles and wars from centuries past'.

Sometimes, admittedly, certain students are bewildered by this approach to history. Occasionally it makes even our faculty colleagues uneasy. That is because, as Devisse (1984) points out, it presents an unprecedented methodological challenge. At the same time, it opens up infinitely productive possibilities to researchers unafraid to reflect on political realities and to conduct new studies.

We have kept our working methods in this seminar simple, just as they were in February 1981 when Adande and I began our first historical and technological study of ceramic production at Sè in the Mono area of south-west Benin. At that time we were exploring answers to the following questions:

- What do the potters themselves remember about the origins of pottery?
- What traces, old and new, has the craft of pottery left in the village environment?
- What techniques do potters use in their work?
- How do they obtain their raw materials?
- What are the different forms of pottery produced?
- How are ceramic products marketed, and how important are they in daily village life?

- Where are there likely to be promising zones for archaeological study, with potsherds near the surface?

Two subject areas were highlighted in the 1985-86 academic year: handicrafts and nutrition. Studies of the following handicrafts were conducted:

- Ritual pottery at Sô-Ava;
- Pottery at Toffo;
- Pottery in the Porto Novo region, with Trako serving as a case study;
- Aluminium smelting in the city of Cotonou.

The nutritional studies were as follows:

- *Sodabi* alcohol distillation from palm wine;
- The making of palm oil in Gadome township, Mono province;
- The making of palm oil in Ouémé province.

In 1986-87 we extended our research to a number of new sectors, including housing. Twenty-one reports were produced that year, dealing with food technologies, handicrafts and housing. Studies were also conducted on the following topics:

- Cassava processing techniques at Banté in Central Benin;
- Salt-making techniques at Djègbadji, Ouidah region;
- Yam processing techniques in Savalou: a case study of *libo* yam flour;
- *Sodabi* distillation techniques in Abomey-Calavi;
- *Néré* processing techniques in Northern Benin;
- Palm oil and palm nut oil production techniques in Agonlin region, Central Benin;
- Groundnut processing techniques in Azovè region, Mono province;
- Coconut processing techniques among the Popo of Grand Popo region, South-West Benin;
- Metal recycling: the making of finished products and iron and aluminium processing in Cotonou;
- Copper-working techniques in Abomey;
- Gunsmithing techniques among the Fon of Agonlin;

- The production and use of *gèlèdè* masks in Sakété;
- Contribution to the study of the manufacture of selected musical instruments: a case study of the Igue family, Porto Novo;
- Weaving techniques in Abomey;
- The manufacture and use of fishing equipment among the Aguégué;
- Clay processing techniques for pottery in Lokossa;
- Granary building techniques among the Fon of Abomey;
- Traditional architectural techniques in Benin: a comparative study of two regions — Ouémé and Mono;
- Berba housing construction techniques in Materi district North-West Benin;
- The manufacture of products for everyday use: oilcake-making techniques in the Adja area of Honton, Mono region.

Research conducted in the academic year 1987-88 provided data on nutritional, handicraft, housing and fishing techniques. Individual topics were as follows:

- *Féijoada* preparation among the Afro-Brazilians of Ouidah;
- The manufacture of cabbage palmetto oil in Abomey;
- Preparation of *bolu-klaklu* maize and shrimp tarts;
- Preparation of *ablo*, sweet, steamed or baked maize meal cakes, among the Mina of South-West Benin;
- *Gari*-(cassava meal) making techniques in Dassa-Zoumé;
- *Acandji*-(corncake) making techniques in Adjara-Adovié, Pahou region;
- Research on monuments in the rural township of Agblangandan, between Cotonou and Porto Novo;
- Studies on traditional housing in the Dendi-Songhai area: the *Sijifa* case study;
- Studies on rural housing in Zangnanado region, Central Benin;
- *Kossile* mat making from stripped palm branches in Gakpe township, Ouidah region;
- Mat-making in Godomey, Cotonou region;
- The construction of maize granaries in Sakete;

- Traditional shrimp fishing in the Porto Novo lagoon.

Up until that point, then, the organizers of the seminar on the archaeology and history of material cultures focused on three main sectors. There was obviously no shortage of topics. The main problem confronting students was how to identify an efficient methodological approach and then to master it. In the first quarter, we presented them with a range of information designed to enable them to come to grips with the central problem-solving approach of the seminar. Students then selected topic foci, after which we went through with each individual student the draft questionnaires they planned to use in their field work. The general impression from the reports was that students had a hard time using information obtained during their field work as a basis for posing fresh questions, adopting new approaches and generating new ideas about history.

Research on nutritional technology was also conducted at the Polytechnical University College. Examples of work done include a historical study of *chukutu* (millet beer) brewing techniques. Liliane Okoumassoun (1984) conducted a study entitled Chapalo: Technological Study and Qualitative Analysis of Glucides Using Chromatographic Methods on Thin Film. After pointing out that maize is a nutritional staple in Southern Benin, Okoumassoun indicates that the crop has multiple uses, one being the brewing of *chapalo*, a malt beer. Millet and sorghum can also be used to make this beer.

The study on the preparation of *chapalo* in the Dassa-Zoumé area is divided into three parts: the technological process; the application of fine-film chromatology in a study of the glucide component of *chapalo*; and experimental studies, findings and discussions.

While findings from such research may only be of indirect interest to historians, the advantage here is that they incorporate information furnished by expert technicians capable of offering practical recommendations for technological improvements. In the specific case of *chapalo*, Okoumassoun (1984:52) shows that production can only be expanded after the solution of several problems connected with grain quality, ratios of crushed grain, chaff and water, cooking time and the total control of fermentation.

Scholars who link research on traditional African knowledge and techniques with the continent's development are sometimes accused of irrelevant antiquarianism. The assumption in such situations is that only economists, planners, engineers and people in that league can initiate serious change. Accumulating experience proves, however, that if Africa is to emerge from its 'underdevelopment', all branches of knowledge have to be involved in an organized, systematic, interdisciplinary process. In any case, it seems patently absurd to study endogenous knowledge and technologies while staying hooked on external methodologies. For our part, this is the approach our archaeological research team has been following so far at the National University of Benin.

The study of traditional knowledge and techniques as a component of African culture has direct implications for the future development of generations on this continent. It is therefore important, right from the start, that we choose methods designed to lead to the most accurate, dependable results, and that we take pains to clarify our choices.

The Issue of Methodology

The French palaeontologist André Leroi-Gourhan (1974) makes a key point in saying that history before writing is the history of humanity in the process of self-realization through prehensile skills, in the sense that it is the history of mental constructs given external, manual form. In plain words, it is the history of human beings as tool-makers.

This statement opens up undreamed methodological possibilities, in Africa more than anywhere else. It is reassuring to have it come from a scholar of the calibre of Leroi-Gourhan. It is nothing less than an invitation to study the history of the technological traditions of various peoples. It is, after all, hard to comprehend human experience in its totality while shirking research on the knowledge and techniques of different peoples. What is necessary is to approach such a study with appropriate methodological tools capable of yielding fruitful findings.

I am put off by methodological preconceptions. It seems to me that often we have to adopt specific approaches tailored to individual cases. Success in the solution of one problem does not make any single method the ultimate solution to all problems. I distrust off-the-shelf methods. For that reason, I am perfectly comfortable with research techniques emphasizing trial and error. I have taken pains to spell out my position because we are dealing with a discipline in which change comes so slowly as to be hardly perceptible within a single lifetime. For that reason it is advisable to proceed cautiously, step by step, through trial and error.

Researchers conducting field studies in Africa encounter an extra problem that some might call specific: the problem of sources. A great deal of information on African traditions is preserved in the memories of living human beings. Since the 1960s there has been widespread debate about the usefulness of oral traditions from the viewpoint of historians. Here we do not intend to enter that debate (Vansina 1961; Ki-Zerbo 1969; Laya Dioulde 1972; Person 1962; and Diabate 1980).

In a paper addressed to French historians on perceptions of other people's history, Devisse (1985) suggests a series of highly interesting methodological approaches. His ideas on writing, in my opinion, offer extremely useful insights likely to enhance the appreciation of the role of oral traditions:

> Writing acquired superior status because of the uses to which ruling power structures and classes put it. Not surprisingly, the dominant perception of history today, to which we subscribe, has conferred absolute authority on written documents, going so far as to make them the sole acceptable source for the reconstruction of the past. From this perspective, any people who, for whatever reason, did not opt for the use of written documents as the repository of memory could have no history. Everyone, from the Mediterranean to China, has acquiesced in this sanctification of cold, formal, written text. And those whose business it has been to hand down historical or technical knowledge, as well as those actively involved in political affairs, have all accepted these presuppositions uncritically (Devisse 1984:63).

To get an accurate understanding of Devisse's statements, we need to recall the phenomenon Joseph Ki-Zerbo (1972) so aptly called 'the barrage of myths'. In the name of the written word and the absolute power conferred on it by Europeans, Africa, or at any rate Black Africa, was excluded from history, and major French historians felt justified in writing, without even cracking a smile, that Africans had played no part whatsoever in the construction and management of the world.

One might forgive scholars with no specialist grounding in African studies for publishing such bromides. But it is disappointing and shocking to find so-called Africanists repeating them. In his recent work, François de Medeiros has exposed the operational mechanisms of 'Africanism', showing how dangerous this ideology has been and continues to be in the field of African historical research (de Medeiros 1989).

Jean Devisse (1984:63) gives a clear account of the long route travelled in the effort to gain recognition for oral traditions as credible sources.

> In the beginning, there was little chance of meeting the legitimate aspirations of Africans to reconstitute their past — either by projecting their own conception of history or by coming to terms with a historical tradition still exploring paths and making compromises in its effort to achieve universal validity — as long as the written word continued to enjoy the overweening supremacy accorded it....It has taken a generation for scholars to devise and polish critical methods for the study of oral sources. It was necessary to overcome the arch-conservative resistance of those who thought oral sources should be above critical analysis because they expressed popular truths. Simultaneously, the variously expressed skepticism of all those who thought it unacceptable to give any credence to oral sources, on the grounds that they were unreliable, had to be dealt with.

Important as oral traditions are, they still cover only a fraction of Africa's historical record. It is an axiom that oral traditions have little to say about the scientific and technical experience of Africans. That is probably one reason why ignorance of Africa's technological traditions is so widespread, sometimes among Africans themselves. As a matter of fact, there are areas of the continent where people have not the faintest idea of the scientific and technological heritage left them by their ancestors. So we need urgently to marshall the resources necessary for conducting an inventory of every mechanism devised in Black Africa for the solution of everyday problems. This kind of research is of vital importance, since there are so many Africans still convinced that all progress has come to the continent from abroad, and that their own ancestors were never able to invent anything.

Ki-Zerbo (1969:11) has roundly condemned the myth of a do-nothing African people, a standard feature in most texts produced by major European historians covering Africa. According to these European savants:

> It was the Caucasoid Hamites who, pushing southwards into Africa, brought Africa the technical skills required to domesticate nature. Gold mines, *cire perdue* sculptural techniques, the naturalist art of Ife, Aggrey beads, the concept of State organization, everything positive came from whites. Occasionally the source could be red or brown people, but invariably even those turned out, on more detailed identification, to be white.

Robert Cornevin asserts that it was probably the Arabs who introduced *cire perdue* techniques, known throughout Eurasia from the Bronze Age on, into Africa across the Sahara. Furthermore, he says:

> The prevailing working hypothesis now is that certain Arab craftsmen must have arrived at the courts of black kings where they were put to work teaching the excellently gifted races of Southern Nigeria their techniques.

Here we come face to face with the most harmful myth produced by ethnocentric Europe concerning African history. Unfortunately, the myth has nine lives. No doubt the colonial and neo-colonial context in which the first books on African history were written made their authors feel they could get away with such stupidities. But now the time has come for us to stop decrying this negative situation while still continuing to approach the discipline of history as if it were some objective, neutral ground instead of a field deeply pocked with multiple subjective standpoints and positions.

Apart from addressing methodological issues, we also need to sort out priority issues for Africa today and tomorrow. African historians should recognize that this is their vocation. To accomplish it they should not hesitate, when necessary, to tap inspiration from foreign sources. On this issue, Devisse (1984:62) raises a number of questions of interest to most historians. He thinks Europeans should re-examine their conception of history, especially their historical approach to the sciences and technology, material production and the development of social structures. 'What serious historian', he asks:

> can remain mute about the great advances achieved by, using techniques we can still admire through recent texts Chinese science long before the 16th century; the Indian record of refined iron production stretching over two millennia; the scientific contributions of the Arab world, whose discoveries in mathematics and astronomy advanced and developed the knowledge of antiquity, helping to set

> the stage for the technological and scientific take-off of the West after the 13th century? And what historian can fail to wonder at the technological intelligence of African peasants, capable of accomplishing quiet but extremely effective revolutions by the reasoned adoption of plants imported from the Americas? Which historian can pass over the skill of craftspersons who in past ages produced the copper and iron works and tools they needed?

Increasing specialization in the field of historical research on Africa, especially with regard to the continent's technological traditions, makes it necessary for historians to work together with researchers from various other disciplines (Devisse 1984:64). Because we have an archaeologist in our team, we are able to alert our audiences to the pivotal role this discipline can play in providing information on the history of peoples without writing systems. Here I agree with the following opinion expressed by Devisse (1984:64, 66).

> Not so long ago, archaeology was a discipline specializing in the discovery and study of inscriptions and monuments. The leading practitioners were not French scholars but English, German, Polish and American. New methods went through various name changes as they got developed, but the main aim of the discipline was to restore the material history of peoples without writing systems or coherent historical traditions. Since then, the focus of archaeological research has shifted. In the effort to retrieve the material culture and history of societies without writing systems, greater emphasis has been placed on the study of stone artefacts, iron, copper, traces of foodstuffs, and the study of problems. In principle, the scope of chronological studies opened up by these new methods is infinitely vast, given the new chronology of human history.

Devisse's work brings us to the core of the methodological debate, and there is every reason to treat the author's statements seriously. He knows Africa both through his coverage of publications in African studies, and through his own direct experience of field research.

We return, then, to the key point that archaeology can be extremely helpful to African history. It is one of the main guides to the exploration of the past. In this role it is highly demanding:

> Imposing a need for at least a working knowledge of human and animal palaeontology, palaeo-zoology, physical anthropology, pathological anatomy, laboratory techniques for the study of metals,

> ceramics, textiles, organic chemistry, nutrition, geology, geography, meteorology, linguistics and cultural anthropology.

This is a far cry from the old set of 'ancillary disciplines', as Devisse (1984) himself concludes. The fields mentioned give us an idea of what researchers today have to understand, at least in outline, in their effort to restore the history of societies supposedly without writing systems.

To further clarify the role of archaeology in historical research in general, and in the exploration of Africa's past in particular, let me paraphrase a statement made by Adande in December 1988: every human group produces knowledge, skills, attitudes and aptitudes, in addition to labour. Knowledge and labour together work on ecofacts — the sum total of nature's produce. Some of this produce may be useful to human beings. Labour and knowledge are transmitted through techniques applied to natural objects to produce artefacts, defined as products of human activity designed to satisfy consumption needs and other material requirements of society.

When archaeological researchers examine traces of past technologies, what they have to work on, as a rule, is a collection of natural objects preserved in the form of charcoal, etc. The only surviving artefacts, generally speaking, are weather-resisting objects such as sculpted stone, bones, buildings, etc. In order to reconstitute intellectual, labour and technological history from such elements, researchers quite often find themselves having to rely on a new branch of knowledge: palaeography or palaeobotany. One step leads to another, and ultimately, techniques and data from all modern science come in useful.

Artefacts, then, are studied in laboratories, while sites are excavated and their contents examined. The result is the reconstitution of ancient techniques, along with that of the science underlying the invention of these techniques and the exploitation of resources in the interests of human welfare.

Obviously, the approaches of Adande and Devisse converge on a number of issues. Both keep up with current archaeological research, while doing their share of work in the field, each in his area and in his own style. What is refreshing in their statements, as far as I am concerned, is their emphasis on the interaction of multiple disciplines. Modern science is becoming increasingly specialized. This has made interdisciplinary approaches a must in scientific research. One is in fact tempted to conclude that the scholars of antiquity followed a multidisciplinary approach, to the extent that they were interested in all human experience and everything in the cosmos. Herodotus, father of history, certainly worked close to that pattern. To be more precise, however, I agree perfectly with the point made by Hountondji at the December 1988 seminar already referred to:

> Herodotus was not a scientist if we go by current definitions of the term. He was not a researcher but a learned man, at a time when it was possible to play that role. We no longer have learned men these days; instead we have researchers, each focusing on a specific sector of reality. This is quite a recent development, an outcome of modern, post-Galilean scientific advances. As recently as the age of Descartes, it was still possible for individuals to straddle all known branches of learning simultaneously. Since then, the division of intellectual labour has grown increasingly pronounced, specialization has grown increasingly narrower, and the status of the single encyclopaedic intellect is no longer possible. Herodotus did not, strictly speaking, follow an interdisciplinary approach. What he did was to master a whole field of knowledge as it existed in his age.

Nowadays, only interdisciplinary approaches guarantee solutions to methodological problems encountered by African historians, especially those doing research on traditional techniques and know-how.

The Distillation of *Sodabi*: A Historical Case Study

Prior to the discovery of the technique of *sodabi* distillation from palm wine, people in Southern and Northern Dahomey already knew how to brew alcoholic beverages from maize and other cereals. The following is a description of *sodabi* distillation in Gbokou, a neighbourhood in Porto-Novo, Benin's political capital, 30 kilometres from Cotonou.

The group that specializes in *sodabi* distillation in Gbokou is the Tolinu group, originally from Toli in Allada region. According to information collected in June 1986 by Katina Agueh, then a fourth year history student, *sodabi* has long played a role in the trading relationships of several population groups in southern Benin. As we shall see, the drink is consumed on different occasions in the daily life of south Benin, especially during funerals and certain festivals.

Ordinarily, *sodabi* is distilled from palm wine, which comes from the sap of felled palm trees growing 'wild' in many parts of southern Benin. According to the Ministry of Rural Development and Cooperatives, palm trees grow over more than 130,000 hectares, an area far greater than that covered by other oil-producing plants such as groundnuts and shea (Adamand Boko 1983:48). Apart from palm wine, palm trees also yield oil and a variety of by-products much used by the people. There is no space here for a detailed treatment of these various products. We need only point out that palm wine is a sweetish, refreshing drink whose alcohol content, initially quite low, increases with fermentation over a number of days.

Among the Toli of Gbokou, palm wine is known as *atan*. In the Mono area of South-Western Benin it is generally known as *déhan*, meaning palm wine. Peasants, however, classify palm wine into a number of categories depending on quality. In their judgement, the best *sodabi* is made from a type called *hankou*. In the Sè area, the very first drops of palm wine are called *dideta*, meaning ant-head. The reason is that these drops are so sweet they attract ants, which, losing their heads under the palm trees, die. This supersweet palm wine is never used for distilling *sodabi*.

People here have yet to adopt a method of extracting palm wine from palm trees without destroying the trees. Agueh conducted a survey of various reasons why peasants cut down their palm trees. Some do it to make money. In other cases there are legal reasons, as in situations where the trees concerned are situated on disputed ground. Palm trees are also cut down when they grow too old, or to clear fields for food crops. In countries as Nigeria, the Ivory Coast and Senegal, there are techniques for extracting palm wine without killing the trees. But the above information indicates that in Benin, such techniques are not automatically applicable.

It seems altogether likely that Dahomey, now called Benin, was the country in which *sodabi* was first distilled. According to an article whose author, unfortunately, is unnamed (La Croix du Bénin 1976:3), this 'alcoholic drink made from palm wine by local handicraft methods was first distilled by the brothers Gbehalaton and Bonou Kiti Sodabi, from the village of Sèdjè-Houégoudo in the district of Allada'.

The same article informs us that Bonou Kiti Sodabi served in the rifle corps recruited from all countries of French West Africa but synecdochically known as *tirailleurs sénégalais*. These infantrymen fought for France during the 1914-18 war. While in France, Bonou Kiti Sodabi learned to make alcohol from fermented bananas. On his return to his country, he and his brother Gbehalaton built makeshift stills with which they proceeded to distil alcohol in their village, Sèdèj. Using fermented bananas, they were able to distil a drink called *ahankou* or *anko* from 1919 until 1925. In 1926 the brothers hit on the idea of using fermented palm wine. The result was a drink with an altogether special kick. Friends loved it. Soon, people were coming from neighbouring villages to buy it from the brothers. Its fame spread, and in time the drink came to be known simply as *sodabi*, after its distillers (La Croix du Bénin 1976).

We think it important to draw attention to the fact that it was during their trip to France that the Sodabi brothers learned to distil alcohol. That fact is a direct challenge to some prejudiced perceptions and judgements of black soldiers published by certain French officers. Among books and articles written at the time on the so-called Senegalese rifle corps, there was a small volume entitled *Coulibaly*, by a French Sub-lieutenant called Léon Gaillet, published in 1917. This 153-page volume was widely read in all French colonial circles, and it is quite probable that quite a few French colonialists were influenced in their thinking about black people as a result of absorbing information from Gaillet's little book. The author starts by explaining that the name Coulibaly applies to the typical black, the African in general.

> I could just as well have used other names such as Kamara, Diarra, Sissoko, Traoré, names extremely common among our Senegalese and our Sudanese. Somehow, though, in ways mysterious to me, the name Coulibaly attracted me most strongly. I have become accustomed, when I think and speak of blacks in general, to using that convenient name, to the point where I am now quite devoted to it.

Having thus set the tone of his book, Gaillet proceeds to give a detailed description of the daily life of African soldiers in France. For the purposes of this chapter, the most interesting chapter is the one on Coulibaly's intelligence, taken by the author, in his own words, to exemplify the intelligence of black people as a whole. Gaillet grants black people a measure of intelligence, but takes care to stress that they lack abstract reasoning powers. In his opinion, black people are incapable of isolating relationships from objects, and making deductions from them (Gaillet 1917:35). 'Coulibaly's practical intelligence is quite limited', the author says:

> At home he satisfies his basic needs as best he can. He is entirely lacking in that advanced form of practical intelligence that makes use of scientific knowledge, industrial intelligence. It would be pointless to expect any glimmering of scientific intelligence from Coulibaly. The reason is simple: he is devoid of curiosity, and it would seem that he was denied the faculty of wonder. Contemplating such inventions as the telephone, the cinema projector, the aeroplane, all our modern inventions, in fact, he remains apathetic, quite without surprise (Gaillet 1917:45).

Now it is perfectly possible, as it was at the time, to prove Gaillet's assertions baseless. His blithe statement that black people lack the faculty of wonder is particularly absurd. The fact that two Dahomeans, having travelled to France during the war of 1914-18, learned the use of alcohol distilling stills there, and that on their return they set up their own makeshift still, is a convincing rebuttal to the French officer's opinions on the intelligence of all black people, encapsulated in the name Coulibaly.

According to Agueh's research, the Toli of the Gbokou neighbourhood in Porto Novo learned to make *sodabi* in the village of Ouémé-Djigbé on the Porto Novo-Dangbo road through the Ouémé valley. Palm trees might be cut down at any time of day throughout the year, the only exception being the harmattan season, on account of its extreme dryness.

Palm wine is tapped in the field. The sap is poured into huge clay jars. In the past these were brought in from Sè, but later they were also obtained from around Porto Novo. Traditional clay jars proving rather brittle, peasants gradually switched over to barrels imported from Europe.

Whatever the container, palm wine is left to ferment for five to eight days. Distillation begins after the wine is thoroughly fermented. The process takes place in the palm grove or in some hidden part of the peasant moonshiner's home. The fermented palm wine is poured into a barrel, which is then placed on a fire. A stilling tube measuring five to seven metres leads from the barrel through two or three jars three-quarters filled with water, to a funnel into which the *sodabi* drips. The first three or four litres drawn are super proof. Connaisseurs call it top grade or *aku*, which means pure *sodabi*. It costs twice as much as second-grade *sodabi*. Near the end of the distillation process, the last few litres, of very poor quality, are known as *bélo*. In the Mono area, it is customary, as soon as palm wine gets tapped, to set aside the lowest grade, known as *odofouin* around Sè, for making *bélo*. In Gbokou, as in other parts of Benin, *bélo* is used to distil new *sodabi*. The normal practice is to mix fresh, good quality palm wine with old *bélo* in a 5:1 ratio.

Sodabi got a rousing reception from the moment it appeared on the market in 1926. To this day it is still in great demand in numerous areas of Southern Benin, because it is an indispensable item at funerals and during various ceremonies that punctuate the daily lives of large numbers of the rural and urban population. In the face of stiff competition from imported European drinks, backed by repeated banning orders, *sodabi* continues to sell strongly. Villagers use it as an antiseptic. Traditional healers use it regularly to speed up the healing effects of roots and leaves. For several reasons, then, it would be in the interests of the nation's economic authorities to promote the development of *sodabi*. Ghana offers an example here: in that country the local equivalent has been produced under license for some years now.

We have already cited the article on the history of *sodabi* published in *La Croix du Bénin*. It concludes with a query: 'What, in practical terms, does the Benin Revolution plan to do about *sodabi*?' The question is on target, because in the body of the article, the author recapitulates the tribulations visited upon the Sodabi brothers by the French colonial administration, which banned the distillation and marketing of the drink in the 1930s.

In 1931, the French administrator Jean Jarton, acting on a report from the local chief Agoundafo Sékou, arrested the two Sodabi brothers and jailed them. A local newspaper, *Le Phare du Dahomey*, took up the matter, publishing a photo of Sodabi the inventor along with a detailed article. Still, the two Sodabi brothers were kept in jail for six months, and did not get out until after the departure of the administrator Manget from Allada, and the payment of a fine totalling 6,000 francs, a heavy sum in those days (La Croix du Bénin 1976:3).

This episode brings us straight to the core of one of the real obstacles blocking development in Africa. We have already touched on this obstacle: the extroverted nature of the continent's economy. In many areas of life, the French and English colonialists forced Africans to give up any attempt at imaginative thinking and invention, and instead to wait for foreigners to bring them solutions to their problems. I think Europeans who today assert that Africans lack inventive intelligence add insult to injury. Their jibes should motivate us to achieve greater self-knowledge and self-confidence. Sadly, though, often that is not the case. Ever since I began working with the research seminar on the history of material cultures, I have become aware that the tragedy of Africans is that they are sublimely ignorant of the achievements of past generations of Africans, assuming that Africa has made no scientific and technological contributions to humanity. The time has come to correct this anomaly.

Today, the central field for African historiography embraces knowledge and techniques, know-how and traditional technologies, material culture, in short. Material culture comprises the whole range of vestiges and traces handed down by past human societies to future generations. There is a communal aspect to the concepts of techniques and technological traditions. Serious, credible European researchers (Brand, Roger 1971) have suggested that material culture — in the form of objects — facilitates our understanding of humanity, and that art works are especially helpful in this regard, since they mediate between human beings and the world.

Those who study the technological traditions of a people learn what these men and women destined to live together sharing time and space have conceived and produced in the way of appropriate solutions to their everyday problems. This type of history differs fundamentally from the tale of royal reigns, kingdoms, political parties and outstanding personalities. Outstanding personalities and grandiose entities are respectable enough, but it is inaccurate to present them as if they were the only actors in African history.

Because we are dealing with a new, practically untouched branch of African historiography, we have to resolve the thorny problem of methodology as rapidly as possible. I have described the experience of our archaeological research team. We are fully aware that ours is a constant search for information. I have repeatedly quoted, every time with pleasure, an extract from the address delivered by the late Professor Georges Dumezil on his accession to the French Academy.

> In Literature and the Arts, a man can show you a work, sincerely claiming it is his own, and expect you to give him the benefit of the doubt. Matters are different in our archaeological work. It is a field in which each practitioner, in his brief tenure, extends by a few meters the area of knowledge opened up by predecessors, with tools tested by others, before disappearing after leaving his findings for those to come.

I am deeply persuaded that our research and theoretical work in the seminar on the history of material cultures, prolonged and enriched in the seminar on the sociology of knowledge, is the kind of research the late Professor Dumezil advocated for the Humanities. Our study of the history of techniques, traditional technologies and material cultures is the culmination of a long and dynamic process of historical scholarship. In times past there was a dualistic tendency to split material activity from intellectual activity, establishing a dichotomy between material production and intellectual production. One positive contribution the history of knowledge and technology can make is to reunite the two aspects of human activity. Researchers who achieve this healing juncture make common cause with humanity in its most ordinary and intimate strivings. Such an objective can only be achieved through the joint efforts of multiple scholarly disciplines. We hope this seminar on the sociology of knowledge will help convince university academics in Benin and Africa as a whole of the need for such interdisciplinary work.

Notes

1. Most of the ensuing section is a revised version of an article by this author published in the magazine Entente africaine, No. 75, December 1988 and No. 76, March 1989.
2. On maize and its uses in Southern Benin, Adande (1984) has this to say: 'Peasants distil alcohol from maize beer, using moonshine stills. Beer heated in a container turns to steam, which then passes through a coiled metallic tube immersed in cold water. The condensed stea to let drip into a gourd or bottle. Alcohol produced by this technique is inflammable'.
3. This information is corroborated by the research of our colleague Felix Iroko of the National University of Benin, who, after an inquiry conducted in the village of sédjé, came up with practically identical findings.

2

'Traditional' Iron Metallurgy in West Africa

Alexis B.A. Adande

We cannot even make a needle or a simple nail, yet we presume to want independence. On 28 September 1958, on the initiative of General Charles de Gaulle, then President of France, a referendum was organized throughout the French African colonies including Madagascar. A yes vote would mean continued French tutelage, a no vote independence. The argument about the inability of Africans to make needles or nails was used by politicians pushing for a yes vote. The assumption was false. But it reflected a widespread opinion concerning the technological level of black Africans. Certain members of the *évolués* elite, especially those colonial intellectuals who held various political and administrative posts, in the years following the granting of independence, subscribed to this negative attitude.

Among colonial scholars and 'metropolitan' researchers, the issue was framed differently. They knew perfectly well that black Africans had in the past known and mastered iron-working technology. For them the riddle was about the origin of that technology. Was it invented on the African continent? Or was it transferred here after being developed elsewhere?

Today the focus of iron metallurgy research has shifted, and methods have changed. Standards are more exacting, and more rigorous procedures are followed in field work, thanks to the development of specific research programmes. These changes were possible only because of the emergence of a new generation of researchers, and the training of African researchers, who have been exercising a growing influence in the field of archaeological research.

Research in West Africa has progressed quite vigorously in countries like Ghana and Nigeria which have substantial research facilities. Lately, Burkina Faso, Mali, Senegal, Mauritania and Togo have also seen increased activity (see Figure 1). In Benin, scientific and scholarly research in general, and archaeological research in particular, are handicapped by a chronic shortage of financial and other resources. Nevertheless, thanks to the efforts of such individuals and groups as the Benin Archaeological Research Team of the National University of Benin, there is now an accumulation of interesting data.

This chapter, focused on West Africa, addresses three questions: What is iron metallurgy? What do we know about the practice of iron metallurgy in ancient times, and how was this knowledge acquired? Why study this socio-economic activity?

What is Iron Metallurgy?

Metallurgy might be defined as the process of extracting minerals from ores, transforming them into semi-finished products, and moulding them with a view to turning them into useable artefacts. The process comprises two phases: primary and secondary metallurgy.

Primary Metallurgy: The Extractive Phase

Primary iron metallurgy involves the extraction of iron from iron ore. To accomplish this, the iron-worker uses a furnace (see Figure 2). In the African context, iron-workers developed and used low firebox hearths and low-shaft furnaces. Low-shaft furnaces are not necessarily small. In some areas of Africa they used to be very large. They are called low-shaft furnaces in reference to the highest temperature in the furnace during smelting operations.

Iron melts at 1536°C. In low-shaft furnaces the temperature at the heart does not rise that high. High-blast furnaces can reach that temperature or go even higher. African ironworkers normally used direct iron-making methods, designed to yield metal without going through the intermediate foundry stage. The indirect method appeared in Asia (China) from the twelfth century and in Europe between the sixteenth and seventeenth centuries. To make steel or wrought iron, it is necessary first of all to adapt the molten metal by decarbonizing it (Gille 1966:21 and 31-33).

Figure 1: Map of Ironworking Sites in West Africa

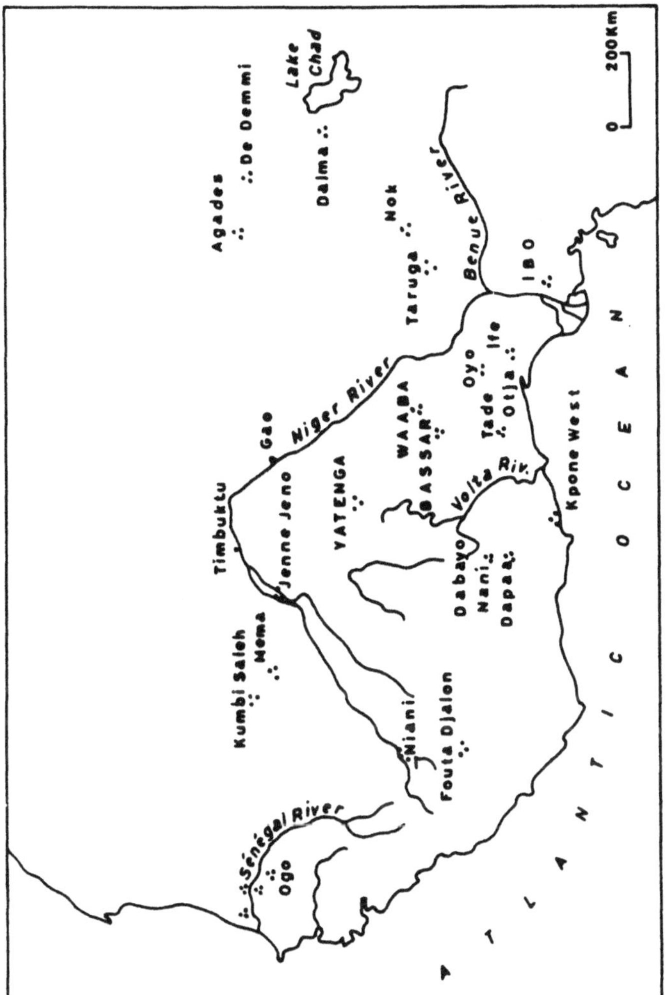

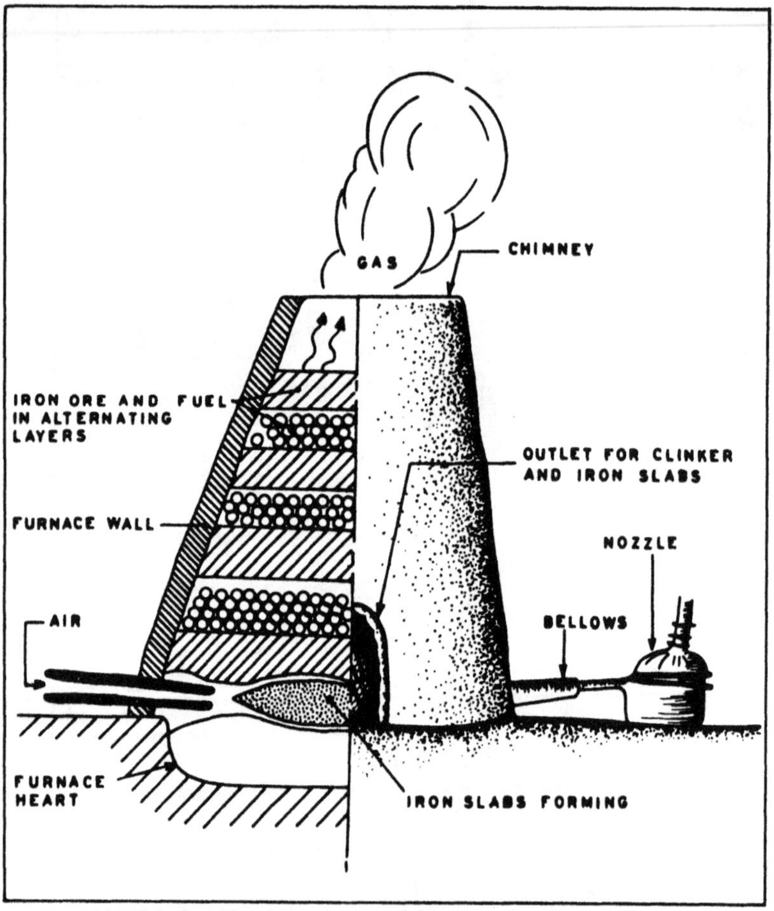

Figure 2: Diagram of an Iron-smelting Furnace

Secondary Metallurgy: The Processing Phase

The purpose of this phase is to extract raw iron in a purified form fit for forging. This means it has to be free of impurities, especially ash and clinker. In that state it is hammered into shape. This is also the phase in which iron is worked into instruments and artefacts used for a variety of socio-economic, military, religious and other purposes.

Anthropologists have published several monographs on West African ironsmiths. Recent studies have also enriched our knowledge of the development of smelting techniques (Wantchecon 1983; Godonou 1985). New studies have expanded coverage to include smelting instruments, their level of efficiency and their potential for development.

Thanks to these refinements in ongoing research, it is now possible to classify the various types of smithies as well as to identify a certain degree of specialization among them. For instance, a recent ethnographic study in the township of Bassar, North-Central Togo, shows that bellows used in the area were powerful enough to enable ironsmiths there to purify pig iron and to make it workable after beating it with stone hammers of different sizes at different stages in the processing of the metal and its shaping into various objects. These smiths used a special type of tong, with large hunks of granite serving as anvils. Kotokoli ironsmiths in the same area used iron anvils set in blocks of timber, and their bellows were lighter, while their tongs were designed for more delicate handling. Today, Kotokoli smiths get their iron from the Bassar ironworkers, or recycle scrap. They have a reputation for skill in such fine-grained, artistic work as the manufacture of rings, bracelets and knives. Their Bassar counterparts, on the other hand, are specialists in the manufacture of hoe blades. The two groups are entirely different from smelters, but they form complementary links in the metal-working process. Bassar ironsmiths build permanent smithies, while Kotokoli workshops are portable.

One question that has long worried archaeologists is the determination of the origin of extractive metallurgy in Black Africa. A great deal of controversy has surrounded the issue.

The Controversy about the Origins of Iron-working Technology in Black Africa

The first colonial administrators and missionaries to do research in the field were struck by the array of processes employed in primary metallurgy. They were equally impressed with the diversity of furnace types. Their conclusion was that extractive iron metallurgy originated in Black Africa, from where it got diffused into Europe. Some argued for a Near Eastern diffusion path, others for a different route (Rattray 1916:431; Boeuf 1937:403-404; Porteres 1938:463). In the 1930s and after, other colonial researchers began to challenge this view. In their opinion it was inconceivable that black Africans could have invented primary metallurgy. They thought this metallurgy, or in any case the basic technological knowledge that made it possible, must have come to Africa from the Middle East by way of the Nile Valley or Carthage (present-day Tunis). The precise points of contact were hard to establish, but then the colonial researchers fell back on the notorious concept of 'chariot routes' (Mauny 1970:62).

That, in fact, was the only 'palpable' proof brought up to shore up the notion that extractive iron technology came to Africa from abroad. True, certain 'Africanist' researches put forward a third version, claiming that the technology came to East Africa from India. The strongest refutation of these theories of external origins for African metallurgy came from a French researcher, Henri Lhote, and most conclusively from Professors Louise-Marie and Cheikh Anta Diop. They pointed out that given the overwhelming weight of ethnographic, archaeological and even historical evidence in favour of African origins, the theory of external diffusion was untenable (Lhote 1952; Diop 1968; Diop 1973, 1976). We shall clarify the issue by outlining current information on the issue.

The State of Knowledge about Iron Metallurgy in Ancient Times

Up until the 1950s and the early 1960s, very little was known about primary metallurgy, apart from such information as was contained in the writings of colonial military officers and administrators who had witnessed the death throes of iron-working technology in various parts of West Africa. On the other hand, thanks to numerous publications from anthropologists and historians of material culture, available information on secondary metallurgy was much more plentiful. In the last few decades, interest in ethno-archaeological studies and archaeological research has boomed, and the urge to reach a greater understanding of the metallurgical history of Sub-Saharan Africa, with a special emphasis on iron, has intensified accordingly.

A Methodological Approach: Ethno-Archaeological Surveys and Archaeological Studies

Ethno-archaeological surveys differ markedly from ethnographic surveys, strictly defined. They involve observations of structures as they exist now, a look at of the way they were designed to operate, an examination of the process of their breakdown, and, where possible, an examination of their sedimentation. This inquiry goes hand in hand with the recording of oral traditions from elders who still remember the technology formerly used for extracting iron.

This type of research has been carried out in Nigeria, Ghana, the Ivory Coast, Burkina Faso, and more recently, in North-Central Togo. In Burkina Faso, for example, over the past few years our colleague Jean-Baptiste Kiethega has been organizing a vast programme designed to draw up an inventory of known sites of extractive iron-working technology in the country and beyond (Kiethega 1981). In Ghana, apart from the orthodox ethnographic survey conducted in the north (Pole 1975), there has also been a full-fledged experimental survey led by Professor Merrick Posnansky on and around the Begho site in the West-Central area. In addition to technical aspects, one of the goals of this research was the assessment of the ecological impact of the socio-economic activity involved over time (Goucher 1981). Members of this American team conducted similar research together with archaeological excavations on metallurgical sites in the Bassar areas of Togo (Goucher 1984; Barros 1985). Findings from these surveys should lead to a more accurate understanding of ancient structures dug up during the excavations.

Ancient Metallurgical Sites in West Africa

Let us point out right from the start that the following descriptive report gives only a faint idea of a much richer reality. Archaeological research is a recent undertaking in West Africa. Centres of activity are very unevenly distributed in the area, and patterns of resource allocation are just as unbalanced. In spite of these drawbacks, research in the field has already yielded extremely valuable findings.

A number of archaeologists have suggested the division of Africa's Iron Age into three periods: the Early Iron Age, from still indeterminate beginnings to 650 A.D.; the Later Iron Age, from the 7th to the 16th century; and the Recent Iron Age, involving only certain sites, from the 17th to the early 20th century. So far there are only a handful of known sites from the Early Iron Age. At the moment, three zones have been identified in West Africa: the Nok culture complex between the Niger and Benue Rivers in Central Nigeria; the Aïr area in Northern Niger, and the area around Daboya in Northern Ghana.

Detailed findings from the Daboya site are as yet unavailable. However, samples dated there indicate the use of iron as far back as the first millennium B.C. (Sutton 1982:297). Available data on the Nok civilization are much more plentiful, and they provide conclusive proof that Nok belonged to the Early Iron Age. The Taruga site in particular, where excavations were conducted by the British archaeologist Bernard Fagg, provided tangible proof of dynamic metallurgical activity. A total of thirteen furnaces were excavated there, together with fragments of nozzles and wall linings, clinker and coal. Radiocarbon dating techniques indicate that the sites were active between 790 B.C. and 70 B.C.

There are two Early Iron Age sites in Northern Niger. One is situated on the foothills of the Tigidit cliffs south of Agadès. Iron-working sites there date back to the 5th century B.C. and the first century B.C. (490 + or - 100 B.C, and 60 + or - 90 B.C.). South-east of Agadès, on the Termit plateau, studies have been conducted on a low-shaft furnace at Do-Dimmi, apparently dating back to the 7th century B.C. (678 + or - 120 B.C.).

Iron-working sites dating back to later periods are more numerous, and they seem to have developed around large agglomerations. A good example is the steel-making site at Hani near Begho. Others include Dapaa, close to the oldest known Akan settlement, Bono Manso; various metallurgical sites near Niani, capital of the Mali Empire; Kumbi Saleh, capital of ancient Ghana; and Ile Ife, the holy city of the Yoruba people. Other regions were famed for the sophisticated skills of their iron smelters. Of these the best know were Mema in ancient Ghana, various sites in Mossi country, sites around Bandjeli in the Bassar area, sites in the Waaba region, the Atacora highlands of Benin, and the Yoruba sites around Otta and Oyo.

It would seem, from the evidence, that iron-making developed throughout the entire West African region, including the forest zones

(Porteres 1938:463-4). This is a region with abundant iron ore reserves, generally speaking. Iron content varies widely from location to location, of course, but extractive iron metallurgy was known in the southern areas of the Ivory Coast and the Gold Coast (present-day Ghana) as well as in the Gulf of Benin, long before the arrival of the first European navigators (Adande 1983). Traces of primary metallurgical industry have, for instance, been found at Tado near Aplahoué (de Medeiros, Metinhoue and Adande 1981; Bertho 1945). Yet in the course of history, all this activity died after steadily intensifying contacts with Europe. What were the reasons for this loss of extractive metallurgical traditions?

Known Causes of the Disappearance of Extractive Iron-working Traditions

There may well be a few isolated places where iron-smelting operations are still conducted in the ancient style, but they represent the dying remnants of an activity that was once widespread. In the Gulf of Benin, which at one time came to be known as the Slave Coast, iron metallurgy seems to have vanished quite early, some time between the 17th and 18th centuries. The first reason is obvious enough: the impact of the Slave Trade. This region was among the principal suppliers of human merchandise, exchanged for iron bars and various metal artefacts which slave dealers used to procure new supplies of captives. Furthermore, the permanent war of attrition installed by the hunt for captives must have upset iron-working activities in these zones for very long periods, and there is every reason to think that ironsmiths were themselves often kidnapped for sale. Proof of this possibility is the fact that iron metallurgy appeared in South America with the arrival of African slaves in a tropical environment that was less alien to them than it was to their European masters. On this issue the Brazilian researcher Gilberto Freyre, in his well known book *Masters and Slaves, The Formation of Brazilian Society,* writes: 'As Eschwege points out, in Brazil iron-smelting was learned from Africans.... Africa provided 'housemistresses' for settlers without white wives, technicians for the mines, craftsmen for the smithies...' (Freyre 1974:287-290).

Before the Americas were colonized, the indigenous population knew how to work gold, copper and bronze, but not iron. It was enslaved Africans who brought their metallurgical knowledge across the Atlantic.

This is an example of technology transfer passed under silence by historians writing on the world-wide diffusion of knowledge. It is not beyond the bounds of possibility, in this connection, that some European slave traders may specifically have asked their suppliers for African iron-workers, and the practice might conceivably have contributed to the rapid disappearance of this activity from the Gulf of Guinea.

Farther inland, primary iron metallurgy vanished in gradual stages, the principal causes of its demise being the establishment of the trading economy and the imposition of colonial rule. After breaking the resistance of Africans to colonial penetration through brutal 'pacification' campaigns, the colonial authorities banned the practice of primary metallurgy by Africans. Evidence from North-Central Togo, the Bassar area and the Waaba country of North-Western Benin indicates that the few primary ironworkers who continued in that profession had to work underground.

The net result is that nowadays all secondary metal-workers use imported iron. Often they simply make do with scrap metal salvaged from a weird assortment of wrecked vehicles and containers. The quality of this metal is not necessarily better than that of raw iron formerly extracted in local furnaces (Goucher 1984:13-14).

Reasons for the Study of the Ancient Socio-economic Practice of Metallurgy

Form a researcher's viewpoint the reasons for studying ancient metallurgical traditions in Africa are self-evident. This is the stuff of basic research. The deliberate cultivation of ignorance is a devastatingly harmful activity. We have seen the damage done by African politicians fundamentally ignorant about the underpinnings of their own people's cultural heritage. Their ignorance impinges actively on the way they judge human beings and objects. A similar ignorance inspired the colonial scholars who had the overweening ambition of reconstructing history on the basis of flimsy, fanciful scraps of misinformation. The issue, at bottom, is epistemological.

In addition, knowledge of ancient metallurgical practices can be of practical, utilitarian benefit to technicians and scientists today.

Knowledge of a Basic Technical Production System

The study of iron metallurgy is an important pursuit, marking as it does the entry of African societies into the Iron Age after the long pre-historic period of the Stone Age. In addition, mastery of the technology for extracting and processing iron played an important part in shaping the salient features of Africa's agrarian civilizations and cultures.

That being so, there is no way any scholar can acquire a solid grounding in the history of Africa's peoples without an accurate understanding of the knowledge and know-how of the continent's iron-workers, these technicians who invented ingenious and relatively straightforward operations for extracting iron. The knowledge they accumulated over centuries has been disappearing too rapidly. Yet today, it is drawing the interest of modern technicians eager to borrow ideas they can use in the development of new techniques capable of yielding workable iron directly from iron ore, as in the ancient African style, without first having to pass through the pre-steel foundry stage.

Forms of Social Organization of Production: An Analysis

There is no doubt that one of the effects of the development of metallurgy was to help diversify production and promote social differentiation or socio-economic specialization. Numerous ethnological studies on ironsmiths have focused on the definition of their status in West African societies. The status of smelters, however, remains hazy for lack of detailed studies. It seems clear enough that smelters were not invariably ironsmiths as well. There were communities in which specialization was pushed to such extremes that all the men worked exclusively to make slabs of iron for sale. Examples include the Waaba of North-West Benin (Tiando 178:188-192), and a number of Ibo communities in South-Eastern Nigeria (Anozie 1979:119-134).

Recent studies have clarified differences between societies in the Sudano-Sahelian zone and those more to the South, in attitudes towards iron-working technicians. In the Sudano-Sahelian belt iron-smelting and iron-working specialists, while being feared, are regarded as socially inferior. Their status in the Southern areas of the West African region is diametrically opposite. There they are honoured members of society, and some actually belong to the aristocracy.

According to the historian Djibril Tamsir Niane, it was during the emergence of the Mali Empire in the 13th century that professional groups in the region, including iron-workers, were transformed into professional clans or castes. 'Sundiata Keita,' Niane writes, 'codified the system of professional clans, making professions hereditary. Earlier, in the Ghana Empire, it would seem that individuals were free to practice the profession of their own choice. Henceforth, however, sons would have to do the work their fathers did' (Niane 1985:158-59). The evidence suggests, then, that the creation of endogamous socio-professional groups began with a historically identifiable process. Apparently, the social model established by the founder of Mali after his famous victory over the iron-smith King Soumaoro Kanté was adopted in many neighbouring kingdoms. Some adopted it after they were conquered, while it came to others (Jolof, Tekrour, Songhay, etc.) as a result of cultural diffusion. In the Yatenga area of the Mossi region, some groups of iron-workers were subjugated through conquest from the 16th century onwards (Izard 1985:254).

In the more southerly communities and kingdoms of the transitional savanna woodland zones, and in the forest regions along the Gulf of Guinea, craftspersons were organized in urban professional guilds whose representatives normally sat on the ruling councils of state. The kingdoms and chiefdoms of Borgou, Oyo and old Benin were examples. Closer to present-day Benin, in the kingdom of Xogbonou/Ajacé (Porto Novo kingdom), between the 18th and 19th centuries, the Sayi community supplied the State with a number of items including arms, because its men were iron-workers. The same community provided the commanding general of the armed forces. Women of the community normally worked as potters. Incidentally, the coupling of male iron-workers with female potters brings to mind the same widespread practice in the Sudano-Sahelian zone. In Benin, however, the group was not endogamous, and it was so close to the ruling dynasty at Porto-Novo that it was in fact part of the aristocracy.

An analysis of the influence of iron production on social stratification shows that there is no justification for sweeping generalizations about the part played by iron-making technology in the emergence of ruling classes and expansionist centralizing States. West Africa provides a very wide range of socio-political structures. We have already cited the Waaba and the Ibo, and we can add the Bassar of North-Central Togo (de Barros 1988:III). These are communities which developed the production of iron artefacts to an advanced degree. Yet they do not seem to have tried to impose relationships on their neighbours other than those appropriate to trade, the exchange of services, and marriage (Tiando 1978; Anozie 1979:129; Neaher 1979). Furthermore, it was quite possible for specialization within the iron-working profession to reach advanced levels. Evidence of this possibility comes from a recent study in the Bassar area which reveals that some specialized in making raw iron, some in the refinement of raw iron, while others specialized in working iron into specific tools or everyday artefacts (Dugast 1988:31-33).

Professional groups of this sort also enjoyed a measure of less clearly defined power in society, quite apart from that accruing from the use of their technological know-how. It was generally believed that they possessed magical and religious powers. This was the factor that attracted the enthusiasm of the initial crop of anthropological researchers. To this day the connection of religious cults with iron-working skills remains a fruitful field of study inviting in-depth research (Soglo 1987:82-98).

The Impact of Iron Production: An Assessment

Beyond its impact on social and political life, iron metallurgy caused changes in the natural environment as well as in economic relationships between human groups and societies. The ecological impact results from the fact that three indispensable natural resources go into the making of iron: the ore itself, which is normally expected to be of high metal content; fuel in the form of charcoal made from selected woods, and air. It is the use of the first two resources that can cause ecological problems. Iron ore reserves are widespread in West Africa, but in metal content the distribution is highly uneven. Areas containing high-content iron-bearing reserves therefore became important. But the decisive factor in the location of metallurgical sites seems to have been the availability of high-quality fuel. Increased metallurgical production naturally destroyed parts of the environment. Archaeologists studying this activity have recently focused more attention on this factor.

For instance, Randi Haaland, a Norwegian archaeologist, has described the impact of metallurgy at the time of the Ghana Empire on deforestation in the region of Méma, in the North-West area of present-day Mali (Haaland 1980:31-46). Along similar lines, Professor Merrick Posnansky and his team conducted a series of experiments and took measurements to determine the impact of metallurgical iron production in the Begho area of what is now West-Central Ghana. Archaeological research findings indicate that ironworkers in Hani apparently tried to attenuate the ecological degradation caused by their industry by increasing furnace capacity through the use of higher furnaces with thicker walls, and by exploring ways of increasing productivity (Goucher 1981). These findings indicate that African specialists in the iron industry did not react to the effects of their work in the same way, and that in some areas they tried to counter the risk of irremediable ecological damage.

Economic historians writing about Africa in general and West Africa in particular, just as much as anthropologists specializing in exchange relations, can no longer pass over the role of metallurgical products in intra-communal relationships or in transactions between socio-economic groups. We touched on this point in our comments on the Waaba. Here we would like to stress the fact that this community of iron-workers and smelters played a central role in their society. They supplied neighbouring ironsmiths and farmers (the Sekonbu Baatonbu of Kouandé and the Bétammaribè) with unworked iron. In return they obtained foodstuffs and livestock. Stimulating studies have been devoted to the dynamic Ibo ironsmiths, the Awka, who specialized in secondary metallurgy. One of the findings is that their working range went beyond Iboland (Neaher 1979:352-366). Metallurgical products were sometimes marketed on regional circuits. Metallurgical centres in Bassar areas, for instance, were linked to towns in the southern zones of present-day Togo. Some of their products went as far as the Ashanti region of present-day Ghana (de Barros 1986). We still have a long way to go before we can get precise data on all trading circuits along which products travelled to the main markets where the continent's metallurgical artefacts were exchanged. Now that detailed local studies are getting done, we are beginning to get an idea of the quality and quantities of iron produced. So far, what we know about the volume of trade in metallurgical products throughout Africa is merely tentative.

The study of African technological traditions is in its infancy. It would be premature to offer conclusions at such an early stage. At the end of this chapter, then, what I can offer is a set of ideas.

We hope we have begun a debate in this volume that will spill over the walls of academia to reach all members of society at large, to whom many of the topics discussed here are likely to be relevant. We hope that debate will plunge us into deliberations on our current problems, starting with an understanding of their historical roots. And we hope, too, that this debate will look forward to the future of the peoples of this sub-regions, and of the entire continent.

A study of ancient iron metallurgical technologies in Africa shows how our people came to lose the technological initiative. It makes a deep background against which our ignorance of our own cultural heritage stands out in its immense and blinding clarity. This rift in our knowledge is gradually getting filled in by archaeological researchers, and their work indicates that our ignorance of our intellectual traditions is no accident. It is part of an organized process, though we still have no clear understanding of the political, ideological and even economic stakes involved. That is the point made recently by our Burkinabe colleague Jean-Baptiste Kiethega (1988:3):

> In the first place, the political and ideological issues involve the international debate on the origins and world-wide diffusion of iron. This remains a matter of controversy. We still use textbooks containing poisonous diffusionist theories that continue to preach the notion that we never invented anything, that all we do is copy others. Yet every new day now we find conclusive proof that these notions are false...

Obviously none of us can advance serious plans for the future unless we first take the trouble to achieve an accurate and profound understanding of the history of the people we claim to want to mobilize and lead towards 'economic and social development'. We therefore need urgently to spark a revival of research in the Humanities along with research on ancient technologies, made relevant through the incorporation of contemporary scientific resources. To achieve this goal with optimum efficiency, we have to cultivate an interdisciplinary approach through the creation of multidisciplinary teams working on a series of national, regional and international programmes, serially or in parallel.

Discussion

Ignace Djenontin: 'Considering the fact that African metallurgists had no education, how did they find iron ore and what criteria did they use to recognize it?'

Abel Yakpa: 'In your discussion of caste societies, you mentioned that in Mali, the blacksmith caste was placed at the very bottom of the social hierarchy, and you referred to Soundjata Keita who defeated the blacksmith king Soumaoro Kanté. But I would like to point out that in some societies, blacksmiths were highly respected and considered. For example, in Savé, in the center of the Republic of Benin, the hunters paid great respect to the blacksmiths'.

Rogatien Ségla: 'Have modern researchers reached a consensus on the origin of metallurgy in Africa?'

Geoffroy Botoyiyé: 'You claim that colonisation was responsible for the loss of many metallurgical centers. But why did Africans themselves let those sites be completely wiped out after independence? And what good does it do us now to know whether we were the first to produce iron or not, since we don't know how to make iron nowadays?'

Félix Hodonou: 'What is the precise definition of the term "caste"?'

Seth Akplogan: 'You say that iron smelting originated in Africa. Don't you think that its decline there was caused by the rise in the use of gold?'

Alexis Adandé: 'There are several justifications for the historical study of metallurgy, not the least of which is that it is an area of scientific research and as such, is not necessarily grounded from the outset in utilitarianism. Nevertheless, modern technologists are interested in ancient techniques in order to study the solutions our ancestors found for a number of natural or technical problems. These solutions could be adapted or improved using the powerful scientific and technical tools available to us today. Hence, we can see that traditional technology contains a wealth of important data attesting the inventiveness of Africans and other peoples thousands of years ago, and their capacity for adapting to available resources. For that reason alone, it is vital that African researchers take an active part in assessing these forms of ancestral knowledge which are disappearing along with the social structures that used to ensure their perpetuation'.

'Using a similar line of reasoning, it should be remembered that education is not necessarily dispensed by formal structures, such as schools, since metallurgists were also able to teach their young apprentices knowledge such as how to find and identify ore. My distinguished colleague Jean-Baptiste Kiethega has explained the means and methods used by metallurgists or blacksmiths in Burkina Faso to detect or identify underground veins and determine the quality of the ore. They include using a long iron bar, examining certain visual, tactile or taste clues, and using certain plants. Naturally, traditional ideas about the origins of raw materials are very different from those held by modern geologists and mineralogists. Certain peoples believed that veins of ore were like tremendous snakes moving about underground, and that a person needed special skills to locate them'.

'The concept of "caste" denotes an endogamous social group made up of individuals who generally practice a common, hereditary activity. Before we apply this notion to societies in our region, we should first make sure that all these criteria are present in the social structures we are studying'.

'As for the origins of iron smelting, I never stated that Africa was the primary source for that technology in the world. After reviewing the theories put forward by African research, I tried to address the state of the question. Need I point out that knowledge in scientific research is a temporary matter ; there is no way of predicting future research findings, especially in archaeology which is a newly-developed discipline on the African continent. Many claims and a priori ideas about African cultures have been questioned in light of discoveries made by recent scientifically rigorous archaeological digs'.

'Finally, the decline in iron metallurgy cannot be explained by the increasing use of gold. Geographically, ancient gold production was much less widespread than iron production, since iron technology was highly developed before contact with Europe. Obviously, the marginalization of local and regional handiwork and industries in African countries should be seen in the context of the enforced dependence of local economies on the industrial economies of Europe and America. The fact that even now, no real effort has been made to reverse this trend, is hardly the result of a lack of studies and plans. One example being the essay *Fondements culturels, techniques et industriels d'un futur Etat fédéral d'Afrique noire* by Cheikh Anta Diop, in which precise proposals were made for the establishment of an African industrial base using the resources of the continent. What is lacking is the political will of our leaders, who despite their enthusiastic reception of the Lagos Action Plan have taken no steps toward its execution'.

Paulin Hountondji: 'How did the socio-economic importance of ironwork compare to the use of other metals such as gold, copper, etc.? How can we update traditional knowledge and skills for modern use? It's a matter of development methodology'.

Alexis Adandé: 'Iron smelting was dominant because the production of iron had to fulfil the needs of the whole society. In precolonial Africa, many whole sectors of activity depended entirely on iron tools forged using iron produced either locally or by specialists in neighbouring areas. That is why metallurgists and blacksmiths occupied a central position in our societies, wherever they stood in the social hierarchy. The huge slag heaps they left behind in major iron-producing areas bear silent witness to their importance'.

'Other metalworkers generally had a smaller role to play, either because the metals they used were rare or they were limited to a small geographical area. Gold in the form of gold dust was used only for transactions with the Berber Arabs of the Sahel and the Persian Arabs, and later the Europeans, along the coasts. Nuggets were the exclusive property of sovereigns, particularly in the Empire of Ghana, where only the Kaya Maghan was allowed to possess them. This custom was carried on by the Mansa of Mali. The working of gold into jewelry or "regalia" was reserved for specialists organized in castes or corporations, under the control of royal or imperial power. The same applied to silver, although to a lesser degree since silver seems to have been much more widely used than gold, and, like copper it was used in popular jewelry. However, copper was very much in vogue, especially when copper alloys were imported in huge quantities by Europeans who exchanged bars or shackles of brass or bronze for services, goods or slaves on African coasts. Copper in its pure or alloyed form was already known and used in certain regions before the European traffickers arrived. For example, in Shaba, in modern-day Zaire and Zambia, it was melted and shaped into crosses of different sizes for use as coinage. In historical Benin, in Edo country, and in Ile Ifè, skilled artists poured it into clay moulds to produce the famed "bronze" heads and plaques which decorated the temples and royal palaces of those legendary cities. In other regions of Africa, copper was more highly prized than gold. This subject was very well covered in Eugenia W. Herbert's recent book, *Red Gold of Africa, Copper in Precolonial History and Culture* (1984). In African societies, each metal had a symbolic value and occupied a rank in the hierarchy of earthly goods or religious objects which varied according to the scale of values. In fact, this is a matter which anthropologists are very interested in studying'.

'But how can we bring back traditional knowledge and skills? This question cannot even be asked unless we first resolve the issue of whether it is worth our while to study them. As paradoxical as this may seem, only countries equipped with state of the art laboratories can properly analyse ancient or traditional technologies. Because in order to reproduce and understand these apparently simple processes, we often need sophisticated scientific tools and modern techniques'.

'But this does not mean it is impossible to develop a real "development methodology" in countries that want to reintegrate the traditional knowledge and skills of their peoples. I have only pointed out the obstacles that need to be overcome. This sort of methodology has its requirements, including the choice of locally centered development and optimization of our universal scientific heritage, with all the attendant rigor in resource and skills management'.

3

'Rain-makers': Myth and Knowledge in Traditional Atmospheric Management Techniques

Gbnoukpo Bodhou Dah-Lokonon'

The rain-makers' craft is a rather arcane subject. Little wonder, then, if even the boldest researchers think twice before tackling it. Researchers are likely to find a minefield littered with problems. Why, for instance, should specialists in the management of atmospheric forces be eager to reveal the secrets of their trade to casual snoopers? A close-mouthed set, they open up only to initiates or to the few lay persons who gain their confidence. Which is what, happily for our research, we were able to do.

This chapter is not a study of the state of the rain-maker's art in Benin. First, that would be an overweening ambition. Second, those interested in such a study would be well advised to turn to the work of Michel Boko, which is excellent in more than one regard. What we intend here, instead, is to present a selective description of procedures used by rain-makers in Benin in their work, which is the management of the atmosphere. In the process, we shall also analyze and discuss the operative mix of myth and knowledge from which rain-makers ply their trade.

After Dah-Lokonon's analysis, a transcript of the discussion which took place at the Cotonou seminar at the National University of Benin in 1987-88 is included in this chapter. An examination of traditional rain making from a hydrologist's view point, Abdel Afouda, then follows.

Functional Procedures

In all African traditions, myth enjoys a central status. Gods, goddesses and other supernatural beings are ubiquitous, and they play pivotal roles in the understanding, explanation and control of the cosmos. These divinities are immanent in such natural phenomena as water, stones, iron and trees. It is in the gift of human beings to emulate divinities in all their activities, but in this enterprise there are prerequisites to success. Aspiring humans must follow prescribed rituals and procedures in the invocation of Vodun and other intermediary spirits. These spirits are then committed to transmit expressed human wishes to the invisible powers that be. The latter, after evaluating the seriousness and scope of each request, may then grant or withhold its fulfilment.

For our purposes the relevant question is: by what means do expert rain-makers manage to influence the atmosphere in order to precipitate rain? In this chapter we shall focus on two types of procedure, both based on the manipulation of stones. The first uses stones called *Aklan-kpen,* found in the entrails of the red monkey. The second uses stones called *Tunvi-kpen,* found in ponds where tunvi fish breed.

Aklan-kpen Stones

Hungry red monkeys have a habit of waiting for farmers to finish their work and go home, whereupon they descend on the crops and ravage them. But when a farmer stays on the farm longer than expected, the waiting monkey vomits the *aklan-kpen* stone. The moment the stone hits the ground, it begins to rain. The farmer is thus forced to seek shelter off the farm, leaving the monkey free to pillage the farm crops. Now the *aklan-kpen* is a two-tone stone, half white, half blue. If the white half hits the earth first, the resulting rain is heavy and lasts several days. That gives the monkey and its tribe ample time to eat their fill. But if it is the blue part that hits the ground first, the rain, though heavy, lasts only a couple of days.

Tunvi-kpen Stones

Tunvi is the name of a type of catfish related to the fish known in the Fon and Gun languages as ason. Votaries of the Vodun cult consider the flesh of this fish taboo, because it is from its head that they obtain the lagbla, a gill-like formation that members hold up when entering a possession trance. The *tunvi-kpen* is a natural stone found in large ponds where the tunvi fish live. In times of drought, when water supplies get short, the fish, needing cool, fresh water to counter the irritating heat, turn the tip of the tunvi stone skywards. Immediately, rain begins to fall. Falling thus for days on end, it restores the familiar, balanced environment of the fish.

Origins of Rainmaking Procedure

Aklan-kpen

The following is an account of the discovery of rainmaking practices based on the *aklan-kpen* stone.

> Exasperated by frequent large-scale devastations of their farms by red monkeys under cover of unusually heavy rains, veritable accessories to the simian food-robbers even in the dry season, men dreamed of inflicting a punishment on the monkeys so severe it would stop them from ever repeating their pillage. The problem was how.
>
> One day a hunter out in the open farmlands came upon a grand parade of red monkeys. Observing them from a hiding place, he saw the monkeys, after a careful look around, close ranks around the leading male, who then proceeded to vomit up the stone known as the *aklan-kpen*. Flabbergasted by the goings-on, the hunter observed the scene more carefully. The stone had fallen white side up, but another monkey turned it blue side up. Immediately, it began to rain.
>
> Now was the time for the monkeys to execute their plan, since no one would come to drive them off in the rain. The monkey horde fanned out and occupied the farm, pillaging to their hearts' content. Angered by the sight, the hunter waited impatiently for the moment to attack, gun at the ready. He did not have to wait unduly long. As the monkeys finished their dastardly romp, they turned back intending to pick up the magic stone. But leaping from his hiding place, the hunter opened fire at point-blank range against the marauding horde. The monkeys scattered in bewildered disarray, screeching in total terror. Then absolute silence. Their feast over, the monkeys fled as far as they could. Calmly, the hunter picked up the *aklan-kpen* stone. And that is how human beings came to possess the stone'.

The Tunvi-kpen Stone

In the lagoon country of Lower Benin, it is usual to see riverside farms called wodji. Once, so goes the story, a farmer cultivating such a field chanced to find the stone known as the *tunvi-kpen*. Since then human beings have used it to conjure up rain or drought. The following are the ingredients used for conjuring up a drought, according to wise initiates: 1) One chimpanzee head, technically known as a lokita; 2) Selected medicinal herbs; and 3) Special incantations.

The procedure is as follows: the chimpanzee head, together with the medicinal herbs, is carefully prepared, to the steady accompaniment of incantations. A large hole is then dug and the entire bundle buried in it. This guarantees that there will be no rain. The drought will be absolute, and will continue as long as the chimpanzee head and herbs remain buried.

Two key factors need highlighting in these procedures:

- Language — or to be more precise, speech — plays a crucial role in the process just described.
- The techniques used for regulating rainfall have an economic impact. Initiates might be requested to use their resources to cause rainfall, especially during droughts. They would thus ensure bountiful harvests, and the population as a whole would be well fed.

It is a pity that in this country, public officials acquiesce in the notion that control over the hidden forces of nature is an aspect of diabolical power, the work of Satan. That is the kind of thinking expressed in the 17 July 1987 issue of the daily newspaper Ehuzu. It is fashionable these days to show contempt for traditional know-how. But I for one am convinced that it is a matter calling for serious study. Time will tell which attitude is right.

Discussion

The following is a transcript of the discussion after the presentation of this chapter at the research seminar at the National University of Benin (See Introduction in this volume).

Jean-Marie Apovo: I wonder why in your presentation you mentioned only procedures based on the use of stones. Why, for instance, did you overlook certain leaves used by rain-makers? After all, they are much easier to find.

Incidentally, it would seem that the issue of virginity is of central importance when it comes to the management of the atmosphere. I remember that during my visit to Senegal, when people wanted to make sure their ceremonies wouldn't get rained on, the custom was to get a pre-pubescent girl to dig a hole. Salt was then poured into the hole, which was then closed up. After that, it was guaranteed that there would be no rain over the area where the ceremony was to be held, even if rainclouds had been gathering just before the ritual.

Recently I met a Geography student specializing in Climatology for a Master's degree. I had a little discussion with him about the matter of hexes and juju charms, known here as *bô*. He told me he had a tiny strip of black cloth, measuring no more than a hand in length. No matter where he went, if he carried this strip on his person, there would be no rain in the area. Several times he had seen it work. He told me that one day, invited somewhere in Mono Province to stop rain from falling, he was confronted with opponents bent on making the rain fall. His opposition had to come to terms with him in the end, because he had his little strip of black fabric with him, so as long as he was in the area it could not rain there. At the time I was writing a doctoral thesis on the *bô* phenomenon, to be presented at my university in France. My acquaintance offered to lend me his strip of fabric to take to France so that when the time came for me to defend my thesis, I could astound the academics by getting it to perform. I declined his offer, arguing that climatic conditions over there in Europe were different, and that it was snow, not rain, that one would have to deal with. He said that made no difference whatsoever, and that the strip could cause climatic changes in any zone.

I remember another case: once, when I was a young pupil in Porto-Novo, I knew a man called Lankpankpan. I am sure lots of other people knew him. He always wore this particular bracelet. Now whenever he raised the arm with the bracelet, it began to rain. When he brought it down the rain stopped. So whenever there was a party or ceremony anywhere in the area to which he had not been invited, he'd simply crash the party. The moment people saw him they'd fall all over themselves to shower gifts on him. I mean, this man, using nothing but his bracelet, made it rain or shine whenever he pleased.

I also know that the warrior group known as *Akodjigbèto*, whenever they concluded a blood pact with each other to ensure peace and prosperity, had ways of making rain fall. That was how they forced their enemies off the battlefield. For the time being, I cannot give detailed information on their procedures. But I would like to point out that rain also serves sometimes to foretell victory or defeat. There is, for instance, a popular belief according to which the soccer club known as the 'Dragons de l'Ouméné' based in South-eastern Benin invariably wins its matches if it rains just before the kick-off. I have so far been unable to determine whether this is true or false.

And then there is this leaf: the moment it is dropped on the ground, it causes not just rain but lightning too. Now the question that arises — and I would like to hear the opinion of Paulin Hountondji himself — is whether this type of know-how can be given scientific formulation. Could we, for instance, say with certainty: this object placed next to that produces rain? The problem is that in every case, rain-makers set conditions we cannot manage to meet, and therefore we are unable to reach a scientific formulation. As a matter of fact, there are times when we follow their rainmaking instructions in every detail and bring together all the ingredients they ask for. And yet we do not get the expected results. No rain falls. Then the rain-makers claim certain feelings were not quite right, or that a number of subjective conditions had not been met. One wonders why the workings of our traditional intellectual practices are always subject to such psychological, individual and climatic conditions. What can we do to get rid of these subjective factors and achieve pure objectivity?

Dah-Lokonon: Admittedly, leaves play an important part in rainmaking as well as in the provocation of drought. In my paper I emphasized the use of stones because stones are practical, useful, handy objects. One can simply pick up a stone and use it. Leaves are more complicated: they require incantations. Besides, initiates are reluctant to reveal incantatory formulae to young people, fearing they will misuse their knowledge. That is the attitude of 75 per cent, even 90 per cent of the initiates. That being the case, we can try out every possible combination of ingredients, but as long as we do not add the correct incantations we cannot achieve any positive results.

As for your geography student, the one who claims he can cause or prevent rain with just a strip of black fabric, I am sure he is holding back some of what he knows. He certainly possesses other ingredients, and the strip of black fabric is merely the final item in his *paraphernalia*. After all, it is not just anyone who can up and make rain fall from scratch. Under certain conditions, if you try to do that, you risk getting struck down by lightning yourself. That is the truth. It is a natural law.

I am going to give you a formula for you to test when you have the time. Just for the fun of it, get hold of a chameleon and a scorpion and put them together in a bottle. Close the bottle and make sure you place it far from any human habitation. The moment the scorpion stings the chameleon, there will be an explosion, and lightning will devastate everything in the neighbourhood.

One last point. Let me repeat that it is not just anybody who can cause or prevent rain at will. Certain conditions have to be met. If you ever meet a soul who from sheer kindness offers to give you the requisite paraphernalia for making rain, free of charge, telling you it is all you need, turn down the offer in all politeness. For that person seeks your ruin.

Ignace Djenontin: You did not go over the general issue of the 'management of the atmosphere'. Why not? Second, what are the sociological implications of the rainmaking and rain-prevention techniques you described? Third, why was your study limited to the use of two methods only, in just one particular province (Ouémé, in South Eastern Benin)? After all, the issue is national in scope. Lastly, is the use of stones for rainmaking effective in all seasons?

Servais Smith: What was the social status of rain-makers in traditional societies? And what is it in modern society? I read an article entitled "Contribution l'histoire du moyen Dahomey", published in *Etudes dahoméenes*, according to which there once were two legendary characters in Ketou endowed with the fantastic power of causing rain whenever they stepped outside. I used to wonder if these stories could be true, but now my doubts have been laid to rest. I figure that these characters probably wore on their persons various objects that caused rainfall whenever they went outside. But do you think this explanation correct?

Satchou: On my way to this hall, I was thinking that by the end of the lecture I would know the secret techniques the wise elders used to make or prevent rain. But I have realized that the lecturer left out certain crucial aspects required for mastering the techniques of atmospheric management. In so doing he did exactly what he himself said the old initiates did, behind the excuse that they thought young people indiscreet and injudicious. I find it particularly frustrating to come to a lecture of such high scholarly status only to listen to half-truths. Anyway, this is my question: since the initiates are said to know how to use certain familiar objects to make rain fall, why do droughts happen? At the very least, these initiates should be able to make it rain on their own farms, and thus beat the drought. Can they do that?

Max Padonou: You say words have a certain power. That means you recognize the effectiveness of incantations. But in the case of our wise initiates, can it not be argued that they use incantations to create a fake atmosphere of mystery around processes that are otherwise quite logically explainable?

Dah-Lokonon: Let me start with the first set of questions. There are close links between psychological and social phenomena, between the power of words and the forces of chemistry. The two are indissolubly bonded. That is why initiates collaborate in this domain. What we are dealing with is not individual knowledge. It is a collective enterprise. That is the sociological aspect of its impact. Initiates complement each other's knowledge in order to achieve accurate results. It was in this vein that recently the District Head of Adjohoun requested rain-makers in the area to combine their energies to make rain fall not simply in Adjohoun but throughout Benin.

As for the unwillingness of initiates to tell us their secrets, let me tell you about the problems we faced when preparing this paper. I had asked students to conduct a study on techniques used by rain-makers. When the students' reports came in, I realized nothing of substance would come out of their investigations. Some of those they interviewed had fed them partial information, withholding the rest. In other cases they had been given a list of ingredients, but the accompanying incantations had been left out. That is when I decided to go back to the village, with the intention of concentrating solely on observable behaviour.

Now as to the question why the elders are reluctant to share their secrets with the young, I think I have already answered it. They do not trust the youth. They suppose young people, once they get hold of such secrets, will misuse them to cause harm.

The reason why I focused on the use of stones in my presentation is that with these stones you get immediate, tangible results. I want it to rain, good. I take out my stone and presto, it begins to rain more or less continuously, depending on whether the blue or white part comes uppermost.

I come now to the social status of rain-makers. These are usually old men. Let us call them elders. Occasionally we find a young one. It should be noted that where there are young rain-makers, they are often of exceptional courage, politeness and integrity. Indeed, it is on account of these qualities that their parents pass on their special rainmaking powers to them, just before they die. It is a reward. So rainmaking powers are not a monopoly of old men. Young people, old people and women can also be rain-makers.

Some of the audience reprimanded me for focusing exclusively on procedures involving the use of stones, thus neglecting other techniques. Right off, let me say I had to make a choice, an unavoidable one. My concern was to produce substantive, specific work that could be monitored and checked for accuracy. Initially, my thesis topic was national in scope. Once I began field work in the north, however, I was compelled to demarcate my research boundaries more clearly. The reason was that all sorts of obstacles presented themselves: language problems, differences in habits and customs, lifestyles, etc. It became clear to me that there was no way I could overcome all these obstacles and still have enough energy left over to produce substantial work. I therefore had to come back down south, where I felt closer to the realities of the field, and where I could study these phenomena in their proper context. And so doing, I had to reformulate my thesis subject limiting research to Southern Benin. The point is that in treating a subject such as ours, we must always make sure that the realities we cover can be studied, tested and checked. We are, after all, in an academic environment.

Someone asked if rain-makers 'could make it rain on their own farms'. I will answer that question by describing an actual incident I saw with my own eyes in Mono Province. In the course of my research I came to Adja Bokpa. The drought was at its height. The heat was sky-high. The sun used to roast growing corn right on the cob. Faced with the prospect of imminent disaster, the wise ones held a meeting. One healer, a fellow from Abomey nicknamed De Gaulle, decided to cause rain. He told me: 'Gbnoukpo, today it is going to rain as much as we want'. No sooner said than done. Enough rain fell to avert disaster. Farms grew green again, harvests were good, and there were no lean times. So yes, rain-makers are capable of causing rain over a specific area. If they decide to make it rain over Cotonou, rain it will.

Ben Johnson: Is the *aklan-kpen* stone real or legendary? Could one snatch it out of the red monkey by slitting its gut? You said the *tunvi-kpen* was a gift of nature. Why is it found only in the habitat of the tunvi fish? What is it there for?

Epiphane Houngnon: Africa today is afflicted with a string of calamities. One is the spread of the desert. If African governments agreed to engage rain-makers to use their skills, could they make rain fall in the desert?

Hilaire Degan: All I want to know is this: is it possible to use lightning rods to keep lightning from striking those who invoke rain without observing the ritual formalities?

Abel Yakpa: How were people able to keep the *aklan-kpen* stone extracted from the monkey's entrails? My second question is: It is reported that if a chimpanzee's head is brought into contact with that of a human being, the latter dies. Now take someone totally ignorant of our culture, or entirely sceptical about this 'law of nature'. If this person placed a chimpanzee's head on his own head, would he die? Third question: what happens if two individuals clash, one determined to make rain, the other to prevent it?

Maimouna Alafi: Last year there was an intense radio campaign against sorcerers keeping the rain from falling. Then suddenly, between August and September, the rain came down in torrents, causing floods and other damage on a wide scale. The situation in Cotonou was particularly bad. Lots of people concluded that rain-makers were using their powers to get back at the political rulers. Can you give a scientific explanation for this?

Mama Bio Saka: You talked only of 'initiate rain-makers', forgetting that in times of drought people also look to Christian priests and Muslim marabouts to help with their prayers. My question is: are the methods used by marabouts and priests any different from those of traditional rain-makers, or are they, in a sense, identical?

Geoffroy Botoyiye: One has an impression that your lecture left much unfinished business. You did not even begin to address the epistemological aspect of the issue. Another point: it would seem that the methods used to prevent rain are much more potent than those used to cause it. Could you enlighten us on that?

G. Dah-Lokonon: I will take the last question first. You are disappointed, and you have the impression that the subject was skirted. I suppose the issue would have been clearer if we had begun with the following questions: what is the best approach to the study of rainmaking techniques? We could have posed a set of similar questions. But the information I presented about the two types of stone, the chimpanzee head, the chameleon and the scorpion, was all aimed at stimulating research. No one is going to do that research for you. I just spoke of the *aklan-kpen* stone, a gift of nature found in the intestines of the red monkey. Before farmers could suspect its existence, and before they could extract it from the monkey's gut, they had to go through a veritable process of research. It is that process we call science, technique. Science is not some manna from heaven. It is a collective invention.

I do not think rain prevention techniques are more potent than rainmaking techniques. These powers are evenly balanced, and it is the same individuals who make and prevent rain. Now when Paulin Hountondji asked me to present this paper, I told him the idea made me somewhat uneasy. The reason is that this is not the kind of topic that can be treated by just anybody. As a matter of fact, I told him I might get up and say nothing at all. When I began my research in this field, my own brother warned me not to meddle in such business. He said I might get into hot waters.

I am aware that in times of drought, people appeal to Christian priests and Muslim marabouts to pray for rain. But I also know their prayers are seldom answered. In the long run, it is usually the traditional healer or vodun cultist who steps in and solves the problem by making the rain fall.

Now when the latter are called in, they do not set about reciting prayers. Likely enough, they go before their Vodun, offer them their allowance of sacrificial oil and water, and recite appropriate incantations. But that is not the main thing. The main thing is a set of real, scientifically verifiable processes. And I can promise you this: next year, we shall make rain fall on this campus.

Someone asked if anyone could go and look for red monkeys and get rainmaking stones from them. Well, I know in our area there is a village called Aklankpé. In all likelihood, there are red monkeys thereabouts. But now the questions is: suppose you find a red monkey. Is it then enough to kill it and tear out its guts, or take a different tack and coax it to give up the stone? The fact is that the monkey only throws up the stone under the right conditions, of its own free will, when it is hungry. Unless it is hungry, it does not vomit up the stone. So you could grab a red monkey, pamper it or manhandle it, or even kill it to extract its stone. Your efforts would all be in vain, and you'd probably end up frustrated. The stone is an endowment given by nature to the red monkey to ensure its livelihood.

Someone asked about the spreading desert. Some time ago, when I was writing my thesis in Paris, my supervisor used to twit me, saying: 'You are a fine fellow, sitting here claiming to know about techniques for controlling atmospheric forces when back home on your continent the desert keeps eating up more and more land. What can you do to make your deserts green again?' My answer was that we could indeed make the desert bloom. If the rain-makers were brought together and asked to do something to make it rain in the desert, or to stop the desert from spreading, they certainly would do it. Take the example of the Israelis. To make trees grow in the desert, they first watered the sand. The Libyans did likewise. When water reaches the desert, the desert disappears. I am personally convinced that the initiates, our rain-makers, with their backlog of experience, would do something similar.

Consider this anecdote: two of our local politicians went blind, so they travelled to France to get cured. French doctors tried their best but failed to restore their sight. So the politicians arranged for traditional healers from Benin to join them over there in France. The healers examined them, diagnosed their disease and promised them a cure. They employed all their knowledge, with the result that our two blind politicians can now see. I saw all this with my own eyes, and I know the people involved well. They are well known politicians here. I shall say no more.

A questioner asked about lightning. Let me repeat: it is not just anyone who can influence the atmospheric forces. No doubt you know the story of Toffa and the Thunderbolt, having heard it before. It is part of the history of the kingdom of Porto-Novo, and it is eloquent. A moment ago, in answer to a question from my colleague Apovo, I advised you to decline the offer if some generous soul gave you a formula for making rain fall, with nothing added. The reason is that gifts of that sort, given without the necessary preparation, can only destroy you. And if you think you can take shelter beneath a lightning rod, as a substitute for the right protective formula, you will surely die, struck by lightning. Einstein, the genius you all know about, was once confronted with these natural phenomena. He was powerless to explain them.

You could, if you wish, conduct an experiment. Instead of taking the correct precautions, you might get under a lightning rod, then invoke rain. You wouldn't live to draw any conclusions from your experiment. But others would register the result, and take a lesson from it.

Abel Yakpa asked about the preservation of the stone. Well, it was wrapped up in a piece of black cloth. The man who discovered these stones did not pick them up with his hands. Instead, he took off his own cloth, then carefully wrapped it around the stones and took them home, where he could use them. That was how these stones came to be passed down from generation to generation, as heirlooms.

Concerning the effect of these techniques on people from cultural backgrounds different from ours, let me give you an example. Suppose I suffer from an ulcer, and that I am taken abroad for treatment. As long as I am convinced that everything necessary for my recovery has been done, I am sure to get healed, even though my cultural background is different from that of the country in question. Regarding the chimpanzee head, you all know what the skull means in Fon culture, and what role it plays. Suppose your enemies, sworn to destroy you, ask the vodun to eliminate you by telling him he upset me, so kill him for me'. What does the vodun do? The very first step he takes is to attack the head. Only later does he go to work on the guts. So whether you share our cultural background or not, by and by the effects will reach you, inevitably. Let us say someone from Burkina Faso, just for the fun of it, puts a chimpanzee skull on his head, claiming he does not believe it will affect him. He will surely reap the consequences. Whoever wants to test this is welcome to try. After all, these are verifiable statements.

It is on account of all these reasons that in our traditional communities, young people are required to watch their behaviour when they are around elders. This is merely the respect they owe the elders. Because if we misbehave, the elders would rather die with their secrets than share them with us. So if we aim to get hold of this esoteric knowledge, to preserve it and to develop it as part of a genuine scientific tradition, we have no option but to humour these 'elders'. Unless we do that, we shall never succeed.

Berba Abou: Listening to you, one gets the impression knowledge has succumbed to myth. At any rate it is hard to identify knowledge here, especially in relation to the origin of the *aklan-kpen* stone. Now I would like to know your personal position. Do you distinguish between myth and knowledge? Another question: your hunter supposedly carried a gun. Guns were brought to the African continent in relatively recent times. So are we to conclude that these techniques go back no farther than that?

In my opinion, we will not achieve real knowledge until we can relate these stones to currently accepted scientific explanations for atmospheric changes. It would be highly stimulating to have an explanation that harmonizes scientific reasoning, cloud formations, and these stones.

Albert Gbodogbe: I have four questions: 1) Considering that information on atmospheric management techniques is secret, to what extent is it possible to get it for the purpose of mastering and using it? 2) I have heard that rain-makers die young. Why so? 3).Is there a god of rain? If there is, why cannot we make sacrifices to him to ensure more regular rainfall? 4).Why do the initiates advise us to pray and sacrifice to Vodun when they know full well that in most cases prayers and sacrifices do not bring rain? There is something fuzzy about their attitude. Could you shed some light on it?

Maxine Houndegla: What is the connection between the rainmaker's props and incantations? What is the difference between colloquial words and the esoteric diction that confers power on such props? How do rain-makers determine how vast an area the rain they cause will cover, and how long it will fall? Is it true that initiates can move about in the rain without umbrellas and still stay dry? Lastly, considering how important traditional knowledge and know-how are, wouldn't it be possible to establish a school run by initiates, and designed to advance these techniques and use them for development?

Ariane Djossou: After eating his fill, does the red monkey again swallow the stone it vomited? If it does, that would indicate it only had one stone in its intestines. If it does not, then it means his organism makes a new stone whenever it gets hungry. If the latter case is true, would it be possible to tame the red monkey in order to get it to produce a new stone whenever necessary? Do you think that in order to harness traditional knowledge to the development effort, it is indispensable to believe in these rituals?

Dah-Lokonon: Do the monkeys retrieve their stones after vomiting them? I say yes. Red monkeys do not vomit up their stones unless they get hungry. Human beings were finally able to obtain these stones only after a long period of observation. People needed first of all to make the connection between the stone and rain, and to understand that it was this stone that helped the red monkey to cause rain, the aim being to force farmers off their farms. Only after the painstaking observation of these phenomena did human beings decide to act, tricking the red monkey in order to snatch the stone from it. As far as the domestication of the red monkey is concerned, I doubt it could be done. All other monkeys may be tamed, but the red monkey is an exception. In this connection, it is generally reported that if it pisses in a house, the urine causes a disease called *Azon ve*, a name for which I do not know the French translation. It is said that once you catch this disease, it stays with you for life. You can go to all the state-of-the-art hospitals you want, but none of them can ever cure you. In any case that is what I have heard from respectable, trustworthy elders. The gist of all this is that no one can simply get up and tame red monkeys. The cost is high. However, if you are bent on experimenting with them, I can tell you exactly where to find them, in an area close to my village.

Now let us talk about the power of speech. As you all know, when we say 'good morning', 'good evening', 'how are you?' or 'how's life?' we are not, strictly speaking, tapping the power of speech. We are simply communicating. When I say: 'Go to such-and-such a place', I am communicating. It is possible, though, to want to impart some power to communication. When that happens, there is a shift from simple communication to the realm of potent speech. Right now, all I am doing is communicating with you. I am not tapping the power of speech. It is when we use words to cause people to act, whether they want to or not.

To illustrate, let me tell you a story. One day, in the course of a military campaign somewhere in Benin, a brigade commander went up with his troops to confront an elderly traditional chief and ordered him to pay up his taxes. The old chief said his advanced age exempted him from taxation. The brigade commander thought this an insult, so he leapt at the old chief and gave him a slap. The angry old chief unsheathed his cutlass, intending to slash the rude soldier. But the district head, one Adamou Laminou, cooled him down. But the old chief was still upset and feeling vengeful. He conjured the spirits of all the dead kings, calling them by name, after which he ordered the foolhardy soldier to go bathe in the river. Immediately the brigade commander, who had so recently been so bold and omnipotent, meekly took off his clothes, elbowed aside the dense crowd of curious onlookers, and ran under his own steam all the way to the river, where he drowned. Now that is a typical example of what I call the power of speech. It was the district chief himself, the same Adamou Laminou, who told me about this episode.

Let me remind you that this power is not given to just anybody. I know there are young people who have it. Indeed, I know some of our former students who have become past masters. Whatever they order you to do, you have no choice but to obey them. This kind of power comes from two ingredients: the *nudida* and the *kpe*.

There are two types of *kpe*. The first is benign, the second casts an ineluctable spell. Generally, the *kpe* is a crafted object on which two needles are placed, one red, one white. To use it, you have to get up early in the morning, before taking a bath. You ask for whatever you desire, then lick the *kpe*. After that, you rinse out your mouth, to ward off the dangerous effects of the *kpe* from yourself and your loved ones. After that, whenever you desire to harm anyone, you take the red needle, lick it, call the offending person by name, list his or her offences, reciting specified incantations. The targeted persons will then assuredly suffer harm, unless they have protective powers of their own.

In addition to the *kpe*, there are other objects that can impart power to speech. One is called *ahowe* (Gancinia cola), another *avi* (Cola acuminata). A description is contained in my thesis (Dah-Lokonon 1985). The power of speech is not some manna from heaven. Neither is it simply the use of ordinary words. It is contained in the *nudida* and the *kpe*. Without them, the words themselves would be flat, ineffective.

Turning now to the boundaries of the rainmaker's art in time and space, I have already cited an incident that happened at Bokpa. I am going to have to go back to it. At that time, Bokpa had been hit by such a severe drought that it was feared the worst was imminent. That was when De Gaulle (not the Frenchman; this one was from Zou), an adept rainmaker, promised his people he would do something. He asked them how long they wanted the rain to fall. The inhabitants replied: 'Just long enough to make our fields green and give us good harvests'. De Gaulle lived behind the secondary school in my village. I was right there when he used the *tunvi-kpen* to bring down the rain. It lasted a few days, falling only in Mono Province.

Someone wondered if we should not create a school where young people would get trained in the mastery of this knowledge and know-how. I know there were plans to mount some such project for the teaching of Fa divination. If they have so far not been implemented, I suppose that it is because the ruling Marxist regime, with its materialist leanings, cannot accept the idealistic philosophy behind the science of Ifa divination. In my opinion the problem is entirely ideological.

The aspect of divination was also brought up in the discussion of traditional knowledge. Someone asked how the knowledge could be retrieved. On this point, I shall tell you about an episode that I witnessed myself. One day, two lecturers on the Abomey-Calavi campus got into a long discussion. The first thought it absurd that people could worship the earth. The second agreed, going even farther: he said he had stopped talking to his father because the old man was full of such diabolical superstitions. As the two lecturers got into the swing of their discussion, piling up arguments and making fun of traditional practices, I asked if I could join their conversation and slide in my point of view.

My point is this: there is no way we can gain the confidence of the elders and initiates with a view to gathering data, if we begin with attitudes like those of the two lecturers. Vanity, pride and irreverence are qualities sure to block our way to that goal. The initiates do not confide their secrets to young people they cannot trust. I know I might get called a feudalist for saying this, but I think they are quite right. It is a matter of principle. If you come to me for help, the least I expect is some respect and good manners. Otherwise I have nothing to do with you.

Someone asked why rain-makers have such short lives. Let me answer with a precise example. It is about a man who was once my neighbour. His name was Yahoutcha. This man was a renowned expert in the art of atmospheric management, a professional in great demand. One day, as he was attempting to cause rain, an enemy of his was bent on preventing it. His enemy won out, and Yahoutcha, struck by lightning, died. This means that those who aspire to make rain or prevent it from falling have to have special powers. If not, they're likely to get killed by a thunderbolt.

When the initiates say sacrifices have to be given to some Vodun before it rains, I think they are simply throwing dust in people's eyes. It is a way of protecting their knowledge. In addition to the pouring of oil, there are other rituals. In pure science, the accepted formula says A + A = 2A. In our traditional knowledge, however, A + A is not always equal to 2A. The reason is that one has to factor in such natural phenomena as speech, rivers, the earth on which we live. Each has its own force. To control them, all one needs to do is to understand their language, but that is not a skill accessible to just anyone. That is why, in the universe of our traditional knowledge, A + A gives a vast array of possible results. Hence the opinion that the black man's culture is complex, and that the black man is deep and dense.

Paulin Hountondji: I would like to thank our friend who, as you have noted, is well versed in all sorts of mystical and non-mystical learning. Whatever one might say, this is a man of conviction, profoundly committed to the local culture, and widely informed of the most secret aspects of that culture.

I have deliberately held back from joining the discussion, even though I had an urgent contribution to make. But before we adjourn, I would like to make two or three observations.

The first is this: Lay persons, when they talk of secret techniques like those just discussed, invariably present their information in an indirect mode: I know someone who knows someone who says some other person has the power to accomplish such-and-such a wonder. The chain of intermediaries is long; there is no direct observation of the acts described by the lay person recounting them. And the hearer has no direct access to primary sources of information. All this makes the resulting knowledge and know-how utterly esoteric, secret, confidential.

Second, a number of protective stratagems are used to reinforce the confidentiality of this type of knowledge and know-how. The idea is to keep it from public knowledge. Thus, you might be told: If ever you attempt to check on the truth of these assertions, something terrible will happen to you. Or if you try to verify this or that item of information (instead of taking our word for it) you will be struck by lightning, or you will catch an incurable disease. I think we have to say plainly that these are tricks to intimidate people. That said, it should be recognized that they are used for a precise purpose. They operate as techniques for protecting knowledge, in much they same way that the industrialized countries use other techniques to protect their nuclear secrets.

In France, Great Britain, the United States or in the former Soviet Union, atomic research is strictly protected, and access to laboratories subject to stringent rules. Each major power tries to snatch the other's secrets, and the result is a series of well-organized spy and counter-espionage networks. From time to time some incident makes the headlines: France expels Soviet diplomats accused of spying; the Soviet Union hits back by expelling the same number of French diplomats. All this is only the visible top of a gigantic iceberg that remains largely hidden from the public at large. A book by Pierre Pean, (1986), gives a good idea of such goings-on. In the industrialized countries, every sector of scientific and technological research linked to national defence is closely guarded by parallel police organizations along with powerful military or paramilitary organizations.

The protection of knowledge in our oral cultures has to be understood as something rather similar. The purpose is the same: to prevent knowledge, along with the power it confers, from falling into enemy hands. It is the methods that differ. Here at home, I think the method most often used is to surround even the most positive and verifiable information with mythical and religious rhetoric. That rhetoric serves to cover up tracks. In a similar vein, threats and other intimidating methods are used to discourage the curious from testing and experimenting with possible technical discoveries. It is a rhetoric that sustains fear, presenting knowledge as something dangerous. It was among the methods invented by our ancestors to ensure the protection of intellectual property rights.

Against that background, we come to a crucial question: by what ways and means, in our time, can we test, check and verify this knowledge, so as to retrieve it for active use? The primary condition for such experimental testing is that the processes on which traditional knowledge is based should be repeatable. If an experiment is to be made generally accessible, one prerequisite is that it should be repeatable. The problem is to find out to what extent the traditional knowledge locked up in the esoteric mode can be rendered subject to repeated experimental testing. That is, in a way, the issue raised by Jean-Marie Apovo. It is an important one.

Knowledge is dangerous. That was the bottom line message the lecturer kept repeating throughout his presentation. For instance, speaking about the possibility of taming the red monkey, he warned: 'Careful. It is dangerous! And if you try, you will see what will happen to you'. Again: 'To make rain, you have to get chemical protection (sic)'. I think what is involved here is more like alchemy, not chemistry. People keep saying: one has to have protection, obtain bullet-proof accoutrement. The idea is to cover oneself with all imaginable sorts of mystical shields.

Last Friday I asked Madame de Souza, after her presentation, how she distinguished between medicinal effects and magical effects produced by particular objects and processes. Remember her answer? She spelled out three scenarios: First, results are magical when observers cannot see the link between cause and effect. Second case: the effect is medicinal when essences from plants, fruits or seeds are absorbed, producing an observable cure. Third case: the effect is medico-magical when one cannot explain the linkage between cause and effect, even though the effect (the cure) is observable.

In the last instance, research should enable us to go farther, to explain what has hitherto been unexplainable. I believe this response should be generalized. From a methodological point of view, it is extremely important. In each case, research should make it possible to establish the same distinctions. That in turn will lead to the clarification of confused situations, and to the precise recognition of the border line between rational realities and mythical fantasies. For example, one of the first things research should help us do is to establish accurately the identity of the 'red monkey', assuming it exists, and its relationship to other monkeys.

Whenever Madame de Souza, during her presentation, mentioned medicinal seeds or fruits, she gave us their names in the local languages, in French, in Latin. She also gave us their conventional botanical names, citing the plant family to which each ingredient belonged. I have a feeling that if our zoologists could identify more precisely the monkey in question, devise experiments for studying it, and carry them out, we would understand a lot more about this wonderful stone.

At the same time, while making enquiries and performing such experiments, we should be careful to avoid rubbing traditional learned men and 'wise men of the bush' the wrong way. In our approach, we need to observe a minimum of modesty and honesty. We need to develop a policy for the management of traditional knowledge and know-how. There are approaches we have to avoid. Dah-Lokonon gave us some very precise examples just a while back. We could cite others. For instance, the launching of huge witch-hunts is certainly not the way to deal with the problem of witchcraft in Benin. That method is especially senseless when promoted by a regime which calls itself Marxist but is absolutely ignorant of the vast body of scholarly writings, most of it from a Marxist point of view, devoted to precisely that problem. Similarly, it is not by castigating those supposed to prevent rain from falling, or by mounting a full-scale media attack on them, that we can make rain fall. Such ill-advised onslaughts have been among the most serious political mistakes made in this country. Scholars and scientists should be bold enough to say that. We need to develop a different approach, to establish a different policy approach to the management of traditional knowledge. Further research is needed to help define this approach.

Third, we need to ask if rainmaking is peculiarly African. In our discussions this question has not arisen. It should have arisen. And a similar query applies to the problem of witchcraft, or, to be more precise, the problem of belief in witchcraft. All too often, we delude ourselves with the notion that these phenomena comprise the parameters of our cultural identity. The truth is quite different. American Indians have their rain-makers, as everyone knows. Anthropological literature teems with instances of rainmaking. And we know that in Europe and America, in the heartlands of the most highly industrialized countries in the world, belief in witchcraft and magic, and in occult forces in general, is not just an archaic souvenir of the early middle age but also an important phenomenon in society to this day. Here, too, a series of comparative studies would throw much needed light on the issue.

A Hydrologist's Viewpoint

Abel Afouda

No one involved in the effort to reassert the value of traditional knowledge and know-how could be indifferent to the discussion following the presentation of the paper entitled "'Rain-Makers': Myth and Knowledge in Traditional Atmospheric Management Techniques". I am a working hydrologist. It is in that capacity that I would like to make a number of specific contributions on points raised during the discussion. The main questions I aim to address are the following:

a) Is it possible, today, to come up with scientific explanations for this type of knowledge, as part of a dynamic process of retrieval?

b) Is rain-making a peculiarly African phenomenon?

One of the basic principles of modern science is hinged on the idea that to shift a given system from a known point of departure to a projected destination, one must be able to impact on the energy within that system directly or indirectly. In plain words, in order to produce a given effect, it is necessary for one distinct object to impact on another. The key question, then, is just how that impact occurs. The answer should be verifiable through repeatable experimentation, and the effects predicted or observed should occur whenever the experiment is repeated. Now it is a matter of notorious record that the mythical and religious rhetoric enveloping traditional know-how is much keener to focus on the question 'why?' than on the question 'how?' The former question leads only to pre-scientific explanations for natural phenomena. Because they are inherently imprecise, such explanations can neither be proven nor refuted. Together they make up a corpus of esoteric lore.

In Dah-Lokonon's paper on rain-making, the experimental equipment consisted solely of a stone which could be turned right side up or down. Any approach designed to explain how the processes described happened would have to include a list of physical and chemical properties of the stone in question. At the very least, it would have to describe the experimental sequence in which such properties came into play. To answer the questions arising from the presentation, then, it would be necessary to take a fresh look at the way a traditional rain-maker operates. The following account is based on an experiment to which I was an eye-witness.

The Experimental Equipment of a Rain-maker

The following events took place in 1978. Widespread drought in Africa had devastated hundreds of thousands in the Sahelian countries. Survivors had been forced to migrate en masse. Wild life and domestic animals had died in large numbers. Some questions then addressed to hydrologists are still asked to this day. The most frequent were: 'When will this disaster end? Can anything be done to alleviate the crisis through traditional methods?'

I expressed my worries to a friend, Mr. Bernadin Viou, then Director of Hydraulic Services, and he introduced me to a rain-maker in Godomey. The procedure used by this rain-maker is an alternative to the one described in the presentation under discussion.

The rain-maker's experimental equipment, as shown to us, comprised a huge wood fire underneath a capacious jar filled with a blue liquid. Beside the fire lay a packet of blue dye of the kind commonly used by housewives. It was therefore easy enough to surmise how the liquid in the jar got its colour. Other ingredients included sodium chloride, also known as common salt, and various herbs and green leaves. I knew neither the local nor the scientific names of these leaves and herbs, and it occurred to me that the proper study of the matter would require the presence of a multidisciplinary team.

The experiment began in earnest when the blue liquid began to boil. The rain-maker commenced to utter incantations, took a pinch of salt plus a sample from each heap of herbs or green leaves, and dumped the lot on the fire, sending a thick billow of smoke up into the sky. He repeated these steps several times, before declaring the experiment a failure. He said his enemies had found out what he intended to do, and worked to block his success.

For my part, what stuck in my mind was the fact that there was a mixture of smoke and vapour rising towards the clouds. It would seem, then, that the stimulation of rain need not be an instant performance. It is possible to establish a cause-and-effect relationship. It was perfectly clear, in effect, that to the naked eye the only visible link between the rain-maker's experimental equipment and the clouds was the mixture of smoke and water vapour rising skywards.

Hydrological Interpretation of the Experiment

Leaving aside the incantations as a subjective, non-rational aspect of the situation, I tried to come up with a hydrological interpretation of the event I had observed. The mixture of smoke and vapour could contain an active substance serving as a catalyst for the condensation of cloud into rain. Indeed, smoke contains fine particles of carbon or other chemicals which could constitute a nucleus for the condensation of water vapour or droplets.

To give a clearer idea of how such particles might catalyze rain, we shall have to look into some basic concepts of atmospheric physics. For the purposes of the present discussion, it might be adequate to note that to understand rain, whether natural or artificial, we need to think in terms of the atmosphere. It is therefore necessary to stress the circulation of masses of air on a synoptic scale, and to have a clear idea of differences between rain-bearing and non-rain-bearing cloud formations.

Very broadly speaking, clouds are made up of droplets of water capable of remaining suspended in liquid form at relatively warm temperatures, with intervals of a millimeter between them. Because they are extremely light, they are buoyed up by rising draughts.

Rain-drops are considerably larger. They range from 0.5 to 2 millimetres in size, and their weight is therefore from a hundred thousand to a million times that of droplets constituting ordinary clouds. To produce precipitation, then, it is necessary to increase the size of droplets by as much as one hundred thousand to a million times. This can be achieved in one of two ways:

- by the direct accretion of several droplets; or
- by condensation, produced when water vapour, ice crystals and droplets of superheated water are brought together. In such situations, ice crystals serve as condensation nuclei, and as droplets evaporate, the vapour collects on the crystal nuclei. Accretions of crystals then form snowflakes which eventually drop earthwards when they get heavy enough to fall past the rising air currents that buoyed them up before. Fusing as they drop past warmer strata of the atmosphere, the flakes eventually turn into drops of rain.

It is important to understand that it is the presence of natural nuclei within superheated clouds that provokes the formation of ice, which in turn leads to rain. It is generally thought that in our tropical regions, large raindrops may form around salt nuclei, probably sodium chloride from sea spray whipped up by rising currents of air.

It would seem that the rain-making experiment I witnessed was an attempt to apply this principle of physics. The huge fire sent up billows of smoke containing fine particles that could have served as nuclei. It is possible that the smoke would have been rendered suitably water-absorbent by the fine particles produced by burning salt, herbs and leaves. Steam from the bubbling coloured water could have helped to start the process of nucleus formation around the fine particles as rising air currents wafted the billowing smoke up into the clouds.

Assuming that the nuclei thus formed reached the superheated cloud strata, they would doubtless be effective in causing rain precipitation in a situation where natural conditions alone would have been insufficient.

Compatibility with Modern Scientific Findings

To find out the local names of herbs and leaves used in the experiment described above, I would have had to repeat it in my own ethnic area. I contacted certain persons with that aim in view, but for reasons impossible to explain within the context of this discussion, the experiment never took place.

Having failed to obtain local confirmation, I turned to accounts of similar experiments in the available scientific literature. It became clear to me that a great deal had been written on the subject, and that far from being some mythical practice, traditional rain-making actually has a universal scientific content. Local rain-makers know this, but they suppose, wrongly, that their knowledge is a secret to be revealed only to a handful of deserving initiates.

For example, a French scholar, Henri Dessens, Professor of Global Physics at the University of Toulouse and Director of the Observatory at Puy-de-Dôme, presented an insightful paper on these African practices in a lecture entitled 'Physicists and Rain-Making Sorcerers', delivered at the Palais de la Découverte on 25 May 1963. Speaking of the advice given by rain-makers, he said:

> While we were busy gauging the sizes of our miserable little cumulus clouds, these natives showed us clouds of a different origin, which they had generated with their bush fires. The results they obtained ranged all the way to full scale storms complete with pouring rain and strokes of lightning. Realizing there was no point sticking to our exclusive little patches of superheated air, we also turned to studying convection currents and clouds created with help from fires.

Referring to his experiences in tropical Africa, Dessens concludes:

> In these regions, winds blow steadily at low velocities. The relative humidity of the lower atmosphere is high, and convection currents abound. This makes the area highly suitable for experiments designed to increase rain precipitation through the use of artificial ice-forming substances such as silver iodide.

Several tests have been conducted on the basis of these ideas, with the Lannemezan Physics Institute founded by Dessens and sited near Toulouse playing an active role. In the 1970s, a team from the Institute, led by Jean Dessens, son of Henri, mounted a set of experiments using ground-based generators to seed clouds with silver iodide particles. The experiment took place close to the Ayame Dam in the Ivory Coast. The team's cautiously phrased report said it was probable that particles of silver iodide sent up by the generator had played a part in provoking the rains that fell over the Ayame area at the time.

A 1972 bibliographical study conducted by Louis Lemoine for the General Secretariat of the Inter-African Committee on Hydraulic Studies (CIEH) summarized known cases of artificial rain-making in Africa and the world to that date. In a 1978 article in the Hydrological Series of the *Cahiers de l'ORSTOM,* Louis Serra analyzed the potential and limitations of artificial rain-making techniques. As far back as 1981, a wide range of literature on the subject recorded the fact that the American Senate had appropriated $9,000 for the purpose of conducting officially supervised experiments in artificial rain-making. Contemporary reports indicate that 'the experiments, conducted in the driest areas of Texas, produced positive results'. From that point on, the progressive discovery of natural laws, supported by a research process that was no longer a matter of trial and error but of basic science, opened the way to technological applications of artificial rain-making techniques.

Industrial-scale cloud seeding is performed from flying planes spraying carbonated ice, silver iodide or sodium chloride particles. In the United States, a summary report of findings from experiments conducted in 1966 was presented at the Academy of Sciences. It analyzed data from fourteen projects of varying duration conducted in the Eastern states of the U.S.A., together with findings from four long-term projects conducted in the Rocky Mountains. The Eastern projects indicated experimental increases in precipitation levels ranging from 0 to 57 per cent, with an average 18 per cent increase. The Rocky Mountain projects yielded experimental increases of 6 per cent, 7 per cent, 14 per cent and 18 per cent.

A number of experiments indicate that experimental success rates vary greatly depending on local natural conditions. Cloud temperature, for instance, is a key factor. Wind also plays a pivotal role. Cloud seeding has in numerous instances been known to produce increased precipitation beyond the target area. Sometimes the effects are felt as far as 300 to 350 kilometres downwind.

Artificial rain-making experiments conducted in the USSR by the Ukrainian Hydro-Meteorological Research Institute sited in the Dniepropetrovsk region as well as in other areas indicate that artificial rain-making techniques can yield precipitation increases from 10 per cent to 15 per cent. The most common technique is cloud seeding with carbonated snow. The findings did not seem sufficiently successful to justify industrial applications of the technique.

In Israel, a vast six-year programme lasting from 1961 to 1967 yielded average rainfall increases of 19 per cent over the experimental area as a whole, and 27 per cent over the central target area.

In France, apart from the work done by Dessens, Reminieras has reported a small number of experiments conducted by the French Electricity Corporation over selected Massif Central basins. The findings indicated increases of about 10 per cent. As in the USSR, these yields were not considered economically satisfactory, especially since rains in the area are quite evenly distributed.

In Chile, experiments were conducted in the arid northern region in 1969. Over a two-year period, there was a significant increase in rainfall levels, 40 per cent.

Experiments conducted in India have mainly been designed to provoke artificial rain from warm cloud formations. Seeding is done with sodium chloride in solution or powder form, sprayed from ground-based throwers. It would be worthwhile to pay greater attention to detailed findings from the Indian experiments, because they involve monsoon clouds. West African clouds form under similar conditions. Unfortunately, the literature from Western sources gives very little information on the subject.

It would seem, then, that even though there might still be large holes in our knowledge of different phenomena, artificial rain-making processes have nowadays gone far beyond the stage of laboratory research and field tests. The techniques are sufficiently developed to allow practical applications. In temperate climates there may be some hesitation concerning their economic profitability. But countries in those areas (Western Europe and the Ukraine for example) are blessed with relatively well distributed rains. It is significant that countries like Israel and Chile, situated in arid zones, and confronted daily with the problem of drought, have concluded that the techniques are economically justifiable, and have proceeded to apply them on an industrial scale.

In Africa, the CIEH member States acknowledge the potential benefits of rain-making techniques. Within the CIEH framework, they have conducted a series of tests in Madagascar, Northern Cameroon, Senegal and Burkina Faso. Lemoine reports various findings indicating that cloud seeding techniques are indeed applicable under African conditions. As a matter of fact, programmes had been scheduled, and the CIEH had offered to raise funds. But, as is the case with most development projects in African institutions today, no one has any idea of the implementational status of these programmes.

The Role of African Intellectuals

In conclusion, we might say, on the basis of the information given above, that the traditional atmospheric management techniques described earlier have an undisputably scientific basis. For the use of ground-based smoke producers requires a thorough knowledge of various meteorological factors ensuring the distribution of particles within clouds. For example, wind speed, the existence of ascending draughts and isothermal levels all have to be understood. On this basis, then, we can assert that it is possible to come up with a scientific formulation for this type of traditional know-how. If we Africans do not take the trouble to appropriate that knowledge, Western scholars will appropriate it, and it will come back to us bearing new patent tags or labelled as imported technology.

While artificial rain-making is not peculiar to Africa alone, African methods might have their peculiar features. It would be most worthwhile, for instance, if we could identify the properties of the herbs and leaves used, and find out if when burned they produce iodides. In the same vein, we need to take a closer look at the function of incantations. For it is quite possible that incantations uttered in well-chosen tones could cause vibrations leading, in the manner of the moth-and-candle chain reaction well known to those familiar with the theory of chaos, to atmospheric disturbances conducive to an increase in rising air currents carrying condensation nuclei. Alternatively, and in a simpler, profounder sense, incantations of this sort could also be an aspect of an African vision of nature, according to which each natural phenomenon has a spiritual double (which we could call its symmetrical counterpart), and is linked with all other phenomena in an established hierarchical order.

As for the stone described by Dah-Lokonon, it is intriguing from many points of view. Most interestingly, it seems to produce its effects immediately. To use it, the rain-maker does not need to recite incantations. All that he has to do, if we are to believe the report, is to turn it right way up in order to make it rain copiously. The description suggests a process of remote control, the achievement of a result with no intervening physical contact, at any rate none visible to the naked eye. From a modern, scientific point of view, however, nothing happens instantaneously. No data can travel faster than the speed of light. So one possible explanatory hypothesis could be based on field theory. But in that case we would have to find out if the stone can radiate electromagnetic waves capable of modifying the static electricity of clouds (since it causes thunder). But there is a preliminary point: we have to be ready to challenge our own assumptions. We have to adopt towards our own statements and beliefs that scrupulous skepticism which is the hallmark of the questioning scientific mind.

The present state of knowledge in the discipline of atmospheric physics may be incomplete. But it provides adequate explanations for rain precipitation mechanisms, whether natural or artificial. We need to develop traditional applications of such knowledge in greater depth, and to analyze them critically. Since 1968, Africa has been living through a devastating drought. It is not over. Various causes have been suggested, none entirely plausible. It would be great if the current generation of African intellectuals could bring traditional knowledge to focus on atmospheric management techniques in a search for solutions to this problem. To achieve that, we would have to adopt a universalist attitude emphasizing the mathematical formulation of hypotheses concerning nature, and capable of dealing with all the attendant hi-tech implications.

For the time has come for the river of African science to flow, like all other continental rivers, into the ocean of modern science. It is time for Africa to tread again the paths along which the scientific heritage of Humanity is created. One possible stage on the way to this goal, I think, is the clash of ideas within the context of national (or continental) seminars on traditional methods of atmospheric management, where rain-makers, sociologists, philosophers, geographers and natural scientists as well as scholars from various disciplines could share their experiences.

Part Two

Conceptual Structures

4

Traditional Number Systems and Modern Arithmetic

Toussaint Yaovi Tchitchi

Introduction

Let me approach the topic of traditional number systems and modern arithmetic from a linguistic angle, basing my argument on observations of the way human beings use language. This is an approach probably different from that of a philosopher, a sociologist or an anthropologist. My aim is to show how number systems operate in our societies within the context of languages giving them their codified meaning, in the service of speakers using them in their everyday lives.

To begin with, a few definitions are in order. By the term component' I mean a linguistic sign formalized to fulfil a syntactical function. A `statement' is a set of linguistic signs coherent enough to enable two communicating actors to understand each other. A statement can be reduced to a schema, which is a graphic representation thereof.

For example, when, speaking in the Fon language, I say `mɛ̌sì Hùntɔnji ɖɔ̀ xó', meaning `Professor Hountonji spoke', I use sounds connected in such a way as to enable me to establish a relationship with you. Now let me isolate each component and identify its syntactical function:

- mɛ̌sì Huntɔnji is a group of words, a (nominal) syntagm here performing the function of a subject. This group of words belongs to the category of nouns, symbolized by N. Because its function is that of a subject, S, we may give it the symbolic label NS.
- ɖɔ̀ is in another grammatical category. It is a verbal lexeme, symbolized by VL.

- xó is a noun with an expansionary function, sometimes referred to as a direct object complement.

The schema for our statement, then, would be:

$$\frac{N}{S} \qquad \frac{LV}{P} \qquad \frac{N}{X}$$

where S stands for the subject, P for the predicate, and X for the expansion.

In semantic terms, a determination is `a process designed to produce meaning by relating a set of signs to an already established support base' (Houis 1981:5). And the term syntagm will be used here to refer to any combination of words.

This chapter is, organized around two main points: first, we shall examine traditional number systems, using as our principal reference a set of findings from research on `Systematic Structure in the Ajá Language'. Second, we shall be examining the issue of decimalization, starting with the probe: `Do our accounting systems need decimalizing? What are the limitations of decimalization?'

Traditional Number Systems

At this point, let us introduce the concept of numerical components. Numerical components constitute a subset within a main category, that of nouns. Ajá, our reference language in this presentation, contains two principal classes of components: nouns and verbs. The noun class comprises nouns, pronouns and numerals. And the numeral component contains all items used in the accounting system.

In our examination of this number system, we shall take up the following topics in succession: cardinal numbers; ordinal numbers; and iterative numbers. We shall then observe the ways in which these numbers interconnect, and also look at the various operators used by speakers to make the system functional. The analysis of operators will enable us to judge whether the traditional accounting system is functional or dysfunctional.

Cardinal Numbers

Cardinal numbers are used to indicate quantitative values. In expressing quantity, that is to say, in the enumeration of numbers, care must be taken to distinguish between two processes: one is the counting of a series of numbers; the other is the assignment of a number to a fixed quantity. With this distinction in mind we shall describe the use of cardinal numbers for two purposes: enumeration and quantification.

In analyzing data, we shall see that Ajá speakers make use of two morphemes for both purposes of enumeration and quantification. However, it is important to point out that these two morphemes are not used in the first nine numerals.

Ordinal Numbers

Ordinal numbers, to recapitulate, express the position of an item in an ordered sequence. In the Ajá language this is indicated through the use of two suffixes, /-tɔ̀o and /-gɔn/, which, when attached to cardinal numbers, transform them into ordinal numbers. The expression for `first', however, is an exception to the general rule, for in that case only one of the two suffixes is used, that is to say, /-tɔ̀/ together with /ɖèká/ or /èɖé/. Thus, an Ajá speaker wishing to indicate that something is `first' says /ɲukɔtɔ̀/; /ɲùkɔ̀/ here meaning `in front of', while /-tɔ̀/ might be translated as: `that which is'. Hence our conclusion that when Ajá speakers talk of `the first' they mean the person, entity or object in the first position.

In grammatical terms, /-tɔ̀/ when pronounced in a low tone belongs to the category of approximative pronouns. That is the value we usually give it. It is translated as `that which is'. When /-tɔ̀/ is attached to cardinal numbers from `two' on up in order to indicate ordinal numbering, there is a change in tone. The low tone becomes a high tone, and the resulting pattern is as follows: low-low-high.

Table 1: Two Types of Cardinal Numbers (Tchitchi 1984:379)

Numerals Arabic	Enumerations	Ajà language Designation
1	èɖé	ɖèká
2	évè	àmɛvé
3	ètɔ̀n	àmɛ̀tɔ́n
4	ènɛ̀	àmɛnɛ̀
5	átɔ́n	àmátɔ́n
6	adɛn	àmáɖɛ́n
7	adrɛ	àmádrɛ
8	èyí	àmɛ́nyi
9	àshiɖéké ou nyíɖe (8 + 1)	àmáshiɖekɛ́
10	èwó	àmɛ́wo
11	wíɖèkâ	àméwìekâ
12	wivè	àmɛ́wivè
13	witɔn	àmɛ́witɔn
14	winɛ́	àmɛ́winɛ̀
15	wiatɔ́n	àmɛ́wíatɔn
16	wìadɛn	amɛ́wiadɛn
17	wiadrɛ	amɛ́wiadrɛ
18	winyí, èvè tó lè wimɛ	amɛwinyí, amɛve to lè wimɛ
19	wiashiɖekɛ̀, ɖèkà tó lè èwimɛ̀	àmɛ́wiashiɖekɛ̀, ɖèkà tó lè èwimɛ̀
20	èwì	àmɛ́wì
21	èwì vɔ̀n ɖèkà	àmɛ́wì vɔ̀n ɖèkà
22	èwì vɔ̀n vè	àmɛ́wì vɔ̀n vè
23	èwì vɔ̀n tɔ̀n	àmɛ́wì vɔ̀n ɔ̀n
24	èwì vɔ̀n nɛ̀	àmɛ́wì vɔ̀n nɛ̀
25	èwì vɔ̀n àɔ̀n [wìvàtɔ́n]	àmɛ́wì vɔ̀n àtɔ́n [àmɛ́wìvàtɔ́n]
26	èwì vɔ̀n àdɛ́n [èwìvàdɛ́n]	àmmɛ́wì vɔ̀n àdɛ́n [àmɛ́wìàdɛ́n]
27	èwì vɔ̀n [èwìvàdrɛ̀]	àmɛ̆wì vɔ̀n adrɛ [àmɛ́wìvàdrɛ́]
28	èwì vɔ̀n nyí, èvè tò lè ègbànmɛ́	àmɛ́wì vɔ̀n nyí, àmɛ́vè tò le ègbànmɛ̀
29	èwì vɔ̀n ashiɖekɛ̀ ɖekà tò lè ègbànmɛ	àmɛ́wì vɔ̀n ashiɖékɛ̀, ɖèká tò lè ègbànmɛ̀
30	ègbàn	àmɛ́gbàn
31	ègbàn èhò ɖèká	àmɛ́gbàn èhò ɖèká

(continued on next page)

32	ègbàn èhò èvè	àmɛ́gbàn èhò vè
33	ègbàn èhò ètɔ̀n	àmɛ́gbàn èhò tɔ̀n
34	ègbàn èhò ènɛ̀	àmɛ́gbàn èhò nɛ̀
35	ègbàn èhò àtɔ́n	àmɛ́gbàn èhò àtɔ̀n
36	ègbàn èhò adɛ́n	àmɛ́gbàn èhò adɛ́n
37	ègbàn èhò adrɛ́	àmɛ́gbàn èhò adrɛ́
38	ègbàn èhò ɛnyí, èvè tò lè èkamɛ̀	àmɛ́gbàn èhò nyí, àmɛ́vè tò lè èkamɛ̀
39	ègbàn èhò ashiɖékɛ̀ ɖékà tò lè èkamɛ̀	àmɛ́gbàn èhò ashi ɖékɛ̀, ɖékà tò lè èkamɛ̀
40	èkà	àmɛ́kà
41	èkà èhò ɖékà	àmɛ́kà èhò ɖékà
42	èkà èhò èvè	àmɛ́kà èhò vè
43	èkà èhò tɔ̀n	àmɛ́kà èhò tɔ̀n
44	èkà èhò ènɛ̀	àmɛ́kà èhò nɛ̀
45	èkà èhò àtɔ́n	àmɛ́kà èhò àtɔ́n
46	èkà èhò àdɛ́n	àmɛ́kà èhò àdɛ́n
47	èkà èhò àdrɛ́	àmɛ́kà èhò àdrɛ́
48	èkà èhò enyí, èvè tò lé èkà hòwómɛ̀	àmɛ́kà èhò nyí, àmɛ́vè tò lè èkà hòwómɛ̀
49	èkà èhò ashiɖékɛ̀	àmɛ́kà èhò ashiɖékɛ̀ ɖèká tò lè èkà èhòwómɛ̀
50	èkà èhò wó	àmɛ́kà èhò wó
51	èkà èhò wó èhò ɖèká	àmɛ́kà èhò wó èhò ɖèká
52	èkà èhò wó èhò èvè	àmɛ́kà èhò wó èhò vè
53	èkà èhò wó èhò ètɔ̀n	àmɛ́kà èhò wó èhò tɔ̀n
54	èkà èhò wó èhò ènɛ̀	àmɛ́kà èhò wó èhò nɛ̀
55	èkà èhò wó èhò àtón	àmɛ́kà èhò wó èhò àtɔ́n
56	èkà èhò wó èhò àdrɛ́n	àmɛ́kà èhò wó èhò àdɛ́n
57	èkà èhò wó èhò àɖrɛ̀n	àmɛ́kà èhò wó èhò èhòàdrɛ́
58	èkà èhò wó èhò ènyí, èvè tò lè kàtàkpúmɛ̀	àmɛ́kà èhò wó èhò nyí, àmɛ́vè tò lè kàtàkpúmɛ̀
59	èkà èhò wó èhò ashiɖékɛ̀ , ɖèkà tò lè kàtàkpúmɛ̀	àmɛ́kà èhò wó èhò nyí, ashiɖékɛ̀ , ɖèkà tò lè kàtàkpúmɛ̀

Thus, by using the suffixes /-tɔ̀/ and /-gɔ̀n/, we can obtain the following ordinals:

èvètɔ̀	or	èvègɔ̃n	`second'
ètɔ̃ntɔ́	or	etɔ̃ngɔ̃n	`third'
ẽnɛ̆tɔ́	or	enɛgɔ̃n	`fourth'
àtɔ̀ñtɔ́	or	àtɔ̀ñtɔ́n	`fifth'
ãdɛ̆ntɔ́	or	ãtɔ̀ñtɔ̃n	`sixth'
ãdrɛtɔ́	or	ãdrɛgɔ̃n	`seventh'
ènyìtɔ́	or	ènyìtɔ́n	`eighth'
àshiɖékɛ̀tɔ́	or	àshiɖékɛ̀gón	`ninth'
evotɔ́	or	ewogɔ́n	`tenth', etc.

In a given context it is possible to use terms based on these combinations.

E.g.: n kpɔ̀ èví wiɖekàtɔ́ló

I/ have found/ child/ the eleventh

`I have found the eleventh child'

ɳusu witɔngɔnió cí àhwà

Man/ the thirteenth/ remained/ war

`The thirteenth man fell on the battlefield'

Such is the reality of ordinal numbers. In speech they function like nouns, playing the primary and secondary roles assigned to nouns: as subject, expansion, complement.

Iterative Numbers

Strictly speaking, there is some question as to whether we are dealing here with numbers or instead with terms identifiable as iterative. Our information, based on analysis, is that the prefix /zè-/ attached to the numerical component is used to express repetitive action. The combination makes up the iterative number, i.e., the element which introduces a repeated action in any linguistic process.

E.g.: Kɔ̀kú yì ashimɛ̀ zètɔ̀n

/Kɔ̀kù/ went/ market/times three/

`Kɔ̀kù went to the market three times'

n kpɔ̀ hùntɔ̀jí zènɛ́ lè ɛ̃xwɛ̃cɛ̃mɛ̀

/I / saw / Hountondji / times four / is / year-this-in/

`I have seen Hountondji four times this year'

The prefix /-zè can play a different role in speech when combined with /-nɛ̀ní in an interrogative phrase, as in the following example:

E.g.: zènɛ̀ní wò xò ètòmɛ nɔ ɖàjɛ́lɔ́ɔ̀

/Times how many / they / beat / ear / of / young / man / that / pdm?/

`How many times was that young man slapped?'

Clearly, /zè-/ and the other terms that may be connected to it are used as part of a determinative linguistic unit with a numerical function. The prefix is a relational morpheme that plays the role of complement to the numerical component expressing repetitive action. By itself, /zè-/ cannot play the primary role of a noun. It is invariably connected either with /nɛ̀ní/ or with a numerical component.

The evidence of daily life suggests that one motive for the invention of numbers was the need to count money. In pre-colonial society cowries were the units of currency. They were used for exchange transactions in the market place until quite recently. This is, I think, an appropriate point for a bit of numismatic analysis: a look at the way monetary values are expressed in the Ajá language.

Currency

Today the Ajá word /èhò/ clearly means, in semantic terms, `money' or `currency'. In times past, however, /èhò/ by itself, or /èhòɣí/ meant `cowry'. The language has a complement /-èɣí/, meaning white, on account of the colour of cowry currency. We might deduce from this the possibility that there was or still is money of a different colour. Whatever the uses to which /èhòɣí/ may have been put, we have reason to believe that some time in the past the art of copper processing made it possible to produce tokens named /ègàjɔn/, from /ègà/ meaning `iron' and /èjɔn/, meaning `red'. We need to find out the most likely periods when these different monetary values first appeared in our societies. That would enable us to understand the resulting nexus of relationships, and their impact on economic, social and cultural life.

It may be worthwhile, at this point, for us to identify and understand a set of monetary values formerly used in Ajá society, whose equivalent value in French currency was established by a research team based at Azové and led by the Reverend Father Harguin Deguy (1969). The values are as follows:

-/hòkagɛ/ or `two and a half centimes'

-/kàtɔ́n/ or `one hundred centimes'

-/hɔ̀cú/ or `fifty centimes', etc.

These are examples of local monetary values that were supplanted by foreign monetary values during the imperialist period. Hence the fact that the currencies used in our markets today are derived from the Franc, the Dollar or the Pound. We should be careful, however, not to make imperialism the sole reason why our languages use these borrowed monetary terms. Such borrowings may also result from friendly relations between various peoples. The fact that I use the terms `biyé', `dola', `kpono' or even `flan' does not necessarily imply that imperialism committed aggression against my ancestors. The primary point of interest here is the fact that these borrowed terms have been integrated into the lexical system of our target language. Our focus is on the semantic transfer and the exchange value assigned each foreign currency.

Thus, with the adoption of the English `pound' into the Ajá language, we find such resultant modifications as:

/kpɔ̀nɔ́/ or /kpɔnɲú /or/ kponɔ́ɖeká, equivalent to 25 francs CFA;

- ɖɔlaɖeká or biyedeká equivalent to five francs CFA;
- biyejinɖeká equivalent to a hundred francs CFA;
- flan or flanɖeká equivalent to one franc CFA.

E.g.: biyevè hwè do ǹ

/notes two/ lacking/ to/ me

`I am ten francs short'

n xlwè mɔ̀lú ɖɔlaɖeká

/I /have bought/ rice/ dollar one/

`I bought five francs worth of rice'

wò nú nɔ n b nyɛ le ná biyejinàtɔ́n

/they / said/ I / should/ give notes red five/

`I was asked to give five francs'

In general, the reference currency for all the various terms is the French franc, which clearly dominates economic transactions. And as in the case of the local currency, the colour is regularly mentioned when the monetary unit is cited.

Ajá speakers, like speakers of every language in the world, use operators for handling figures and numbers. In the main, these operators facilitate the addition and subtraction of numbers.

Operators

Ajá number systems, whether they operate on a base of five or on a decimal base, are invariably made up of the first nine numbers and their derivatives. The terms used to designate these derivatives make up the category of operators.

In analyzing data from our target language, we find that the identification of these operators follows a set of regular rules governing the determination of nouns. Composite nouns are obtained by joining two nouns in a direct, non-mediated relationship.

E.g.: efyɔxwé

/king/ house/

`The royal palace'

ashinɔ̀

/wife/ mother/

`Mother-in-law', etc.

In the Gùn language as in the Fon language, the same relationship is both mediated and unmediated. In the Gùn language, for instance, we have:

àxɔ́lúxwé = efyɔ́xwé, or àxɔ́lú sin xwé; here /sin/ is a grammatical particle identified as a connector. It is also present in the Gon language in the form: /bé/. Ajá speakers do not use this form.

Now let us see how the numerical relationship functions. What types of operators are active in this function? And is the relationship solely unmediated?

Unmediated Numeral Determination

This type of determination can be observed right from the formation of the expression `eleven'. In the coupling of numbers from 11 to 19 there are no associative or coordinating terms whatsoever. The result is exemplified in the expressions: wiɖeka, wivé, witɔ̀n, ... wiashiɖekɛ̀ (19), and èwì (20).

Here, care must be taken not to confuse the /wí/ in wiɖeka and the èwì that stands for `twenty' in the language.

Bearing in mind the lexical bases of the language, along with our brief explanation of unmediated determinative relationships, it becomes clear that the /wí-/ in wideka and wivè is a result of a process of vocal assimilation. It is a proven linguistic fact that when two nouns in this particular language form a complementary group, both the final vowel of the main noun and the initial vowel of the complement are dropped in pronunciation. Neither is sounded. There are cases, however, in which contact between two vowels might lead to the formation of a third through a process of vocal harmony. On this point Dubois et al (1973) offer the following observation: `Vocal harmony is a phenomenon of vocal assimilation that may affect several vowels within a single word. Whether the change affects one or several vowels in a given position is not a question of arbitrary happenstance; it is automatically determined by the presence of some other, specific vowel'.

That, in our opinion, is the explanation for the morphology of the numbers we have just described. Within this framework, it is perfectly clear to us that the main noun in these composite numerical nouns is in fact /èwó-/, and that the first nine numbers play the role of complements. This means that wivè = èwó kódó évè, literally, `ten with two' = `twelve'. The word kódó, translated into French as `and' or `with', is a recognized coordinate in Ajá syntax.

Unmediated Numeral Determination

For purposes of enumeration and designation, the Ajá counting system makes use of two operators. One is `vɔn', which connects numbers from 21 to 29. The other is `hò', which connects numbers from 31 on. This is what we observed in the tables presented above.

E.g.:

21 = ewí vɔ̀n ḍèká

22 = ewí vɔ̀n vè

31 = ègbàn hò ḍèká

33 = ègbàn hò tɔ̀n, etc.

These operators, however, are not always functional when it comes to enumeration. For instance, when enumerating the number 60, instead of saying ekà hò wì, which is literally `forty' and `twenty', the counting system uses a different element: /-tàkpú/ which in the language also means èwì, that is to say, 20. Thus, to enumerate 70, 80, and 100, for instance, the following elements might be used:

- 70 kàtàkpú hò wò
- 80 kàvè (40 x 2) or kàtàkpú hòwì
- 100 kàvè hò wì or kàvètàkpú.

An examination of the information presented above leads to the following conclusions:

- Addition is particularly important in counting operations within the language. For purposes of enumeration, noun forms such as /vɔ̀n/ and /èhò/ seem to function as unavoidable operators.
- Addition, understood as an operation using modern arithmetical computations, relies on another operator: /kó / /kódó. Thus, eka kodó ewí wà kàtàkpú (40+20) = 60. In our opinion, this operator is used for designation.
- Addition in the sense of an operation involving unmediated numeral determination and the use of the first nine numbers

for quantities between 10 and 20 should not be confused with multiplication, which we shall discuss in the next section.

Other Operators

Such is the preponderant role of operators used for additions (computations of sums) in the conceptualization of terms within our target language that a casual listener might conclude the language has no other operators. That would be a mistake. In their own quiet way, other operators, specifically for multiplication, subtraction and division, also exist.

Multiplication

Multiplication occurs in two forms: mediated and unmediated.

Unmediated multiplication involves the use of an operator that functions only with specific numbers. Only the number `forty' can combine directly with the first nine numbers to give a set of ever larger numbers. E.g.:

80 = 40 x 2 or èkàvè

120 = 40 x 3 or èkatɔ̀n

160 = 40 x 4 or èkanɛ̀

200 = 40 x 5 or èkatɔ́n, etc.

The practice is to add `forty' to each lower number to make up the higher number, or to use unmediated multiplication.

Mediated multiplication is accomplished by the use of a link word /dònù/. The evidence suggests that this word means `a heap of ...'.

E.g.:dònù nɛ̀ wà ekanɛ

40 x 4 = 160

- ègbàn hò àtón dònù nyí wà èkatɔ́n kódó èkàvè
- /thirty-five/ which/ multiplies/ eight/ equals/ two hundred and eighty.

Here the verbal lexeme /wà/, normally translated as `to make', expresses the concept of equivalence.

Substraction

Here we find a striking similarity between the Ajá and Latin counting systems. Both systems designate certain numbers by subtracting `one' and `two' from selected reference numbers. In Ajá these reference numbers start from twenty and increase in steps of ten at a time. Thus:

- 18 = winyi or èvètòlèwimɛ̀, i.e., `two subtracted from twenty'.
- 19 = wiashiɖekɛ́ or ɖèkátólèwimɛ̀, i.e., `one subtracted from twenty'.

These statements expressing subtraction reminded us of the equivalent expressions in Latin for these same numbers: `duo de viginti' for eighteeen, `un de viginti' for nineteen. Hence our observation about that specific similarity in the two languages. For Ajá speakers, subtraction is a mental operation facilitating the reduction of a higher number by a lower.

E.g.:

nɔ́ wò ɖè biye adrɛ tí lè

kponɔvèmɛ

/if/ one/ subtracts/ thirty-five francs/ from/ fifty francs

ɖe nɛ̀ni á kpɔtɔ̀ɔ̀

/?/ how much /(future predicate)/ will remain?/

`how much will be left?'

To sum up, we would simply use the following expressions: /ɖè tó/ tí lɛ̀ ... mɛ̀ or `to take away from, to subtract'; kpɔ̀tɔ̀ or `to remain'; /kpɛtɛ/ or `the remainder'; and /dèdetilemɛ/ or `subtraction'.

These are the codified forms used in the language.

Division

The method for accomplishing this is quite simple. There is only one operator used for division, and it is the expression /mà dó/.

E.g.:

wò sɔ́ ɳuci eka hò tɔ́n sɔ mà dò

enɛ̀, meaning:

`They have divided forty-three oranges by four'.

An analysis of operators makes it clear that the Ajá counting system works not on a basis of five but on a basis of ten. Jean-Dominique Penel (1985) speaks, in this connection, of reference numbers. Our findings agree with his: the Ajá language uses `ten' as the first reference number, in the sense that numerical components from 11 to 19 are formed by the juxtaposition of complementary numbers to the first reference number. eleven is thus counted as 10 + 1, yielding `wiḍekà'.

It might be supposed that the simple juxtaposition of reference numbers and complementary numbers would be sufficient for computations of sums. But this is valid only for numbers between 11 and 19. After that, connecting words such as /vɔ̀n/, /hò/ and /kodó/ are used for computations involving figures and numbers. Juxtaposition within a context of unmediated numeral determination does not necessarily imply addition when the numbers from one to nine are placed next to the number 40. In this case the juxtaposition implies multiplication. This is the form we have labelled unmediated multiplication, in contrast to the mediated form: /dònù/.

It would seem, then, that in the Ajá language both 10 and 40 serve as reference numbers. It is this use of two reference numbers that led the National Commission on the Ajá Language to propose the streamlining of the counting system on a decimal base.

The Issue of Decimalization

One of the papers produced during Benin's National Seminar on Language Education bore the title: `Decimal Number Systems: the Case of the Ajá Variant' (Tohoun 1979). The paper, after a critical analysis of the old number system, proposes a number of new ideas likely to facilitate its modification into an efficient decimal system.

The traditional number system uses two reference numbers: 10 and 40. This works fine for small numbers up to forty. Beyond that point, however, as the paper points out, `the brain must handle batch computations made up of sets of 40 in order to deal with larger numbers' (Tohoun 1979). This causes problems as soon as the numbers involved reach really large magnitudes. The Ajá number system then stalls because it is saturated. Faced with the complexity of figures and numbers, the brain tends to get `foggy'. To solve the problem, metalinguistic techniques were explored, and a set of new concepts proposed.

New Concepts

Following a series of field studies, the proponents of a reformed number system adopted a set of new concepts fitting in harmoniously with the existing system. The number 10, labelled as /àmɛwo/ or /èwó, becomes /etaɖeka/. In everyday speech /eta/ means the head. By a process of linguistic transfer, this lexeme now means a set of ten, so that /etaɖeka stands for a quantitative unit of ten.

Similarly, the number `one hundred', formerly rendered as /èkàvètàkpú/ or èkàvè hò wì, becomes /sanpudi/. The original equivalent of /sanpudi/ was a heap of a hundred cowries. Among Ajá speakers the term stood for a quarter of /èkàwó/ or `four hundred'. Half of /sanpudi/ meant /hòkagɛ/, or 50.

One thousand, traditionally rendered by /èka wí vɔ̀n àtɔ́n/ (40 x 25), is henceforth represented by the term /kotokun/. This last term comes from the name of a sack filled with a thousand francs or pieces of some other substance. Thus, in the Ajá language, /n ɖo kotokun ɖékà/ means: `I have a thousand francs', even though the statement does not specifically mention /èkó/, i.e., money.

The other concept introduced after /kotokun/ is /linlɔ̀n/. It stands for the number one million. Cardinal numbers are developed along similar lines. The word adopted for a million normally means `ants'. Presumably, a million appears to be a difficult number to count and handle; hence the comparison with ants.

The last in the series of adapted terms is pronounced /ayɔ̀/. It stands for a billion. Despite the similarity in sound, it has nothing to do with /ayɔ́/ or /ayɔmɛ́/ meaning `pubis'. History is somewhat more helpful in giving us an explanation for this term. The name the Ajá give their eastern neighbours is Ayɔnù, which means `townspeople of ɔyɔ'. In times past they made something of a name for themselves because of their military conquests, and also because they were so numerous that other groups could hardly resist their onslaughts. For these reasons, the elders proposed that the reformers of the counting system use the term /ayɔ/ for `a billion'. In the popular mind one billion is a huge quantity comparable to the numbers of ɔyɔ warriors. There is indeed a popular saying that dates back to these old wars: /wò sugbɔ̀ wu ayɔhwà/, meaning: `They are more numerous than ɔyɔ warriors'. It is this idea of quantity that is encapsulated in the new term.

Clearly, then, the concepts involved were already codified in the language. Some had dropped out of common usage. But in a dynamic context of evolutionary change, these terms were given a new lease of life through the process of decimalization. Most were adopted through semantic transfers. Now you might ask: was all this intellectual contortion necessary? Would it not have been better to dig deeper into ancient stores of endogenous knowledge and then to transform the data thus obtained?

Limitations of Decimalization

These questions bring us to a critical analysis of the information presented above. From a practical, pragmatic perspective, the new concepts have the advantage of streamlining the number system. To illustrate this point, it is sufficient to compare old and new terms for selected quantities:

100: kàvètàkpú (Old Term) sanɳudi (New Term)

52: eka hò wó hò vè (Old Term) tatón hò vè (New Term)

68: kàtàkpú hò nyí (Old Term) tadɛn hò nyí (New Term)

98: kàvè hò wó hò nyí, or èvètòlé kàvè tàkpúmɛ̀ (Old Term)

tashiɖekɛ hò nyí or èvètòlé sanɳudimɛ̀ (New Term)

On the surface there does not seem to be much streamlining here, except that the new system gets by with a few less syllables for certain numbers. However, if we focus on the new names given to various numbers, the new system is certainly less cluttered. For example, the old kàvè hó wò is more cumbersome than the new tashiɖekɛ̀. Even so, the number of separate syllables used in the new term is greater than the number used in the old term. After all is said and done, the clearest advantage of the decimal system is that it facilitates the handling of large numbers and figures. E.g.:

The Year 1984	= exwe kotokunɖeká sanɲudi ashiɖɛ tanyi hò nɛ̀
56.000 F	= flán kotokun tàtɔ́n hò adɛ̀n
50.006 F	= flán kotoku tàtɔ̀n ci adɛ́n
975.000.000	= linlɔn sanɲpudi ashiɖekɛ tadrɛ hò àtɔ́n
970.000.005	= linlɔn sanɲpudi ashiɖekɛ tadrɛ hò ci àtɔ́n, etc.

In the above examples, there is no risk whatsoever of system saturation. The margin of error is smaller. That is the advantage of decimalization.

Trial runs conducted by Regional Development Centre officials using the new decimal system in Mono Province have yielded promising results. Peasants taught to use the new system are no longer intimidated by the idea of counting millions of francs in their self-managed trading transactions. This proves that the new number system is an improvement over the traditional one. At the moment, the new terms used to represent numbers, as well as the connectors /ci/ and /ku/ used to replace the old computational operators for sums, are still in the experimental phase. But already, decimalization has broken down the old barrier of saturation that in the past confronted those using the traditional system of enumeration and designation.

This is our contribution to the debate on endogenous knowledge. Its gist is that traditional number systems and modern arithmetic are far from incompatible. By this we mean that problems caused by saturation can be solved through in-depth analysis and reflection on these number systems. Only after such reflection and analysis does it make sense to initiate innovations. Once adopted, these innovations will call for the creation of fresh concepts. That in turn will necessitate the use of an appropriate meta-language.

All endogenous knowledge can be transformed for modern use. After all, African languages in their own right offer the necessary potential for conceptualization. The quality of results depends entirely on the kind of practical backing and support made available to researchers in their effort to update and to tap this conceptual potential.

Discussion

The following is a transcript of the discussion which took place after the presentation of this chapter at the National University of Benin research seminar (see Introduction chapter for details).

Serge de Souza: In Part II of his book entitled *Les fonctions mentales des sociétés inférieures,* Lucien Lévy-Bruhl asserted that African languages were incapable of serving as vehicles for logical reasoning because of an overwhelming tendency to get bogged down in particulars and details. This is the tendency you have described as `saturation'. Are you, then, in agreement with Lévy-Bruhl? If you are not, do you have any arguments from your own research that might shed light on his assertion?

Professor Paulin Hountondji (intervening to clarify a point relating to Serge de Souza's question): Let me put in a correction here. What the French anthropologist Lucien Lévy-Bruhl, father of the theory of The Primitive Mind, actually said in his first work on primitive societies, entitled *Les fonctions mentales dans les sociétés inférieures,* was not that African languages in particular were inadequate vehicles for logical reasoning. He said primitive languages (so-called) in general were unsuitable for abstract thinking. What is Mr. Toussaint Tchitchi's comment on that?

Toussaint Tchitchi: Every language evolves within its own environment. The degree of technical or technological evolution of a people speaking a given language depends on the general level of their environment. Here in Benin, for example, we have population groups specializing in agriculture. On meeting farmers from such groups, you are most unlikely to hear them use language suited to a fishing or an iron-working environment. Bearing such considerations in mind, it would be natural to conclude that languages described as primitive are relatively poor. All they do is to reproduce a set of lexical items they have recorded and coded.

In other words, the richness or poverty of a language depends directly on its environment. By the same token, the vocabulary of any language is necessarily dependent on that environment. Take the European languages: Latin, French, Old French, etc. Many items in these languages have been registered and given codified form. But when we come to our situation, what do we know today about ancient forms of the Ajá language? The best we have are a few arcane documents collected by priests. But how far back do they date?

We have no comprehensive descriptions of our languages. Neither have their speakers always used written words to facilitate the visualization of their thought processes. The result is that when these European anthropologists examine our languages, they filter what they hear through the earphones of their own culture. It is up to us, as Africans, to look at our own culture with a clear consciousness of our own realities.

As for the anthropologist Lévy-Bruhl's opinion, I think it is wrong. After all, only practical experience can prove whether our languages are capable of reaching high levels of abstraction or not. There is no way any armchair theory can prove that. I think Professor Hountondji is in a much better position to treat this question than I am.

Paulin Hountondji: Lévy-Bruhl's assertion was made in the context of a general theory of The Prelogical Mind. We all know the kind of historical, theoretical and ideological circumstances under which that style of thinking developed. Today the theory is entirely obsolete, and it would be superfluous to go over the reasons why. Regarding the languages Lévy-Bruhl calls primitive or semi-primitive, it is glaringly clear that his analysis is half-baked. Obviously, Lévy-Bruhl takes no account whatsoever of the potential ability of every language to enrich itself through internal development, which is to say, through the production of fresh terms as and when its conceptual needs make such innovations necessary. He overlooks the capacity of every language to borrow from other languages. He also forgets that of the most highly abstract terms now used by even the so-called advanced languages, a large number come from old terms that originally referred to perfectly practical realities. Invariably, even the most rarefied of such terms refer back to concrete experience.

In this regard I am particularly impressed by Toussaint Tchitchi's observation concerning similarities between the Ajá and Latin languages in their designation of the numbers 18 and 19. The fact had escaped me until he pointed it out.

Now Lévy-Bruhl, in the book mentioned above, presents an example not from Latin but from Yoruba. In Yoruba, he says, people say `twenty minus four' when they mean sixteen, `twenty minus three' when they mean seventeen, and so forth. From that he concludes that Yoruba is a primitive language. How interesting to find the same counting style in Latin.

Now back to Lévy-Bruhl. How does he explain the Yoruba number system? He supposes it is an utterly peculiar system, and argues that the reason is that the number twenty was originally used to refer to a heap of cowries. In other words, the Yoruba number was not, in the purely conceptual sense, the number twenty. In short, to borrow the terminology Mr. Toussaint Tchitchi has just offered us, it was not used for the function of abstract designation. And so, for example, it is in relation to this concrete style of designation, a style the Yoruba mentality cannot free itself from, that Yoruba speakers think of the number seventeen, to take just one instance.

Now we see that the same thing happened in Latin. It might be interesting to find out what concrete referent speakers of Latin used in the past. In any case, the sole logical conclusion we can draw from this knowledge is that this form of counting that occurs among the most different and most widely separated languages is a universal form.

Let me take this opportunity to slip in a question. It is about the theoretical, conceptual difference between enumeration and designation. I would like to know if this is an old distinction, a linguistic innovation coined by Tchitchi, or a distinction already established in linguistic theory.

Second, in his observations on the direct complementary relationship occurring, for example, in the expression wideka, meaning eleven, which brings two cardinal numbers directly together without the mediation of an operator, M. Tchitchi made a passing reference to lexical laziness. Is this really a legitimate concept? Laziness as a psychological concept carries a potentially negative value judgement. So what right have we to use it to account for the linguistic phenomena in question? I would suggest substituting the concept of linguistic economy for that of lexical laziness. After all, it is more economical, and therefore more rational, to use unmediated complementary relations of this sort.

My next question is about the literal translation of évè tò lè èwimɛ. The translation you offer us is: two/are/taken out/are/twenty/in. This caused a spontaneous reaction among the audience. I think this was because they understood the lè not to mean `are' but to have the precise meaning of the French preposition `de', whose Latin equivalent is `ab', meaning the point of departure.

The speaker, however, disagreed, on the grounds that that would be an interpretation based on the French model. In other words, in translating `lè' by `of', we would be imposing a French linguistic structure on Ajá terms. I have a different impression: that it is rather by translating `lè' as `are' that we impose a French translation on the Ajá term, through the assimilation of two Ajá terms which in fact are homonyms. Certainly, `lè' sometimes is used to mean `to be'. But a more accurate meaning is `the place of origin'. In this case, are we not suppressing the homonym because of our self-imposed obligation to find a French equivalent? I have often observed that in their analyses, African and Africanist linguistics scholars tend to segment units in such a way that the original spoken units in the source language come to have verbatim equivalents in French.

It is this tendency that has led certain linguistics scholars (and I know Mr. Tchitchi is certainly not one of them) to say that when Fon speakers say `Mi kú dó gbàdà', the kú means the speaker wishes the one he or she is greeting to drop dead. This is just another instance of the spurious conclusions produced by assimilating, within an African language under study, two terms which in practice are homonyms. The kú in the phrase `mi kú dó gbàdà' in no way connotes death in the mind of the Fon speaker. And one has to refer to the spontaneous act of meaning or signification executed by the speaker in order to understand if the word is the same or a different term. So the reference to a foreign metalanguage often results in the unreal effect of the suppression of homonyms, and the inaccurate use of homonymic terms. I am almost sure Mr. Tchitchi would agree with me regarding the second example I have given. But it does seem to me that in the way he segments the phrase /èvè tò lè èwìmɛ̀/ he falls into the same trap.

Toussaint Tchitchi: It was I who applied the terminology of enumeration and designation to the Ajá counting system. My observations seem to indicate, in effect, that the Ajá themselves are not so sure whether in using numerical expressions they are enumerating or designating. When, in my research, I came up against these observations, I went back to consult some old texts left by missionaries who had studied the language. But the missionaries had not been able to establish the distinction.

Now, in the old system one reaches a saturation point sooner or later. Furthermore, using the concept of enumeration or designation, I was unable to link initial numbers in complementary relationships. I therefore concluded that even though it was possible to count all the way up to a given number, X, the process was cumbersome. This was the thought process that led me to introduce the concepts of enumeration and designation into our counting system. I am sure there is more work to be done. As a matter of fact, I do not know if what I have done so far is all water-tight. But the information before us is based directly on our own realities.

Turning to direct complementary relationships, I agree with your point: it is more accurate to talk of linguistic economy, and again, I agree it is a rational process.

With regard to the literal translation of the phrase évè tò lè èwimɛ̀, I would like to point out that in most languages there are so-called polysemous terms, that is to say, terms with multiple meanings. So lè in this phrase may well mean `place', or be equivalent to the Latin `ab'. However, in identifying verbal lexemes in the language under discussion, we observed that quite often, lè functions as a verb meaning `to be'. It is possible that in implying a direct equivalence between `lè' and the French verb that means `to be', we may have made a mistake. But then research is an unending process. I intend to go back and re-examine this point, bearing in mind the cogent issues you raised.

In the same vein, Professor Hountondji used as an example the phrase /Mi-kùdò gbàdà/. African languages use sets of clarificatory statements that follow a scheme identical to that of the phrase /évè tò lè èwimɛ̀/. But an unusual statement such as /Mi kù dò gbàdà/ is in a different category. It is a special greeting formula. It is an exceptional case because it does not seem to me to fit into any identifiable schema. It is one of a set of stereotypical formulae used in the language. When we encounter the term `kù' in the language, our analysis has to stretch over several semantic fields. The term `kù' is an ambivalent one in the Fon, Gun, Ajá and Gon languages. It can belong to two categories, especially in Fon and Gun usage. In Ajá, however, nouns are always based on thematic derivatives when their structure is of the VCV type.

I think it correct to translate /èkú/ as `death'. Nevertheless, when the word `kù' is transposed into greeting formulae such as /mi kùdó gbàdà/, it is not taken in isolation. It makes sense strictly in combination with `dó'. The relevant unit here, then, is /kúdó/, an indivisible term. Its meaning here is similar to that of /kódó/ in the Ajá statement:/miwo kódó èdo, /miawo èdo/, meaning literally `you and work', which is to say, `Thanks'.

Analytically speaking, /ku/ or /kúdo/ is a coordinating morpheme, a grammatical particle connecting two nouns. So the meaning of the expression /mi kudò gbàdà/ is: `You with the evening'. Here kù has nothing to do with `death'.

Mama Katchon: In most of our languages we use words which are simply foreign loan words, like the American `dollar' and the French `billet'. But we use these words to mean something quite different from what they mean elsewhere. This seems to me a great pity, and I would like to know what causes such incorrect usage.

Toussaint Tchitchi: The phenomenon you refer to is what we know as a semantic transfer. When people adopt a term, they have the option of giving it the connotation they want under the immediate circumstances. This is why speakers of different languages give different meanings to such loan words as æala (dollar) and biyé (billet). In this particular case, we have to remember the European presence on our continent and the consequent transfer of exchange values. The words in question here are new words that got integrated into various African languages at a very early stage.

Micheline Hadonou: I do not recall Mr.Tchitchi mentioning the figure zero. I would like to know if the Ajá number system makes no provision for this concept, zero.

Toussaint Tchitchi: The new terminology we are currently using in our decimalization programme needs to be exhaustively explained, because there are data we have yet to master. But for the concept zero we use the word `tòotù'. In Ajá it means zero.

Paulin Hountondji: Let me interject a point here. Mathematicians consider the figure zero extremely important. It would be worth our while, I think, to invite a mathematician or a mathematical historian to explain to us the origin of the figure zero. The general impression is that the concept is relatively new, and that its invention was a highly important event in the history of mathematics. Now the concept `tòotù', as normally used in the Ajá language, had the same meaning as the mathematical concept, zero, unless indeed we are now innovating by using that old concept to represent zero. To get to the bottom of the matter, I think it would be advisable to consult a mathematician.

Toussaint Tchitchi: I think the moment it is established that the term exists in a language, there is every reason to conclude that speakers of that language were conscious of its meaning: emptiness.

Micheline Hadonou: I asked the question because I read the text by Gnanvo in which he uses the term `voxwí' to represent zero. Is that a new coinage?

Maxine da Cruz: I would like more information on the coinage `tòotù'. Supposing you had to say `empty basket' in Ajá, how would you translate that phrase? Would it not make communication difficult?

Toussaint Tchitchi: I do not think it would pose any problem. All mathematics teachers have to say to their pupils is that `tòotù' stands for zero, nothing, and that in colloquial speech an empty basket is a `kishi tòotù'. That is a matter of conventional usage.

Victor Nobime: In his presentation on systems of enumeration and designation, the speaker discussed operations for addition, subtraction, then multiplication. Division, however, seems more problematic. My question is: why?

Toussaint Tchitchi: I said nothing about division because I rushed ahead a bit faster than planned. In the Ajá language the concept of division is expressed by the term `mà', meaning to share.

E.g.: n mà ɳúcilɔ́ dó èvè

`I have divided the orange into two'.

In the language, then, `mà...dó' is codified to mean `divide by'.

Albert Gbodogbe: I would like to know if in their field work, researchers aim to rehabilitate ancient number systems. Or do they tend to skip over the old systems because they are unnecessarily cumbersome, preferring to invent other systems such as the decimal system?

Toussaint Tchitchi: No. All we are trying to do is to fill in a gap. Used for purposes of designation, the traditional counting system sooner or later reached saturation point, causing the system to stall. That is why all speakers were asked to think in terms of the decimal system. And indeed decimalization makes the counting system more functional. It is not because we want to avoid studying the two systems. The point is that to envisage such issues more rationally, one has to be creative. In our case, the creative work is still in the experimental phase. We get to test our ideas mostly during the marketing of produce such as cotton.

Paulin Hountondji: I remember meeting someone in Germany who said that thanks to current advances in science, the decimalization of number systems was no longer necessary. I am not sure I understood what he meant exactly. But I do think it important that we give sustained thought to this question. Is it true, for instance, that the use of a decimal counting system is a prerequisite for progress in mathematical thinking? All this underscores our need to work together with mathematicians and mathematical historians in our research seminar. It would be extremely useful, I think, if after Mr. Tchitchi's presentation, we could organize a round table conference during which practising mathematicians and linguistics experts would come together to discuss and argue over the issue in greater depth.

Serge de Souza: I would like to ask the speaker if, given the diversity of our languages, the creation of new terms for various realities might not eventually lead to confusion in the arithmetical system.

Toussaint Tchitchi: There will be no confusion. At the present stage in our research, the People's Republic of Benin has made a clear option, summed up in Article 3 of the Loi fondamentale. It reads as follows: `The People's Republic of Benin is a multinational State. Each nationality within it has a right and a duty to use its language'. Now the question that arises is how to determine the territorial boundaries of nationalities. As far as linguistics experts are concerned, diversity is especially pronounced within the Gbè continuum, with contiguous languages mutually comprehensible from one neighbouring group to the next. If the country had decided on a common language to be used in the educational system, we would all have supported that language, and it would have become our practical medium. But so far that has not happened.

Paulin Hountondji: I would like to thank Mr. Tchitchi for his highly useful contribution to our seminar. Perhaps you are aware that in the Gèn language, the expression for `mathematics' is `akɔnta wɔ̀owɔ́'. It would be worthwhile to examine such pointers in precise detail. Needless to say, the problems raised today are inextricable from those of linguistic policy. But they are also connected to issues of linguistic analysis proper, as well as to issues in the history and philosophy of science. If one were asked to sum up the lessons learned from today's session, one might say it has demonstrated that nowadays, more than ever, it is important to promote interdisciplinary work in practical terms, and to facilitate a more effective dissemination of ideas among the various disciplines.

Annex

Some Data Related to Decimalization

10 taḍeka
11 taḍeka ci ḍeka
12 taḍeka ci ve
13 taḍeka ci tɔn
14 taḍeka ci nɛ
15 taḍeka ci àtòn
16 taḍeka ci deɛn
17 taḍeka ci adrɛ
18 taḍeka ci nyi
19 taḍeka ci ashiḍekɛ
20 tave
21 tave ci ḍeka
22 tave ci ve
23 tave ci tɔ
24 tave ci nɛ
25 tave ci atɔ̀n
26 tave ci adɛn
27 tave ci adrɛ
28 tave ci nyi
29 tave ci ashiḍekɛ
30 tatɔn
31 tatɔn ci ḍeka
32 tatɔn ci ve
33 tatɔn ci tɔn
34 tatɔn ci nɛ
35 tatɔn ci atɔ̀n
36 tatɔn ci adɛn
37 tatɔn ci adrɛ
38 tatɔn ci nyi
39 tatɔn ci ashiḍekɛ
40 tanɛ
41 tanɛ ci ḍeka
42 tanɛ ci ve
43 tanɛ ci tɔn
44 tanɛ ci nɛ
45 tanɛ ci àtɔ̀n
46 tanɛ ci adɛn
47 tanɛ ci adrɛ
48 tanɛ ci nyi
49 tanɛ ci ashiḍekɛ
50 taàtɔn
51 taàtɔn ci ḍeka
52 taàtɔn ci ve
53 taàtɔn ci tɔn
54 taàtɔn ci nɛ
55 taàtɔn ci àtɔ̀n
56 taàtɔn ci adɛn
57 taàtɔn ci adrɛ
58 taàtɔn ci nyi
59 taàtɔn ci ashiḍekɛ
60 taadɛn
61 taadɛn ci ḍeka
62 taadɛn ci ve
63 taadɛn ci tɔn

64 taadɛn ci nɛ
65 taadɛn ci àtɔ̀n
66 taadɛn ci adɛn
67 taadɛn ci adrɛ
68 taadɛn ci nyi
69 taadɛn ci ashiɖekɛ
70 taadrɛ
71 taadrɛ ci ɖeka
72 taadrɛ ci ve
73 taadrɛ ci tɔn
74 taadrɛ ci nɛ
75 taadrɛ ci àtɔ̀n
76 taadrɛ ci adɛn
77 taadrɛ ci adrɛ
78 taadrɛ ci nyi
79 taadrɛ ci ashiɖekɛ
80 tanyi
81 tanyi ci ɖeka
82 tanyi ci ve
83 tanyi ci tɔn
84 tanyi ci nɛ
85 tanyi ci àtɔ̀n
86 tanyi ci adɛn
87 tanyi ci adrɛ
88 tanyi ci nyi
89 tanyi ci ashiɖekɛ
90 taàshiɖekɛ
91 taàshiɖekɛ ci ɖeka
92 taàshiɖekɛ ci ve
93 taàshiɖekɛ ci tɔn
94 taàshiɖekɛ ci nɛ
95 taàshiɖekɛ ci àtɔ̀n
96 taàshiɖekɛ ci adɛn
97 taàshiɖekɛ ci adrɛ
98 taàshiɖekɛ ci nyi
99 taàshiɖekɛ ci àshiɖekɛ
100 sanɳudi ou sanɳudi ɖeka
101 sanɳudi ci ɖeka or sanɳudi ɖeka ci ɖeka
102 sanɳudi ci ve or sanɳudi ɖeka ci ve
103 sanɳudi ci tɔn or sanɳudi ɖeka ci tɔn
104 sanɳudi ci nɛ or sanɳudi ɖeka ci nɛ
105 sanɳudi ci àtɔ̀n ou sanɳudi ɖeka ci àtɔ̀n
106 sanɳudi ci adɛn or sanɳudi ɖeka ci adɛn
107 sanɳudi ci adrɛ or sanɳudi ɖeka ci adrɛ
108 sanɳudi ci nyi or sanɳudi ɖeka ci nyi
109 sanɳudi ashiɖekɛ or sanɳudi ɖeka ci ashiɖekɛ
110 sanɳudi taɖeka
111 sanɳudi taɖeka ci ɖeka
112 sanɳudi taɖeka ci ve
113 sanɳudi taɖeka ci tɔn
114 sanɳudi taɖeka ci nɛ
115 sanɳudi taɖeka ci àtɔ̀n
116 sanɳudi taɖeka ci adɛn
117 sanɳudi taɖeka ci adrɛ
118 sanɳudi taɖeka ci nyi
119 sanɳudi taɖeka ci ashiɖekɛ
120 sanɳudi tave or sanɳudi ɖeka tave
121 sanɳudi ci ɖeka
122 sanɳudi tave ci ve
123 sanɳudi tave ci tɔn

124 sanɳudi tave ci nɛ
125 sanɳudi tave ci àtàn
126 sanɳudi tave ci adɛn
127 sanɳudi tave ci adrɛ
128 sanɳudi tave ci nyi
129 sanɳudi tave ci ashiɖekɛ
130 sanɳudi tatɔn
131 sanɳudi tatɔn ci ɖeka
132 sanɳudi tatɔn ci ve
133 sanɳudi tatɔn ci tɔn
134 sanɳudi tatɔn ci nɛ
135 sanɳudi tatɔn ci àtɔ̀n
136 sanɳudi tatɔn ci adɛn
137 sanɳudi tatɔn ci adrɛ
138 sanɳudi tatɔn ci nyi
139 sanɳudi tatɔn ci ashiɖekɛ
140 sanɳudi tanɛ
141 sanɳudi tanɛ ci ɖeka
142 sanɳudi tanɛ ci ve
143 sanɳudi tanɛ ci tɔn
144 sanɳudi tanɛ ci nɛ
145 sanɳudi tanɛ ci àtɔ̀n
146 sanɳudi tanɛ ci adɛn
147 sanɳudi tanɛ ci adrɛ
148 sanɳudi tanɛ ci nyi
149 sanɳudi tanɛ ci ashiɖekɛ
150 sanɳudi taàtɔn
151 sanɳudi taàtɔn ci ɖeka
152 sanɳudi taàtɔn ci ve
153 sanɳudi taàtɔn ci tɔn
154 sanɳudi taàtɔn ci nɛ
155 sanɳudi taàtɔn ci àtɔ̀n
156 sanɳudi taàtɔn ci adɛn
157 sanɳudi taàtɔn ci adrɛ
158 sanɳudi taàtɔn ci nyi
159 sanɳudi taàtɔn ci ashiɖekɛ
160 sanɳudi taadɛn
161 sanɳudi taadɛn ci ɖeka
162 sanɳudi taadɛn ci ve
163 sanɳudi taadɛn ci tɔn
164 sanɳudi taadɛn ci nɛ
165 sanɳudi taadɛn àtɔ̀n
166 sanɳudi taadɛn ci adɛn
167 sanɳudi taadɛn ci adrɛ
168 sanɳudi taadɛn ci nyi
169 sanɳudi taadɛn ci ashiɖekɛ
170 sanɳudi taadrɛ
171 sanɳudi taadrɛ ci ɖeka
172 sanɳudi taadrɛ ci ve
173 sanɳudi taadrɛ ci tɔn
174 sanɳudi taadrɛ ci nɛ
175 sanɳudi taadrɛ ci àtɔ̀n
176 sanɳudi taadrɛ ci adɛn
177 sanɳudi taadrɛ ci adrɛ
178 sanɳudi taadrɛ ci nyi
179 sanɳudi taadrɛ ci ashiɖekɛ
180 sanɳudi tanyi
181 sanɳudi tanyi ci ɖeka
182 sanɳudi tanyi ci ve
183 sanɳudi tanyi ci tɔn
184 sanɳudi tanyi ci nɛ
185 sanɳudi tanyi ci àtɔ̀n

186 sanŋudi tanyi ci adɛn

187 sanŋudi tanyi ci adrɛ

188 sanŋudi tanyi ci nyi

189 sanŋudi tanyi ci ashiḍekɛ

200 sanŋudi ve

201 sanŋudi ve ci ḍeka

202 sanŋudi ve ci ce

300 sanŋudi tɔn

400 sanŋudi nɛ

463 sanŋudi nɛ taadɛn ci tɔn

500 sanŋudi àtɔ̀n

600 sanŋudi adɛn

608 sanŋudi adɛn ci nyi

700 sanŋudi adrɛ

900 sanŋudi ashiḍekɛ

1000 kotokun or kotokun ḍeka

1001 kotokun ḍeka ci ḍeka

1010 kotokun ḍeka taḍeka

1015 kotokun ḍeka taḍeka ci àtɔ̀n

1020 kotokun ḍeka tave

1021 kotokun ḍeka tave ci ḍeka

1894 kotokun ḍeka sanŋudi nyi taàshiḍekɛ ci nɛ

1960 kotokun ḍeka sanŋudi ashiḍekɛ ci nɛ

1973 kotokun ḍeka sanŋudi ashiḍekɛ taadrɛ ci tɔn

1974 kotokun ḍeka sanŋudi ashiḍekɛ taadrɛ ci nɛ

2031 kotokun ve tatɔn ci ḍeka

2469 kotokun ve sanŋudi nɛ taadɛn ci ashiḍekɛ

24004 kotokun tave ho nɛ ci ḍeka

387 954 kotokun sanŋudi tɔn tanyi ho adrE sanŋudi ashiḍekɛ taàtɔ̀n ci nɛ

807 301kotokun sanŋudi nyi ho adrɛ sanŋudi tɔn ci ḍeka

999 999 kotokun sanŋudi ashiḍekɛ taashiḍekɛ ho ashiḍekɛ sanŋudi ashiḍekɛ taashiḍekɛ ci ashiḍekɛ

1 000 000 linlɔn

1 000 001 linlɔn ḍeka ci ḍeka

1 000 010 linlɔn ḍeka taḍeka

1 002 783 linlɔn ḍeka kotokun ve sanŋudi adrɛ tanyi ci tɔn

1 670 259 linlɔn ḍeka kotokun ve sanŋudi adɛn taadrɛ sanŋŋve taàtɔ̀n ci ashiḍekɛ

895 723 417 linlɔn sanŋudi nyi taashiḍekɛ vɔn àtɔ̀n kotokun sanŋudi adrɛ tave ho tɔn sanŋudi nɛ taḍeka ci adrɛ

999 999 919 linlɔn sanŋudi ashiḍekɛ taashiḍekɛ vɔn ashiḍekɛ kotokun sanŋudi ashiḍekɛ taashiḍekɛ ho ashiḍekɛ taḍeka ashiḍekɛ

1 000 000 000 ayɔ̀

1 022 303 108 ayɔ̀ ɖeka linlɔn tave vɔn ve kotokun sannudi tɔn ho tɔn sannudi ɖeka ci nyi

27 574 831 675 ayɔ̀ tave ku adrɛ linlɔn sannudi àtɔ̀n taadrɛ vɔn nɛ kotokun sannudi nyi tatɔn ho ɖeka sannudi adɛn ci àtɔ̀n

5

Fâ Ritual: A Stochastic Process: Understanding the Geomantic Cults of Coastal Benin

Victor Houndonougbo

Scholars working with statistical probabilities are familiar with the word 'stochastic'. It is a derivative form of the Greek stochastes, meaning 'diviner'. Probability analysis involves the study of aleatory or chance processes. The adjective 'aleatory' derives from the Latin alea, meaning 'dice'.

This Chapter examines the casting of kola nuts, cowries, hollowed beads, Asro almonds (botanical name: *irvingia barteri*) and Avi nuts (*Cola acuminata*). These beads, nuts and other objects used in divination are strung out on a cord to make a sort of rosary we call the diviner's beads. Fâ divination is based on observations of random patterns made by these beads as they are thrown onto a flat surface.

We shall create a model, a finite grid of probabilities, using it to evaluate the probability with which various Fâ patterns are likely to occur, and certain events likely to happen, while analyzing the stochastic procedures used.

In the true-or-false framework of a bivalent mathematical logic, it would seem reasonable to pose the question: Is Fâ divination true or false? Such a cut-and-dried approach, however, would rob Fâ divination of its mysterious content, taking no stock of the mystical beliefs associated with it in contemporary society. So I have opted for a personalized analytical approach, not in the sense of an idiosyncratic style but in the sense of an approach that might be followed by any other mathematician taking the trouble to reflect on local sociological practices. My aim, in sum, is to use statistical evidence to show that Fâ divination is a process for the evaluation of probabilities.

In my analysis of Fâ divination processes, I shall keep to the long-established scientific rule according to which all science is based on representational 'models' starting with the simplest and ending with the most complex. The normal trajectory of inquiry begins with very simple, even idealistic hypotheses, which are then developed into more complex forms later on.[1] I have detected the same progression in Fâ divination processes on the basis of the following divinatory models commonly used:

1. Divination using kola nuts: *Vi-kilkã;*
2. Divination using cowries: *Legba-kikã;*
3. Divination using beads: *Akple-kikã.*

At this point I think it necessary to put in a word of warning concerning calculations of probability and the results we may legitimately expect from them. The probability of an event is expressed as a numerical value that assesses the chances of its happening. The question posed is whether a given event is more likely to happen than some other event. In everyday parlance, these probabilities are indicated by adjectives, nouns and adverbs. The resulting expressions are relatively rich, but they also happen to be markedly vague and imprecise. Particular events may, for instance, be described as possible, impossible, likely, unlikely, doubtful, probable, certain, etc.

The extremes of 'impossibility' and 'certainty' are clear enough. But between these limits there are nuances and permutations such as a straightforward yes or no; an emphatic yes or no; yes, but; and no, but. We shall represent these permutations as follows:

(Yes.) for a straightforward yes;

(Yes!) for an emphatic yes;

(Yes...) for yes, but.

All these nuances are present in the Fâ corpus.

It should be recalled that for any given experiment, the totality of possible results is labelled Ω. That means that every component of Ω is an event, so that the total array $P(\Omega)$ representing the totality of parts of Ω stands for the entire range of events. A probability is the application of one instance P within the array $P(\Omega)$ on a scale [0,1].

Where an event A has a probability of zero, that event is impossible: $P(A) = 0 \Rightarrow$ A is impossible.

Where the probability of an event B is 1, that event is certain: $P(B) = 1 \Rightarrow$ B is certain. In other words, the closer the probability of an event is to zero, the rarer that event will be. Conversely, the closer the probability of an event to 1, the more common that event is likely to be in the experimental or experiential context.

In practice, it is agreed that an event is virtually impossible if its probability is lower than 1 in 100, or 0.01. To illustrate this, consider a set of 100 marbles, identical in shape, 99 of which are white in colour, and 1 black (note: black signifies bad luck). Assume, now, that the marbles are thoroughly mixed up in a closed sack. If in reaching into that sack to draw out a marble, you happen to draw the lone black marble, the event might be interpreted as proof of ill luck. This little game of chance might be regarded as a divinatory process that could help determine whether one is likely to have the chances of success in undertaking this or that project, and then be said that leaving aside the ritual consecration of the cola nuts used in Fâ divination, any individual among us could work out a process for determining beforehand our chances of success. Such a process would in all essentials be identical to a divination process. Indeed, this is the reality behind the fact that in our society, some people declare that if, on stepping out of their homes in the morning, they first meet a woman (or a man), they will have a lucky day.

Divination Based on the Use of Cola Nuts (*Vi-Kilkã*)

This is the most common and the most widespread form of divination in our society. It is an aid to rapid decision making. Family heads and elders in charge of compounds use it in their decision-making processes. It is also used to determine the wishes of the familiar departed, fetishes, and the dead.

Divinatory Equipment

The equipment consists mainly of cola nuts of a special variety known as *Avi*. This kind of nut divides naturally into four perfectly identical lobes.

Because of its regular use for divination, it has come to be known as the diviner's nut. Other types of cola are never used for the purpose.

Modus Operandi

The diviner is normally a member of the family, often the grand-uncle or grand-aunt. To start with, he or she takes a diviner's cola nut and carefully separates its four identical lobes, then throws them. A lobe falling with its inner surface uppermost is said to be open. When it falls with the outer surface uppermost, it is said to be closed.

When a throw results in four open lobes, the diviner calls the outcome *Gbe*. Fâ combinations are classified in a hierarchical order, and the *Gbe* is the leading mother-sign. The following is a list of names given by diviners to other permutations:[2]

1 lobe closed, 3 open: *Aklã;*

2 lobes closed, 2 open: *E mã;*

3 lobes open, 1 closed: *Tawa;* for this combination there is no particular assigned Fâ figure.

4 lobes closed: *Yɛku*. This is the second mother-sign in the Fâ corpus.

Interpretation

Generally, patterns resulting from the throwing of the cola lobes are interpreted as follows, at any rate for the first throw:

Yɛku:	A definite yes;
E mã:	A straightforward yes;
Gbé:	Yes, but.... All options, good and bad, are open; a second throw will be needed;
Aklã:	No;

Tawa-Tawa: This is a message, 'Ta é wa we non du', meaning 'Whatever the head does, it accepts the price to be paid'. This is an ambivalent statement; a second throw is needed.

In the interests of greater clarity, we shall use a tree-like sketch (see Figure 1). In the single-column system of notation, the first number is the number of the throw; the second indicates the number of closed lobes.

Examples:

$\binom{3}{0}$ means a Gbe result from the 3rd throw;

$\binom{2}{4}$ means a Yɛku result from the 2nd throw.

Relevant Probability Field

Let us posit a number of hypotheses:

a) The four lobes are perfectly identical and perfectly balanced. Each lobe has an inner surface and an outer surface.

b) The diviner's plate is a perfectly flat surface.

c) There is no psychic or occult influence whatsoever on the position of the lobes in question (with this last hypotheses, practicing diviners wholeheartedly disagree).

Be that as it may, given the above conditions, the total range of possibilities is as follows: {open, closed 1, closed 2} Thus $\Omega = \{\varphi, \pi\}$ where φ stands for open, π for closed. The resultant equation is $P(\varphi) = 1/3 P(\pi) = 2/3$.

Probability Calculations for Various Events:

The probability of Gbe $= P(\{\varphi,\varphi,\varphi,\varphi\}) = P(\{\varphi\})^4 = (1/3)^4 = 1/81 = 0.0123$

Yɛku $= P(\{\pi,\pi,\pi,\pi\}) = P(\{\pi\})^4 = (2/3)^4 = 16/81 = 0.1975$

E mã $= 6.P(\{\pi,\pi,\varphi,\varphi\}) = 6.P(\{\pi\}).P(\{\varphi\})^2 = 6.(2/3)^2 (1/3)^2 = 24/81 = 0.2963$

Akla $= 4.P(\{\pi,\varphi,\varphi,\varphi\}) = 4.P(\{\pi\}).P(\{\varphi\})^3 = 4.(2/3)(1/3)^3 = 8/81 = 0.09882$

Tawa $= 4.P(\{\pi,\pi,\pi,\varphi\}) = 4.P(\{\varphi\}) = 6.(2/3)^2 (1/3) = 32/81 = 0.3951$

Now let us introduce a random variable X, equivalent to the number of closed lobes after each throw.

X = 0: Gbe: Observation: $P(X=0) = (1/3)^4 = C^0_1 (2/3)^0 (1/3)^4$

X = 1: Akla: $P(X=1) = 4.(2/3)(1/3)^3 = C^1_4 (2/3)(1/3)^3$

X = 2: E mã: $P(X=2) = 6.(2/3)^2(1/3)^2 = C^2_4 (2/3)^2 (1/3)^2$

X = 3: Tawa: $P(X=3) = 4.(2/3)^3(1/3) = C^3_4 (2/3)^3 (1/3)$

X = 4: Yɛku: $P(X=4) = (2/3)^4 = C^1_1 (2/3)^4 (1/3)^0$

Figure 1: Tree-Structured Sketch with Single-Column Notation

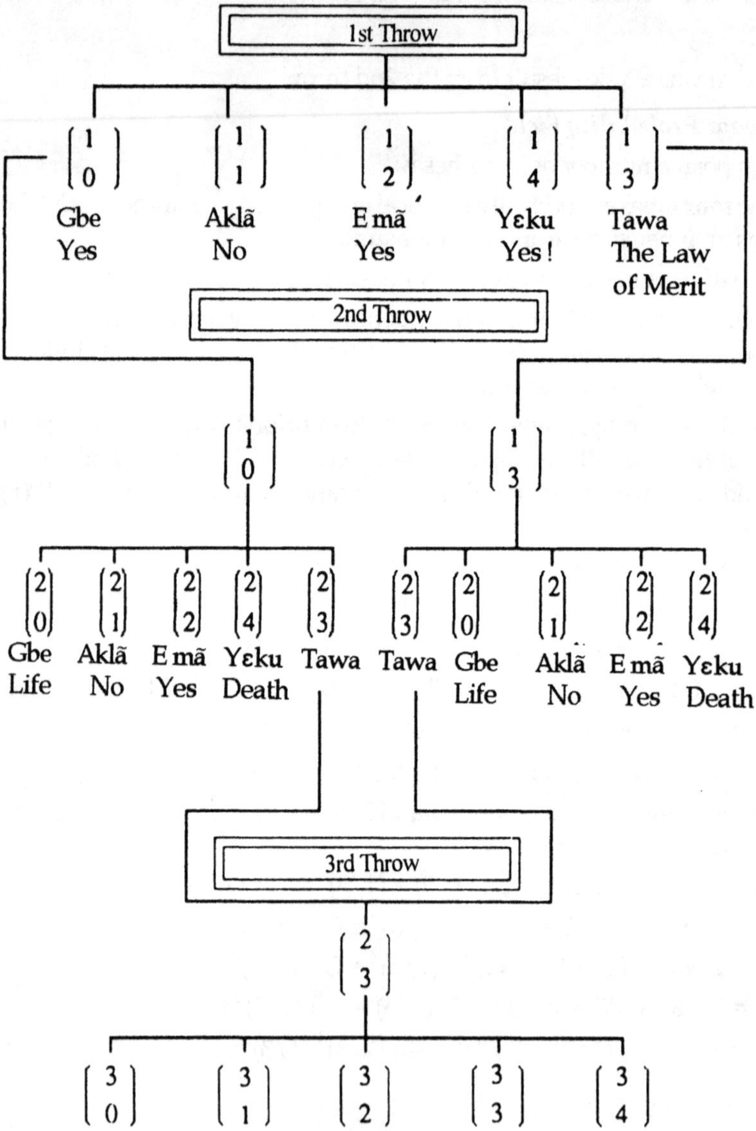

Given the four lobes, I construct a diagram of the factorial structure of throws, as follows (see Figure 2):

Figure 2: Factorial Structure of Throws

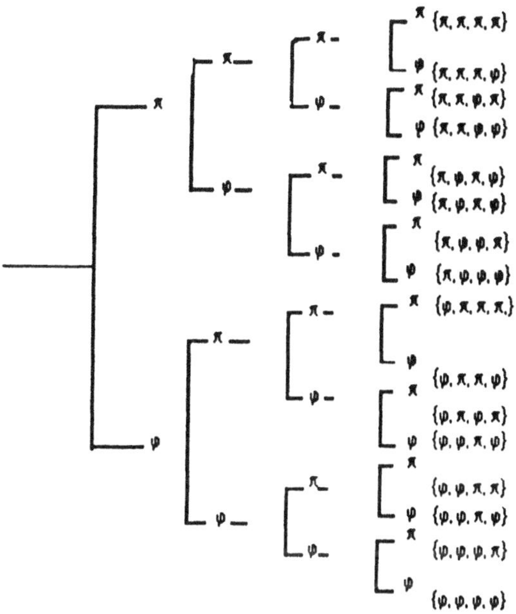

Experts in probability calculations generally agree that this is an instance of the Binomial Law of Parameters: n = 4 and p = 2/3 β (4.2/3).

Result: (Theorem)

During Fâ divination sessions where cola nuts are used, the random variable that corresponds to the number of closed lobes is distributed according to Bernouilli's Binomial Law of Parameters: n = 4 and p = 2/3 β (4.2/3). In other words, Fâ divination based on throws of cola nut lobes conforms to Bernouilli's Binomial Law.

Comments on Figure 3

a) *Tawa*: The probability of this combination occurring is high. For this reason, divination sessions rarely stop with the first throw. This means that the normal verdict after the first throw is that 'Whatever the head decides to do, it should assume responsibility for the consequences'. This is the same statement Jesus made in the evocative sentence: 'As ye shall sow, so shall ye reap'. It is the law of balance, which the philosopher Emerson called the law of compensation. This is the cosmic law of Karma.

b) *E mã*: This is the next highest probability. The frequency of its occurrence invalidates the supposition that Fâ divination is merely a hustle invented by its practitioners to ensure themselves a living. For if the supposition were well grounded, our calculations would indicate that a different method should have been chosen. After all, at the first throw, Gbe, Yɛku and E mã are affirmative forms.

The probability (Yes at the first throw) = P(Gbe) + P(Yɛku) + P(E mã) = 41/81 = 50 per cent. This is much higher than the probability of a No.

The probability (No) = P(*Akla*) = 8/81 = 0.0987 or 10 per cent.

It should be understood that No is not an event precisely contrary to Yes.

c) Let us now evaluate the probability of 'good fortune,' i.e., predict the chances of good fortune, using this divinatory procedure:

Prob (Good Fortune) = Prob (Yɛkʋ or *Gbe* at the 1st throw) = 17/81 = 0.2098 or 21 per cent.

d) The probability of misfortune: To predict misfortune using this procedure, *Akla* must occur at the first throw, followed by *Gbe* or *Yɛku*.

Prob (Misfortune) = P (*Akla*).[P(*Gbe*) + P(*Yɛku*)] = 8/81 x 17/81 = 136/6561 = 0.02072 or 2 per cent.

This occurrence presages imminent ill fortune for the person consulting the diviner. The latter therefore demands a lot of sacrifices to obviate it.

e) Definite Probability of Good Fortune: This requires *Yɛku* on the first throw, followed by *Gbe* at the second throw.

Prob(Definite Good Luck) = P(*Yɛku*). P(*Gbe*) = 16/6561 = 0.00243 or 0.2 per cent. This combination occurs very rarely. Whenever it occurs, therefore, the verdict is: 'Be confident. Nothing evil shall happen.'

Figure 3: Probability Graph

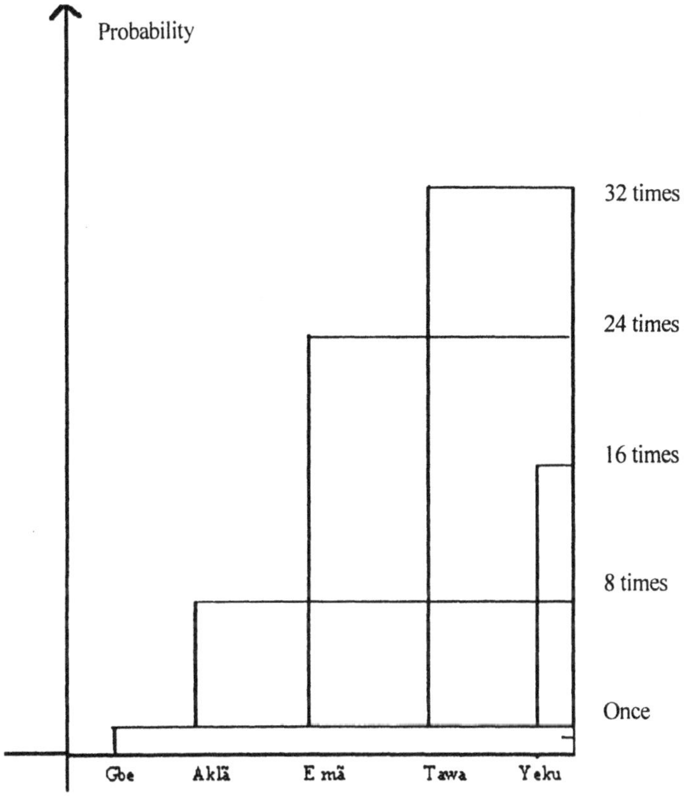

Divination by Means of Cowry Throws (Lêgba-Kikã)

Equipment

Diviners are supposed to derive their powers from an occult power known as Legba-Mahutô. They are often dressed in spectacular garb. On their heads there may be a stylized tuft of hair above the occiput, around the medulla oblongata, considered to be the soul's doorway. A diviner may at times wear a wooden statuette shaped in human form, representing Legba, and to which he offers the blood of sacrificed animals.

Strictly speaking, the diviner's equipment consists of a plate of 16 identical cowries. It is from the observation and interpretation of their positions that he arrives at a message. Here we shall not detail the other accessories such as ingredients used by diviners before divinatory sessions.

Modus Operandi

The diviner begins with a grand gesture, throwing the 16 cowries onto the diviner's plate. He then proceeds to sort them. Depending on the number of open cowries appearing on the plate, he names a Fâ combination called DU. The following is a table of different DU combinations obtained according to this method.

Table 1: DU Combinations with Names

Open cowries	2	3	4	5	6	7	8
DU	*Joko*	*Guda*	*Loso*	*Cɛ**	*Abla*	*Di*	*Jogbe*

Open cowries	9	10	11	12	13	14	15
DU	*Sa*	*Fu**	*Wlin*	*Jila*	*Loso*	*Sa*	*Iba*-*
		Cɛbola	*Lolo*		*Ogbe*		*Egbo*

Note: * These DU combinations are extremely dangerous. They presage imminent misfortune. The following DU are also considered dangerous:
Cɛ (Y = 5), *Fu* (Y = 10), *Jila* (Y = 12), and *Iba-Egbo*, the ineffable Cɛ-*Fu* (Y = 15).

The following values are missing from the above table: Y = 0, 1, 16. The diviners we interviewed considered them so dangerous they refused to give us their names. If in the course of their work, they happen to come up with one of these combinations in a throw, they hastily leave the place where the consultation was held, and proceed to conduct a series of sacrifices (ADRA) to ward off the threat of misfortune.

Relevant Probability Field

Y stands for the random variable equivalent to the number of open cowries in the throw. For any given cowry, the total number of possibilities is two: **open, closed.**

$$\Omega = \{\varphi, \pi\}, P(\varphi) = P(\pi) = 1/2$$

Given the form of the cowries used, a hypothesis of even probabilities is a matter of course, assuming, naturally, that there is no external force directing the cowries.

Results

In divination based on cowry throws, the random variable Y equivalent to the number of open cowries is distributed according to Bernouilli's Law of Parameters n = 16 p = 1/2

$$P(Y{=}k) = C^k_{16}\,(1/2)^k(1/2)^{16-k} = C^k_{16}\,(1/2)^{16} = C^k_{16} / 2^{16}$$

The probability of DU combinations is proportional to the binomial coefficients.

A look at the Pascal Triangle of Binomial Coefficients shows a symmetrical pattern structured around a central space between Y = 8 and Y = 9. Plotted along a graph, this produces a modest Gauss bell.

Comments on Figure 4

A look at the symmetrical form of the Pascal Triangle shows that Prob(*Abla*) = Prob(*Fu*), Prob(Cɛ) = Prob(*Wlin*), and Prob(*Loso*) = Prob(*Jila*). In the light of the above, it is rather surprising that the DU combination called *Jila* is reputed to be dangerous, while *Loso* is not, even though it occurs with the same probability. The same is true of *Fu* and *Abla, Wlin* and Cɛ.

Probability calculations indicate that if two events have the same probability, they have identical chances of occurring in the course of any experiment. However, when I explained my findings to several diviners, they informed me that *Jila* and *Loso* were both controlled by the same divinity, and that this supernatural force could make either combination appear at will, depending on the message it wanted to convey.

Figure 4: Graph of Probabilities

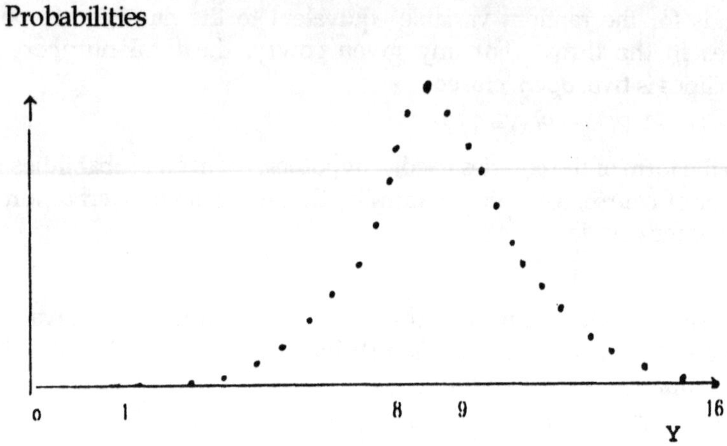

An incidental fact: it is quite remarkable that the combinations considered to be dangerous occur with very low probabilities. For instance, the Ineffable Combinations present the following probabilities:

$P(Y=16) = P(Y=0) = 1/2^{16}$, an extremely low probability,: 0.0000153

$P(Y=1) = P(Y=15) = 16/2^{16} = 1/2^{12} = 0.000244$.

Divination Based on the Use of Beads (*Agunmagã Ki-Kã*)

In our traditional society, people confronted with the unknown and the unknowable rely on this form of Fâ divination in their desire to understand, obtain guidance, find principles on which to base their actions, or seek a way out of drought, famine, epidemics and any other misfortunes besetting the community. Misfortunes that drive people to consult the Bokono or diviner are of many types. They include witchcraft, illness, work-related problems, failure, etc.

The Diviner's Equipment

Various objects are used to structure the course of the divining process: çowries represent wealth; adji-kwi seeds are used to represented persons; pieces of broken calabash stand for poverty, loss of money, an accident or some imminent danger. A small bone serves as a juju fetish, a maize cob for a broken taboo, famine, etc.

These are objects the diviners use to probe divine intentions. We shall not tarry over them here, but move instead directly to a consideration of the diviner's main instrument, the string of beads known as the AGUNMAGA or KPLE. The string is no more than a metre long, and comprises eight beads arranged in two groups of four each, connected by a chain or a string of beads. The eight main items are identical halves of nuts known here as ASRO-KWI (monkey mango; botanical name: *Irvingia Barteri*).

Modus Operandi

The diviner raises the beads in his/her right hand, then grasps the string in his left hand, thus making two parallel halves. After a couple of swings, he throws the string of beads onto a flat surface, which might be the floor. The halves fall in various positions, some open, some closed. The two parts of the string are given gender identifications. The section with a bead is known as male, and is invariably placed to the right of the diviner. Fâ patterns are read from right to left.

The Fâ Graphic Code

Patterns resulting from throws are recorded according to the following conventional rules:

a) each closed half-cowry is represented by two conventional lines: II;

b) each open half-cowry is represented by a single line: I.

The total figure is drawn up in two parallel vertical columns of single and double lines according to the positions taken by the cowry halves. The recording system is called the FA-DU, and it is used both to write down and to facilitate the reading of Fâ patterns. FA-DU writing goes from right to left and from top to bottom, in two columns. It is read from right to left, as in Arabic.

Definition

Let us call each conventional FA-DU sign a mother-sign. The system uses a set of elements, K, each containing 4 items from a set J = {I, II}. As a result, the number of mother-signs equals the cardinal numbers $(J)^K$.

Proposition

There are $2^4 = 16$ geomantic mother-signs in the Fâ corpus.

A Glossary of Geomantic Signs in the Fâ Corpus

The 16 geomantic signs are classified under the following names:

1st sign	2nd sign	3rd sign	4th sign
I	II	II	I
I	II	I	II
I	II	I	II
I	II	II	I
Gbe	*Yɛku*	*Woli*	*DI*
5th sign	**6th sign**	**7th sign**	**8th sign**
I	II	I	II
I	II	II	II
II	I	II	II
II	I	II	I
Loso	*Wlin*	*Abla*	*Aklã*
9th sign	**10th sign**	**11th sign**	**12th sign**
I	II	II	II
I	I	I	II
I	I	II	I
II	I	II	II
Guda	*Sa*	*Ka*	*Trukpin*
13th sign	**14th sign**	**15th sign**	**16th sign**
I	I	I	II
II	I	II	I
I	II	I	II
I	I	II	I
Tula	*Lete*	Cɛ	*Fu*

Domains of Geomantic Succession

Let us recall that each item of FA-DU comprises two geomantic signs.

Definition

In FA-DU terms, the right hand column, a product of the male branch of the string of diviner's beads, is known as a mother-sign in Fâ geomancy. The left hand column is known as a domain of FA-DU geomantic succession. The rule is that each geomantic sign originates in a geomantic domain or house. It is an unfortunate and confusing circumstance that the domain and the sign bear the same name.

Thus, there are 16 geomantic domains: *Gbe*, *Yɛku* and *Fu*, respectively the 1st, 2nd ... and 1-7th geomantic domain.

Conventional Descriptions

The FA-DU comprises coupled signs. If, therefore, I obtain the two signs (A,B), the conventional statement is that B has entered the domain A.

Explanation

Each sign has a specific meaning, symbols and inscriptions. All these, however, are influenced by the domain or house through which the sign happens to be passing. Thus, (A,A) means that A is in its original celestial domain. The name for this is DU-GA, an alternate form being DU-MEJI. Whenever a sign is in its original domain, it is in the ascendant, with its dignity and power at peak levels. It can therefore release and express the totality of beneficial or baneful natural influence in its power. The DU-GA are listed as follows:

Gbe-Meji	*Yɛku-Meji*	*Woli-Meji*	*Fu-Meji*
I I	II II	II II	II II
I I	II II	I I	I I
I I	II II	I I	II II
I I	II II	II II	I I

The 16 geomantic signs transiting through the 16 geomantic domains provide a basis for various interpretations given by expert Fâ diviners. The most gifted initiates make the best diviners. The reason is that it takes a highly retentive memory to register all the symbols, inscriptions and meanings of the entire set of FA-DU.

Proposition

The FA geomantic corpus contains no more and no less than 16 x 16 = 256 FA-DU.

Each sign can transit through 16 geomantic domains. This can be demonstrated by treating a FA-DU as the interaction of a set E containing 8 items with another set J = I, II . The total number of interactions is $\text{Cardinal (J)}^{\text{Cardinal (E)}} = 2^8 = 256$.

Consulting the FA Oracle

Oracular pronouncements are obtained from the interpretation of patterns occurring after three consecutive throws of the FA string of diviner's beads.

The first is the main throw. It is the FA-DU obtained after this throw that completely determines the seeker's quest. From the first throw, the diviner already has all items necessary for an interpretation. Within the worldview of the Bokono or diviner, each of the 256 FA-DU is a divine messenger. Each of them incorporates good and evil qualities simultaneously. They are mischievous, volatile, temperamental, violent and sometimes downright bloody. Accordingly, each FA-DU occasions good luck as well as bad. Hence the diviner's request to know, after each FA-DU, whether to emphasize lucky (*Fâ ivo*) or unlucky (*Fâ win vo*) interpretations. Lucky and unlucky verdicts are the result of a double consultation. The diviner places a cowry to his right, an *adji-kwi* to his left.

The second throw is directed towards the cowries. The third throw is directed towards the *adji-kwi*. For the last two throws, only the right hand section of the diviner's string of beads, the male section, is taken into consideration. The procedure assigns one geomantic sign to the cowries, another to the adji-kwi seed. Which is the stronger sign? Any given sign A is stronger than a sign B if, in the glossary of signs, A comes before B in the order of precedence. And the stronger sign is the one selected.

a) If the item picked up is the cowry, then the verdict of the FA-DU is negative (*Fâ win vo*). The diviner then concentrates on an interpretation of threatening implications of the symbols, inscriptions and mottoes of the FA-DU resulting from the first throw.

b) If the item picked up is the *adji-kwi* seed, then the FA-DU is favourable. The seeker's quest will be fruitful. The diviner concentrates on positive interpretations of the FA-DU symbols, inscriptions, etc. There is no established ranking of FA interpreters, so each diviner interprets the signs to the best of his individual ability and mnemonic powers. But no human memory is capacious enough to contain all the knowledge of the FA corpus.

Computers are certain to come in as an invaluable resource. For the time being, however, even when comparing the potency of two signs, some groups of diviners consider the pairs *Woli + Di, Cɛ + Fu, Yɛku* and *Gbe* as null. In such circumstances, the diviner considers the 2nd and 3rd throws as void, and proceeds to a 4th and 5th throw on which to base a comparison, etc.

Examples of Messages: *Gbe-Meji*

- *Ali nô Sun do Aklasu Aganuga do Felixo*: The road is never traced out for the Great Vulture on the way to Ife (Felixo = the road of life, identical with the road of death).
- *Aklasu Aganuga wɛ je nu kuku ji bo do emije Jogbe*: It is evil for one diseased.
- *Loko Kujo Ava Kudjo*: The iroko tree grows old; so does the lliana (Long life assured, provided health is good).
- *Naki ko gbã nô da Awinya Gédigbaja*: (Hard to cook).
- *So nô jɛ Gidi kpaa-hun do Solome*: Lightning does not strike the guinea pig in the cave (In the teeth of storm and threat, we shall live).
- *Sodokpa jo ma mu*: The wind does not break down the stone wall.
- The egg does not fight the ironstone.

Calculating Probabilities

Ruling Hypotheses Assuming Even Chances of Occurrence

The two halves are perfectly identical and balanced.

The two halves fall independently of each other.

No external force influences patterns resulting from successive throws.

Under these conditions, the probability of each FA-DU occurring is 1/256.

Evaluating the Probability of FA-Ivo Occurring

Prob (Favourable/*Gbe*) = 0 Prob (Unfavourable/*Gbe*) = 1
Prob (Favourable/*Yɛku*) = 0 Prob(Unfavourable/*Yɛku*) = 1
(according to leading diviners)
Prob(Favourable/*Woli*) =2/16=1/8 Prob (Unfavourable/*Woli*) = 7/8
Prob (Favourable/*Di*) = 1/2 Prob (Unfavourable/*Di*) =1/2
Prob(Favourable/*Loso*) = 4/16 = 1/4 Prob (Unfavourable/*Loso*) =3/4
Prob (Favourable/*Wlin*) = 5/16 Prob (Unfavourable/*Wlin*) = 11/16
Prob(Favourable/*Abla*) = 6/18 =2/8 Prob (Unfavourable/*Abla*) = 5/8
Prob(Favourable/*Akla*) = 7/16 Prob (Unfavourable/*Akla*) =9/16
Prob(Favourable/*Guda*) = 8/16 = 1/2 Prob (Unfavourable/*Guda*) =1/2

Concordant Consultations

Let us calculate the probability of two seekers at least out of an array of n seekers, each seeking answers to a different problem, obtaining an identical FA-DU verdict.

In case of Event A, at least 2 seekers get the same FA-DU verdict. In the contrary case, which we shall call A, 'all seekers obtain different FA-DU verdicts.'

$$P(\tilde{A}) = \frac{225 \ x \ 254 \ x \ 253 \ x \ \ldots \ x \ 256 - n + 1}{256}$$

$$P(\tilde{A}) = 1 - P(\tilde{A})$$

For n = 18, we get $P(\tilde{A}) = 0.50425...$ $P(\tilde{A}) = 0.49575$.

Out of a sample of 18 persons, there is a 50% chance that at least two persons will obtain the same FA-DU verdict.

For n = 50, we get $P(\tilde{A}) = 0.00047...$ $P(\tilde{A}) = 0.99953...$

Let us now suppose that $P(\tilde{A}) \simeq 1$. Thus, for a sample of 50 seekers, two persons at least obtain the same FA-DU verdict, even if they consulted the FA about different problems. How, in such a case, does the diviner arrive at specific verdicts? He differentiates between the different problems by using a set of questions.

The Questionnaire

The diviner asks a series of short questions requiring simple Yes or No answers. We have already seen how he uses the diviner's string of beads to obtain answers. Here we come up against a problem in information theory, which is a branch of probability theory. Information theory posits that there are systematic methods for setting up questions in such a way as to ensure that after a number of questions not exceeding a maximum M, the correct answer invariably comes up. The smallest possible number M is called the quantity of information, and it would be interesting to find out which particular methods guarantee it.

Let us recapitulate a theorem in information theory: Given a set of events n all of which have the same probability of occurring, if the goal is to isolate one particular event, then the quantity of information in this problem is $q = \log_2 n$ (logarithm of n on a base of 2).

Here, in consultations where the FA-DU verdict is unfavourable, the diviner automatically accepts the value q = 5. In effect, he poses the question in the following form: *oku, azô, oxuɛ, afo, vodun*. Translation: 'Is this verdict about death, illness, litigation, frustration, or a hex?'

Since $n = 2^q$, the outcome here will be n = 32.

Let us conclude that implicitly, the diviner hypothesizes that in real life, 32 chance events regulate the occurrence of mishaps in human existence. On the theoretical level we are not able to identify these events precisely, the reason being that the technique of most contemporary diviners is typically empirical. Mathematical calculations of expectations should produce enlightening findings.

Let us define the mathematical expectation of an oracle as the product of its utility multiplied by the probability of its occurrence. The point is that the greater the yield from a particular chance event, and the higher the probability of its occurrence, the greater the interest invested in it. Thus, E(*Gbe*) = 1/256 x Gain.

Here, the mathematical expectation is not the same as the Gain. That is the amount to be paid to any person who agrees to bear in place of and on behalf of the principal seeker the impact of the misfortune predicted by the oracle. That is the reason why the diviner takes sacrificial offerings from the seeker, keeping part and placing the remainder at some cross-roads, the expectation being that any animal or person passing that way or takes the offerings will carry away the impending evil. Sometimes, in a ritual of substitution, the diviner sacrifices animals. In such cases the mathematical expectation of the oracle is the quotient of the sacrifice prescribed divided by 256.

$$E = \frac{Sacrifice}{256}$$

This ratio is comparable with the seeker's expectation of gain in case of a successful prediction resulting in the achievement of the predictions in question.

This simple calculation of E enables a seeker to know if he or she is going to win or lose by meeting the stipulations of the Bokonô or diviner. We can therefore easily understand the thinking of Beninois when dealing with life-threatening situations. Life is priceless. The cost of its preservation, if such a price is possible, is always higher than the ratio E, which is invariably a finite quantity.

The question arises as to whether the Bokonô can successfully execute a substitution if he conforms to the stipulations of the oracle. A scientific answer to this question would have to be based on the following calculations:

a) The probability of an individual dying once he knows that the FA has predicted his death;

b) The probability of an individual remaining alive knowing that the FA has predicted his death.

c) The probability of an individual dying knowing that the FA has predicted his survival.

All the above probabilities would have to be calculated for each hypothetical condition, viz.:

a) The individual has performed the sacrifices prescribed by the FA;

b) The individual has not performed the sacrifices prescribed by the FA.

This work can only be done within the context of a programme of statistical data analysis conducted in a multidisciplinary framework, with the participation of sociologists, historians, medical doctors, physicists, mathematicians and computer experts, etc. Such a project would take substantial funding, and is therefore beyond the reach of any researcher working in isolation.

In conclusion, let us observe that in the absence of a comprehensive data bank within an efficient scientific establishment ensuring appropriate guidelines to be followed in dealing with unknown factors considered to be unknowable given the current state of human knowledge, FA divination in this sub-region is bound to remain a method for the assessment and appreciation of chance. In that capacity, it will continue for a long time to resist the stigma imposed on all local beliefs of the black world by the imported tradition of evolution.

Notes

1. Mathematical analysis, for example, starts with a set of natural integers, N, to which cardinal numbers are added or subtracted in simpler cases. The result is a set of relative integers, Z. Through multiplication and division a set of rational numbers, Q, is obtained. This yields a set of real numbers, R, which in turn develops into a set of imaginary numbers, C. Geometry, beginning with points on a straight line, bends them into polygonal shapes and curves, shifts, deforms and transforms them by transferring, rotating, assimilating them.
2. The 16 Fâ combinations are classified according to an order universally accepted by practitioners.

6

Epistemological Reflections on Hausa Zoological Names

Jean-Dominique Penel

The aim of this chapter is to stimulate epistemological thinking about endogenous knowledge in Niger. The production of knowledge and its subsequent systematization into scientific learning comprise a major epistemological issue on a world scale. Yet the issue is seldom given adequate attention in Africa. The usual approach is to make vague pronouncements on folk knowledge. Alternatively, the issue is turned into a Manichean dilemma, and antithetical choices are crudely made, with those asserting that 'endogenous knowledge is altogether false and unscientific' opposing those who argue that 'endogenous knowledge is thoroughly scientific'. Both attitudes are based on misperceptions of endogenous knowledge, its richness and diversity, its positive and negative aspects. Furthermore, they help maintain the erroneous view according to which science is some ready-made commodity produced entirely outside Africa, and the equally wrong-headed notion that science is a form of production no different from other types of knowledge.

The only productive way out of this impasse lies in the serious examination of local knowledge, its identification, explanation and evaluation. The epistemological approach necessarily implies an evaluative outcome, the reason being that knowledge identified is assessed according to a given standard. That implies the making of judgements. The standards applied, being themselves determined by the state of the art in the sciences, are in the very nature of things subject to continuous change.

In order to embark on an applied epistemological study of traditional knowledge in Niger, the most reasonable approach is to select a limited sector within the corpus of knowledge and then to make a precise, thorough study of it within a well defined cultural environment. For every language is endowed with specific structures, and each group evolves within its own peculiar environment, engendering its own specific conceptions. It is therefore impossible, *a priori*, to hypothesize that all aspects of traditional knowledge in Niger covering fauna, flora, pharmaceutical resources, iron-smelting, metallurgy, etc. fit into a unified organizational and constitutional structure. Common characteristics may well exist, but they are likely to become evident only after a comparative analysis of sectorial studies severally conducted within clearly defined cultural limits.

For hitherto, we have fallen too readily for the lure of grand, general statements encompassing all Africa, while philosophic rhetoric has been excessively complaisant in its lyrical and artificial elucubrations on 'African man', 'African knowledge', 'African religious feeling', etc. The time has come to steer clear of such pitfalls. Hence our conscious decision in this chapter to stick to a carefully traced out field, that of zoological names within a specific social group, the Hausas of Niger. We shall be addressing a central epistemological issue: *how to situate Hausa zoological names in relation to the accepted scientific nomenclature in zoology?*

The findings presented in this chapter are not directly derived from field work. They are instead a distillation from previous findings published by experts in the field. Needless to say, there is a risk of error in all work of this nature. The risk is worth running, inevitable as it is, because it would be impractical for a lone specialist in the theory of knowledge to undertake a study of all languages spoken in Niger in addition to drawing up an inventory of all knowledge produced in various fields in each language. In specific cases, then, we are quite aware that we may make mistakes. But reliance on the findings of other specialists is an indispensable aspect of scholarly research. Failing such judicious trust, one is likely to get bogged down in paranoid mistrust, or to sink complacently into sheer lethargy.

The works in linguistics and ethno-zoology on which this study is based were written by authors with definite viewpoints related to their disciplines. Here we shall put forward a different interpretation of the same material, based on a perspective rooted in Epistemology, the philosophy of knowledge. Before we embark on this epistemological analysis. however we cannot avoid making certain preliminary observations on Hausa zoological names as related to the scientific method of zoological nomenclature.

Hausa Zoological Names and Scientific Zoological Nomenclature

General Problems Related to Hausa Zoological Names

According to the published findings of specialists in the field, researchers collecting information on zoological names are faced with the following obstacles. First, there are numerous variations in dialects. Thus, the locust *Zonocernus valetatus* is known as *adindima* in Gidan Magagi, *bwaarat tumfafiya* in Katsena, and *gam* in Kano. Second, names may change from one group of speakers to the other within the same society. Thus, the same locust that is called *adindima* by adults is also called *Kabar mazaa daddahee* by little girls in the same village. Third, animals are called by their names, but in addition they are given what Anne Levy-Luxereau has termed 'epithets'. Thus the scaly ant-eater, known as *dan kunya,* is also called by the epithet *kwaaran kurmi,* which means 'forest animal'. Epithets are sometimes given at the same time as the name, sometimes separately. This may lead to the supposition that the animal has two names, or that there are two different animals. To obviate such confusion in this chapter, whenever we use an epithet, we shall mark it by adding an (E) in parentheses immediately after it. Fourth, a single name might be used for different but closely related animals. Thus the name *wukas sarkis* is used for nearly ten related species of locusts. Similarly, both the wart hog and the water hog are often called by the same name: *aladen daaji*. Fifth, there are a few animals which, even though they inhabit the Hausa environment, have remained unnamed. And finally, from a linguistic viewpoint, zoological names might be classified either as randomly given or as consciously determined, in the sense established by Saussure. The following analysis will be based primarily on consciously determined' names.

We shall also distinguish between simple, iterative and composite names: Zaaki or lion is a simple name; Tawtaw or spider is an iterative name. Iterative terms are a highly regular feature of the Hausa language, and C. Gouffe, in his study on the topic, lists five types of iteration. In this chapter we shall put simple and iterative terms in a single category.

Karan dawaki (literally, cock of horses) is a composite name. It stands for the black-headed ring bird.

Scientific Names

The modern scientific system of zoological and botanical names was developed by the eighteenth century Swedish scientist Carolus Linnaeus (1707-1778). In the system, each name is made up of two parts, both in Latin. The first is the genus name, the second the species name. Hence the name for the horse is *Equus caballus*, while that of the ass is *Equus asinus*. The first term, common to both, indicates that the species *caballus* and the species asinus both belong to the same genus, *Equus*. Within the system it is possible to indicate the existence of a sub-species or variety. For instance, *Equus asinus africanus* refers to an African variety of ass.

This procedure implies a built-in classificatory system. The names for the horse and the ass have a common element (*Equus*), to which a differentiating element (*caballus* or *asinus*) gets attached. This type of nomenclature is part of a general classificatory system built on the assumption that every individual creature in the animal world has its own particular place within a hierarchical scheme comprising interlocking categories whose main components, read from the highest to the lowest, are as follows: kingdom, branch, class, phylum, order, family, genus, species and variety. A few categories also have multiple forms and multiple sub-categories. For example, there may be a super-class, a class, a sub-class and an infra-class, and families and orders may have similar subdivisions.

Each of these categories has to be defined according to precise criteria. In his day, the naturalist Linnaeus had defined such a set of classificatory criteria. Subsequently, other experts concluded that his criteria were 'artificial'. They therefore substituted other criteria, considered more 'natural', for them. To this day zoologists are far from unanimous as to the correct classification of individual animals. They do agree, however, on the overall frame established by Linnaeus. It has therefore been retained, with one modification: to the genus and species names, it has become standard practice to add the proper name of the person who identified the plant or animal, along with the date of identification. Thus, *Orycteropus-afer* (Pallas 1766) means that the genus is *Orycteropus*, that the species is *Afer*, that the animal was identified by Pallas, and that the date was 1766. The animal concerned here is the ground hog, known as *dagbli* in Hausa. To take another example, the manatee, known as ayau in Hausa, is known as *Trichechus senegalensis* (Link 1795). This means that it belongs to the genus *Trichechus*, that its species is *Senegalensis*, and that it was first identified by Link in 1795.

This chapter focuses specifically on the naming system using simple, ad hoc classificatory procedures. We shall not be discussing the general, interlocking system of scientific nomenclature.

Epistemological Considerations

To the question: 'By what means do the Hausa arrive at their knowledge of the animal world?' the answer is doubtless: 'through sense impressions'. Hence the frequent description of the resulting knowledge as empirical. However, it is important to bear in mind the following. First, it needs to be clearly understood that the senses are important instruments in the process of the acquisition of knowledge, and that the observations they make possible are of great value. Second, it should not be forgotten that knowledge is not a product of the senses alone, and that there are other factors at work. These factors include language, which comes with its own structures and intellectual processes such as classificatory procedures based on local ideological concepts, interacting with observation in such a way as to modify or attenuate the resulting findings.

We are dealing, in other words, with a complex reality touching on the history of philosophy, where a rationalist tradition has rather hastily discounted the role of the senses, conferring pejorative connotations on the label of empiricism. In this chapter, we shall use the term 'empirical' to denote the positive and maximal use of sense organs for the purpose of gaining knowledge. By this we do not imply that human beings are simple receptacles for sense impressions, mere passive recorders of sensations. We are far indeed from being just that.

We shall begin with Hausa zoological names as our reference point. After a brief explanation clarifying the fact that all five senses are indicated by name in the nomenclature under study, we shall proceed to a study of observations within the animal kingdom. Second, we shall see how the social life of human beings is projected onto the animal kingdom. Last, we shall look at the way the classificatory processes function. For every one of these three aspects, in keeping with our stated epistemological approach, we shall offer an evaluation.

Instruments of Observation

The senses are organs of the human body available to each individual to provide information on the environment. A study of Hausa zoological names reveals that in their composition, all the senses are in fact used.

a) The sense of sight is the key faculty, and it underlies most of the names studied. It is indispensable in the determination of those names expressing colour, form, etc. On its usefulness there is no need to expatiate. The sense of sight is dominant. That in no way means a total eclipse of the other senses.

b) The sense of hearing: Several names bear the imprint of auditory impressions. For instance:

- Some birds' names are onomatopoeic sounds supposed to reproduce their songs or cries. Thus, the domestic duck is called *agwaagwaa;* the grey touraco is known as *allukuku;* roosters are known as *hututuu,* and the whistling swan is named *kirinjridiya.*
- Certain insects are similarly named. For example, crickets are called *yaraa dada,* dada being an ideophone expressing the sound they make.
- Some names, while not intended to reproduce animal cries or songs precisely, yet manage to suggest sounds. Thus, one type of insect (anthia) is known as *matuusiyao* (the farter); the black-headed tchaya is known as *suudoo,* meaning the talkative one; and the oryx, whose principal name is *walwaaji,* has an epithetical appellation (E): *mais kuukan daadli,* meaning 'the sweet-voiced oryx'.

c) The sense of smell. Some animals are named after olfactory peculiarities. Thus the musk-rat is called *mazuurun jibdas,* meaning musky cat. And the epithet given the skunk, known mainly as buddari, is bunsurun mal waarii, literally, the foul smelling goat. Considering that goats have a reputation for smelling awful even under normal circumstances, this is unflattering.

d) The sense of touch: There is a an ant (*Hymenoptera*) which, however hard it gets hit, is neither crushed nor killed as long as it is in the sand. The name given to it is *Saa kuli*: absorber of blows.

e) The sense of taste: An insect which lives on tender millet grain is called *saa gardi*, meaning: drinker of pleasant juice. Here the human taste for millet is projected on the insect. Indeed, all classifications based on what is edible or potable bring the sense of taste into play.

The sense of sight may well be dominant, but other senses are also active, and Hausa zoological names make explicit references to them. Let us now move on to a consideration of the information involving the use of the five senses.

Observed Characteristics

In normal zoological practice, criteria used for descriptions and classifications are based principally on observations of the animals' morphology (shape and form) ethology (behaviour) and ecology (environment). Hausa zoological names also contain numerous instances of this type of observation.

Morphology and Behaviour

The following is a list of morphological data encapsulated in Hausa zoological names.

General Size and Form

Examples of names here are: *Kwaama faara*, meaning 'A grasshopper would have been better', refers to a tiny bird; *Wukas sarkis*, meaning 'The chief's knife' refers to a long and slim locust; *Yat tandu*, meaning 'The one shaped like a leather skin bag', name of a type of locust; *Dam mazari*, meaning 'little bobbin', refers to a lizard of that shape.

Outstanding Morphological Traits

Examples are: *Kazaazao*, meaning a hump, this is the name of a locust with a hump-like growth on its head, also called *May dooka*, meaning 'One from the hump'; *Ma tukka*, meaning 'the one with a crest', name of the crested skylark; *Buurah hillaani*, meaning 'the Fulani's staff', refers to a fish with an extended snout; *Dan may kunnee*, meaning 'the little one with ears', refers to the hare; *Badbaa da jukaa*, meaning 'the one with the bag', refers to the marabout bird; *May karii*, meaning 'the one who has a needle', name of the scorpion; *Takwaan akuya,* meaning 'the she-goat's heel'. Alternatively, *Kohwa akuya,* meaning 'the she-goat's hoof'. Refers to a locust with an extremely slender femur.

Colour

Several colours are used to form zoological names.

Red is used in: *Jan na suuri,* the red cobra; *Jam baaka,* (red beak): a bird; *Jam biri,* the red monkey and *Jan gaba,* red throat (parrot).

Black is used, as in *Bakin maciiji,* the black snake; *Bakin Kurungugu,* the black kurungugu fish; and *Bakin kiihi,* the black kiihi fish.

White is used, as in *Hwarak karaayaa,* the white karaayaa fish; *Hwaraz zarbe,* the white heron; *Hwarin ageleuuluu,* the white carrion crow; *Hwarin koomoo,* the white vulture; *Hwarin maciiji,* the white serpent; and *Hwarin maiki,* the white bearded vulture.

Green and blue are used, as in *Yas suuni,* the blue bird (Suuni means indigo dye); *Dangae ciyaawa,* green herb, a locust; *Sanwaako,* Blue-green (bird); and *Sanwaakiyao,* the green one (green mamba).

Cries and Sounds

Under this heading come the names cited earlier in the passage on the sense of hearing.

Behaviour

Several examples can be found under this heading, such as *Shaa kymbaabii,* shell eater, name of the wader bird, which lives along waterways; *Tabaa ni ka mutu;* meaning 'Touch me, I die', name of a beetle with a reflex reaction that immobilizes it when touched; and *Karkeeci,* name given to the hyena on account of its ability to tear at prey (keet).

Names Based on Products Derived from Animals

Examples are: *Kujen zumaa,* the milk fly. Name of the bee; and *Mazuurun jibdaa,* musky cat; the civet cat.

Names Based on Observations of Animal Habitats

Very often, animal names derive from places. These may be the animals' habitats, their feeding places, or even places where they might most easily be observed. The following observations are arranged by thematic category.

Natural Environments and Habitats

Water is used in, for example *Karen ruwa,* water dog, the otter; *Kunbaamar ruwa,* water scorpion, water bug; *Kwaaron ruwa,* water beast, crocodile; *Kadangaren ruwa,* water lizard, crocodile; *Raagon ruwa,* water elephant, hippopotamus; and *Giwar ruwa,* water fowl.

Rocks and stones are used, for example *Raagon duuci,* buck of the rocks, wild sheep; *Kaazaa duuci,* rock fowl; *Gada duuci,* rock gadar, cuttlefish; and *Reeman duuci,* rock hyrax.

Bushes and miscellaneous natural habitats are used, as in *Aladen daaji,* bush pig; *Raakumin daaji,* bush camel, giraffe; *Jaabak koogo,* bush bird, shrew; *Bikan kurmi,* forest baboo; *Gadar kurmi,* forest gadar, cuttlefish; *Kiwaaran kurmi* (E) forest animal, pangolin; and *Kaazag geezaa,* bush fowl, rock fowl.

Plants

Examples here are: *Ek kalgo,* kalgo-eating locust; *Faarat tumfaafiyaa,* locust feeding on the clotropis praera; *Kunsun kyamroo,* water rat; *Taaka bado,* 'One who walks on the water lily', the jacana bird; *Shan kawci,* loranthus drinker, the souimanga bird; and *Dan giiwag gambaa,* son of the elephant, son of the gamba plant; the hare.

Animals

Some names are derived from the fact that certain animals live close to others. Examples are: *Na suuri,* of the anthill, the cobra; and *Kujen saanuu,* cattle fly.

Technical Objects, Human-Developed Environments

Examples are: *Eg gidaa* (E), bird of the enclosure, sparrow; *Gurgura tabaara,* the pestle cleaner, sparrow; *Yag gatan turmi,* the bird which haunts the base of the mortar, sparrow; *Taa rumbuno,* the one of the millet granary, grasshopper; *Jeemaagen riijiyaa,* the well-dwelling bat; and *Ceera may gooma* (E), the field fennec, jerboa.

Names Derived from Observations of Time

Observations in the time class are much less frequent. Nevertheless, a few were identified: *Jab bazara,* the one of the period before the first rains, the black miro; *Baa kunkan hanci,* the one who makes people sob in the morning, a serpent; *Dan mii kwaanaa ka baa ni,* son of what will sleep give me? name of a night mouse; and *A ci banaa a mutu baddii;* one eats this year, dies next year, name of a locust.

Even if Hausa zoological names are not all based on such observations, it has to be agreed that on the whole these names and the information contained in them are positive in nature. A number of them are problematic, and they include the names of the giraffe, the otter and the fish named the water buck. But apart from those, Hausa zoological names as a rule contain information potentially useful to zoology in general, and could fit into the overall system.

Incidentally, Latinate scientific names often make use of identification procedures similar to those used in Hausa zoological nomenclature.

Outstanding Morphological Characteristics

The type of hedge-hog known as *Buushiyaa* in Hausa, is in Latin terminology called Alterix albiventris. The Latin word *albiventris* means white-bellied.

The scientific name of the Basiya, a type of ourebie, is *Ourebia nigri caudato*. The last two words in Latin mean black-tailed. The scientific name of the Laahwayaa, a type of nightjar, is *Manodi terys longipennis*. Longipennis means long-feathered.

Occasionally, indeed, the Latinate name corresponds exactly to the Hausa name, as in *Bakin maciiji,* the Hausa name for the cobra, which corresponds to the scientific Nigriocolis, the prefix nigri- meaning black, like bakin in Hausa; *Bakin kurungugu*, a black fish, is known scientifically as *Bagrus docma nigri,* here again, nigri in Latin corresponds to bakin in Hausa and *Hwaraz zarbe,* the white heron, is scientifically known as *Egretta alba,* in this case, the Latin alba, like the Hausa hwara, means white.

Frequent use is also made of place names, as in Kunkun tumii, the Hausa name for the swamp mongoose, which has a Latin counterpart, Atilax paludirsus, the final term here being derived from the Latin paludes, meaning swamp; and Beeram bisa, the galago, is scientifically known as Galago Senegalensis, the Senegalese galago.

As was the case with names derived from morphological features, certain Hausa names derived from animal habitats have precise counterparts in Latinate scientific nomenclature: Haazad duuci, the rock fowl, is scientifically known as Ptilopachya petrosus, here the Hausa ci and the Latin petrosus both refer to rocks.

From the scientific point of view, the factor that makes modern scientific zoological terminology different from the Hausa system is the joint identification of genus and species. Let us take the example of mongooses. In their scientific designation, the first element is the genus name, Herpestes, followed by species names: Herpestes *ichneumon*, Herpestes *fureteus*, (*saaraa* in Hausa), Herpestes *sanguineus*, meaning 'blood-coloured Hepestes', (*mugulmugula* in Hausa), Herpestes pulverulentus, the dusty Herpestes, Herpestes *paludinosus*, the swamp Herpestes, known in Hausa as *Kunkuruu tumii*.

There are other types of mongoose: *bdeogale crassicauda* (bushy tailed; *bdeogale nigripes*, (black-footed); *ichneumia albicauda*, the white-tailed ichneumia, known in Hausa as *tunkuu*.

Epistemological studies may reveal a number of inadequacies, an example being the lack of any connection in Hausa zoological nomenclature between genus and species. A further example is the absence of standard criteria for identifying and classifying animals. But it also has to be recognized that even if Hausa nomenclature is not, strictly speaking, 'scientific', it does present a number of positive characteristics in the wide range of observations on which it is based.

The Projection of Human Social Realities Onto the Animal World

It has been observed that names given to certain animals are based less on straightforward observation of the animals themselves than on a human social conception projected onto the animal environment. The following are a few illustrations.

Animal Names Derived from Human Kinship Terms

Terms describing human social kin relationships are frequently used in animal names. The following are selected examples.

Dan, meaning 'son of': *dan dumi*, fish; dan gari, fish; *dan raguwa*, rooster; *dan gwadarma*, locust; *dan saa raanii*, secretary bird; *dan mazari*, lizard; *dan jaki*, locust; *dan giwang gambaa*, hare; *dan mii kwaanaa ka baa ni*, mouse; and *dan kunyu*, scaly ant-eater.

Mijin, meaning husband: *mijin-kunaamaa*, literally, the scorpion's husband, the galeod.

Maata, meaning wife: *maatak kwaado*, the frog's wife, a locust; *maatan maarai*, the weaverbird's wife, the wagtail.

Uwar, meaning mother: *uwajiyajiya*, yesterday's mother, a bird.

The term *uwa* often occurs in epithets such as *baunaa, uwarshaanu* (E), the buffalo, mother of cattle; *dagee, uwar hwada* (E), mother of quarrels, the badger; *uwar ruwa* (E), mother of meat, the elephant; *gwanmbazaa, uwal yaayaa, me ciki akan ciki* (E), mother of children, (literally, 'the child you carry is already with child', a reference to the animal's reputation as a prolific breeder.

The Vocabulary of Social Relations

Typically human social functions are liberally projected onto animals, some of them being named after social personalities, especially religious dignitaries. Examples are as follow.

Sarkin, meaning chief: *wukar sarkin*, the chief's knife, the locust; *hiri, sarkin banaa* (E), chief of chaos, the monkey; *damoo, sarkin hakurii* (E), master of patience, the monitor lizard; *zaaki, sarkin daaji* (E), lord of the bush, the lion.

Maalam, meaning the Muslim teacher: *maalam buude littaafi*, 'Maalam who works on the book', the butterfly; *maalamin dawa* (E), maalam of the bush, the jackal; *gahiyaa ta maalam* (E), the maalam's rat; *am hudu hudu na maalam*, the Maalam's crest, a bird.

Allah, God: *Baywa Allaa*, slave of God, the swift; *giwa, likwan allaa* (E) power of God, the elephant; *gyaadoo, raagon allaa* (E), God's ram, the wart hog; *kuuraa, dabbar allaa* (E), God's animal, the hyena.

Makerii, the ironsmith: *makerii*, the ironsmith, name of the woodpecker bird.

Mayu, the sorcerer: *zankalalam mayu*, the sorcerer's zankalalam, the locust.

Myths, Legends and Social Repute

There is a two-part division of the animal world. On the one hand there are animals domesticated and integrated into rural life; on the other hand there are bush animals, uncontrolled by humans. Membership in either category determines the way humans react to the animal in question. Wild animals are felt to be a threat because they are powerful and supposedly endowed with magical faculties. Some are supposed to be particularly harmful. The crested crane is said to change shape and form, the cobra to start bush fires, while the orycterope is said to open up the earth by blowing on it, and so forth.

Some animals have derogatory individual nicknames: *caabule kaashi*, he who walks in faeces, the locust; *zankalalam mayu*, the sorcerer's zankalalo, name of a locust *guza me ban haushii* (E), nasty monitor lizard.

Lastly, selected animals figure in specific narratives and beliefs. For instance, the bird known as *jaayaaki*, also known as *gaam da yaaki*, meaning 'the one who pulls in war or confronts people with war', is supposed to signal the imminent incursion of raiders and attackers. The bird *uwa jiya jiya* is said to have sold its mother for potable water. Since then, so the tale goes, it endlessly chants its regret, singing: 'Mother yesterday, yesterday', etc.

The above names, which project human social conceptions onto the animal world, are on the whole valueless from a scientific point of view. Still, it is worth noting that even in modern scientific zoological nomenclature some names bear traces of such social projection.

For instance, scientific zoological names have yet to be completely purged of the distinction between wild animals and domesticated animals. The situation in botany is similar. The dichotomy still helps to separate species within a single genus. Thus, we talk of *Felis sylvestris*, the wild cat, or of *Canis familiaris*, the domestic dog. The distinction is based on a recognition of the objective fact that animals have specific qualities depending on whether they live in a wild or domesticated state.

As for the vocabulary of social relations, we find it cropping up in the classificatory concepts of scientific zoology and botany. Words like family, tribe, phylum and class, used to classify animals into various categories, are obviously derived from human social life. Moreover, within the framework of evolutionary theory, zoological and botanical terms sometimes serve to indicate degrees of kinship and descent. We do not, however, point this out as justification of the Hausa projection of such human social terms as son, husband, spouse and mother onto the animal world.

Within the framework of scientific names for species and varieties, there are occasional instances of the continued use of terms carrying social connotations. The bird known in Hausa as *daalee,* for instance, is called «le Franciscain» in French, after an order of Catholic priests whose garb resembles the plumage of the birds in question. The *malaam,* incidentally, are also similarly named. It so happens that the Latinate 'scientific' name, *Euplectes orix franciscana,* keeps the old social connotation. These are rare instances, however, and in any case the social connotations occur only in the part of the name indicating the species or variety.

The habit of tagging animals with a particular reputation is a very general human attitude. Time was when in Europe the apparatus of witchcraft was incomplete unless it included owls or cats. The role of the serpent in Eve's primal seduction needs no comment in this respect. The Gallic cockerel is almost as famous an icon, and the list is long. In its development, scientific thought, whatever its cultural environment, must necessarily shed such particularistic trappings, but the weaning is not easy, and even scientific names might contain surviving traces of value judgements. Thus, the red-throated bird known in Hausa as *caara,* is scientifically known as *Spreo pulcher,* the Latin pulcher meaning beautiful. Similarly, the galago is called *Galago elegantus,* the Latin word meaning 'highly graceful'. In sum, we find vestigial traces of social projection within the scientific system of zoological nomenclature.

Classificatory Processes

Classificatory procedures call for close examination because they provide evidence of the kind of intellectual activity needed to organize information derived from sense impressions. Whenever we find evidence of such activity, we are able to move away from the notion of human beings as merely passive recorders of sense impressions.

In this chapter we shall not be discussing major classificatory categories for all animal life. Instead, we shall examine selected cases of classification in particular composite names. In the Hausa system of nomenclature, classificatory names of the type in question are unconnected with any overall classificatory scheme. Scientific zoological nomenclature, on the other hand, is a component part of a comprehensive and all-inclusive system.

The Importance of Classificatory Names in Hausa Nomenclature

Classificatory names in the Hausa system are composite names. However, not all composite names include classificatory components. *Ta yaa ni gooyoo*, for instance, is the composite name given to a bird, and it means 'do not cry; I'm carrying you on my back'. It includes no classificatory component. Similarly, the name of the bird *shaara hwagee*, meaning 'sweep the farm', contains no classificatory component. On the other hand, the wild sheep is known in Hausa as raagon duuci, the components being *raagon* (sheep) and *duuci* (rocks). This is a name with a classificatory component, because there is a comparison with a different animal to which it bears a resemblance in some respects, and from which it differs in others. To get an accurate idea of the importance of this type of classificatory name in Hausa zoological nomenclature, it would be necessary to conduct a quantitative study of these names.

In the indexed section of her *Etude ethnozoologique du pays hausa*, Anne Levy-Luxereau presents four categories of names:

a) The name of the animal which forms the indexed title;

b) Synonyms, where applicable;

c) Genus names;

d) Epithetical names.

We have left aside the first three categories, i.e., (a) 218 reference names for the index; (b) 128 synonyms; and (c) 34 genus names, making a total of 380 names. These 380 names, covering only mammals, birds, reptiles and fishes, are divided as follows: simple names: 291 (74 per cent); compound names: 99 (26 per cent), including 32 without classificatory components, 57 with, a total of 15 per cent of all names under study.

The same author's article on locusts in the Maradi region presents 51 names, broken down as follows: simple names: 18 (35 per cent); compound names 33 (65 per cent), including 26 compound names with no classificatory components, 7 with, making 13 per cent of all names studied.

Overall, then, the figures are as follows:

Total names:	380 + 51 = 431
Total simple names :	291 + 18 = 309 or 71.6 per cent
Total compound names without Classificatory components:	32 + 26 = 58 or 13.4 per cent
Total compound names with Classificatory components:	57 + 7 = 64 or 14.8 per cent

Needless to say, in order to get an accurate idea of our subject, we would have to work with much more comprehensive lists, enabling us to establish the percentage of names with classificatory components according to major zoological categories: birds, fishes, insects, etc. The point is that it is possible that names with classificatory components occur with varying frequencies depending on the category of animals in question. Roulon, in his study on Gbaya zoological classifications, demonstrated this. In any case, given the current state of our knowledge, it may be estimated that Hausa zoological names with classificatory components make up about 15 per cent of the total. That would be a relatively high proportion, but the caveat remains: we need to conduct more analytical studies.

Examples of Names with Classificatory Components

The following are examples of naming procedures

Kujen, fly; *kujen-saanu*, cattle fly; *kujen-zuma*, milk fly, the bee; *kujen-zakkuwaa; kujen-galla; kujen-buubawaa, bumblebee.*

Kazzaa; fowl: *kaazaar-ruwa*, water fowl; *kaazaar-duuci*, rock fowl; *kaazaar-geeza*, wild fowl.

Mazuuruu, cat: *Mazuuruu-jibda*, civet; *mazuuruu-twaassa; mazuuruu-junda; mazuuruu-tantal.*

Raago, sheep: *raago-duwa*, rock ram, the wild sheep; *raago-ruwa*, water ram, name of a fish.

Raakumin, camel: *raakumin-daaji*, bush camel, giraffe; *raakumin-kasa*, land camel, *Myrmeleoni planipedes*.

Bardon: turtledove.

Bardon-gude, little black-beaked turtledove; *bardon-juuga*, Cape turtledove.

Zankalalo, locust: *zankalalo-mayu*, *zankalalo*, the sorcerer's aide; *zankalalo-fari*, white *zankalalo; zankalalo-tsamiya.*

Gadaar, cuttlefish: *gadaar-ducci*, rock mollusc; *gadaar- kutmi*, wood mollusc;

Na suuri, cobra: *jan-na suuri*, a type of cobra.

Muujiyaa, the African grand duke (bird): *muujiyaa-karami*, little duke.

Bantaa, the hunter bird; *bantaa-na hwadama*, hunter bird

Alade, pig: *aladen-daaji*, bush pig, warthog.

Karee, dog: *karen-ruwa*, water dog, otter.

Kuuraa, hyena: *kwallan-kuura*, hyena cries, the plover.

Jaboo, shrew: *jaabak-koogoo*, tree-hole shrew, the mocking bird.

Biri, monkey: *jan-biri*, red monkey.

Bikaa, baboon: *bikan-kurmi*, forest baboon.

We have observed that the Hausa style of nomenclature starts with a basic name, to which one or more attributes are then attached. It would be premature to assert that this is a scientific zoological nomenclature. For one thing, such a system presupposes a distinction between genus and species, which in turn has to fit into an overall theoretical framework in which classificatory categories interlock. Nevertheless, the Hausa system presents points of similarity with the scientific system. For instance, the practice of starting with a basic name and adding supplementary attributes, which exists among the Hausa as well as many other groups, is in a sense like the original pattern from which the Linnaean refinement was developed. Hausa nomenclature does not use this procedure for all names. Indeed, some basic names occur alone, with no attributes added at all. Neither does Hausa nomenclature form part of an overarching system organizing the entire animal world into interlocking groups. Still, the occurrence of this base-cum-attribute procedure is a highly positive aspect of Hausa zoological nomenclature.

On further examination of the validity of the resulting classifications as exemplified above, it is necessary to establish the following distinctions.

A number of classifications seem quite justified, examples being those based on *Bardo*, the turtledove, *zankalalo*, locust, *gadas*, mollusc, *na-suuri*, cobra, *muujiyaa*, the grand duke, *bantaa*, the passerine sparrow, *biri*, monkey, *bikaa*, baboon.

A number of classifications are utterly arbitrary, their underlying analogies zoologically unsound, as in the case of the transition from the cat to the civet. Classifications are equally unjustified when the underlying rationale is merely metaphorical or the resemblance simply superficial. Examples are the appellation 'water sheep' for a type of fish, bush camel for the giraffe, land camel for the Myrmeleoni. Similarly, the comparisons of the otter to the dog, the plover to the hyena, and the mockingbird to the shrew, are unconvincing.

As far as content goes, it is patently impossible to reach a comprehensive conclusion. Each name should be assessed on its own merits. At issue is the very nature of analogical comparisons. The transition from mammals to fish, and from mammals to birds brings together animals from very different domains. And in the comparison of the camel to the giraffe, as in that of the dog to the otter, a single morphological characteristic is emphasized to the detriment of others. In the case of the camel and the giraffe, that trait is height. By contrast, the comparison of the cat and the civet is based on several common traits. As a result, the comparison is much more solidly based.

The accurate identification of degrees of resemblance and difference implied in the separation of genus from species often requires the deployment of resources beyond simple external descriptions of animals. Disciplines entering into play include anatomy and physiology, functional analysis and structural analysis. The combined use of these resources enables zoologists to support or disqualify analogical judgements based on simpler sensory observations of animals. We should remember, however, that the prototypical zoological and botanical classificatory system developed by Linnaeus was based solely on selective observations of external traits of fauna and flora. Admittedly, these observations were remarkably detailed and thorough. This is one reason why it would be a mistake to discount the capacity of the senses to serve as a basis for scientific systems. They can indeed perform that function, provided sensory impressions are subsequently organized and developed within a theoretical framework.

After this rapid analytical overview, we can now identify, within the system of Hausa zoological nomenclature, those aspects which tend to bring the local system closer to international 'scientific' standards, those which tend to deviate therefrom, and those which are simply lacking in the scientific spirit. All aspects of Hausa zoological nomenclature incorporating morphological, ethological and ecological observations of animal life constitute a positive step forward. Furthermore, some Hausa zoological names are already organized in a two-part pattern in which the first part is the basic name, the second an attribute. Admittedly, in the Hausa system this pattern is only partially followed, instead of being a consistent standard. To bring the Hausa system into line with the universalized and systematic style of zoological nomenclature, the following modifications would have to be made.

First, concepts of genus and species would have to be formed for all items to be named in the animal and plant worlds. The resulting names would have to fit into a comprehensive classificatory process embracing all categories from genus and species to kingdom and branch. Second, observations would have to be extended and deepened so as not only to cover external appearances but also to examine internal structural details, the performance of biological functions, etc. Third, to carry this analysis to a thorough conclusion, it would be necessary to conduct a companion study on Latinate nomenclature in zoology. One probable conclusion from that study would be the realization that Latin terms do not of themselves make designations scientific; they are merely a useful convention adopted to obviate the friction that might result from conflicts of national sensitivities among scientists if some living language were adopted as the standard language of zoological nomenclature. Latinate names thus contain their share of sensory observations, value judgements and human social projections. In this regard, the language of zoology falls far short of the degree of scientific accuracy attained in other disciplines such as physics or chemistry. Even within the confines of the life sciences, zoology still falls short, in its terminology, of standards achieved in biology. Any study of the meanings of Latinate zoological names, then, ought to go hand in hand with reflections on the general problem of zoological taxonomy. For this is an aspect of the discipline which to this day is subject to continuing debate and adjustment. It is not by any means a comprehensive system of fixed, unchanging values.

This study of Hausa zoological nomenclature has provided an opportunity for establishing within the intellectual context of Niger an important epistemological issue: that of the connection between traditional knowledge and scientific knowledge, through overtly defined comparisons of their respective terminologies. We hope this initial essay will prove sufficiently successful to stimulate further work in other disciplines as well as among other cultural groups in Niger. Interestingly enough, those who talk in terms of dichotomies between folk knowledge and modern science tend to focus on the most modern sciences or on completely formalized disciplines. As a rule, they skirt around zoology and botany. Yet it is precisely in the domain of animal and plant life that local knowledge is best endowed, and the counterpart in modern science relatively underdeveloped. In our opinion this avoidance (or is it a case of deliberate oversight?) has a poignant meaning. It indicates a tendency to forget the beginnings and formative growth of all scientific knowledge. And that is all the more reason why open discussions of these issues are valuable.

Part Three

Medicine and Pharmacology

7

Fruits, Seeds and Miscellaneous Ingredients Used in the Pharmaceutical Practice of Benin

Simone de Souza

From the earliest antiquity, human beings have used various organic and inorganic ingredients culled from the environment to treat the sick as well as to communicate with supernatural forces. The pharmacopoeia of humanity has included fruits, seeds, rhizomes, bulbs and tubers, leaves, bark, roots and minerals extracted from the earth, and shells and the remains of animals, vertebrates as well as invertebrates.

In Africa these ancient practices have retained their vitality to this day. Many of the substances used are supposed, in addition to their medical efficacity, to possess magical powers. Their effects are therefore described as medico-magical. Their use is always accompanied by ritual incantations, the idea being that otherwise they would not work at levels of maximum potency.

In the pharmaceutical practice of Benin, as in that of Africa as a whole, words are of fundamental importance. They help to make individuals psychically ready and receptive, whether they are patients expecting to be cured, or simply individuals seeking to be told their fortunes. Between medicine and magic, in short, the interface is extensive.

For one thing, traditional fetish cults invariably require the offering of sacrifices including leaves, fruits, seeds and miscellaneous ingredients with spiritual powers. In Benin it is only in the urban markets of the South that one finds medicinal plants on sale. In the North, users personally gather the plants they need from the bush, and every family has at least one member who can identify the species used by their local names.

The purpose of this chapter is to present a description of a selective sample of well-known medicinal products found on sale in the markets of Cotonou and Porto-Novo.

Fruits

Acacia nilotica (L.) Willd. ex Dei. (Mimosa)

Yoruba name: *Boonien*. Fon and Gèn speakers have adopted the Bariba name *Gamalwa,* because this savanna tree grows in the Borgou and Atacora region. Concoctions made from the pod alleviate coughing. Scientific studies have demonstrated that the fruit is effective against molluscs in cases of *Bulimus* and *Boimphalaria*. No antibiotic effect has been noted (Bep 1986).

Adenopus breviflorus Benth. (Cucurbit)

Yoruba: *Tagiri*. Fon and Gun: *Yeblikpen*. This plant is supposed to possess medico-magical properties. The reputation is possibly due to its weird, spotted appearance. It is suspended above doors or placed in corners of houses as a protection against smallpox and other epidemic diseases. (Though smallpox has been eradicated in Benin, people still dread the disease). The plant is reputed to have the following powers:

a) It drives off pythons;

b) It protects harvests from thieves, by covering their skin with spots as soon as they commit their theft;

c) It is used for tanning leather;

d) In combination with Trema guineensis and Olax subscorpioidea, it accelerates the maturation of fruits;

e) Infusions or the chewed pulp of the plant added to palm oil can be rubbed on skin inflammations caused by chickenpox;

f) Infusions are drunk as a treatment for gonorrhoea and stomach ulcers;

g) Individuals seeking an antidote to enchantment open up the fruit from the top, hollow it out, replace the pulp with chicken intestines and place the bundle at a crossroads to exorcise the demon from their souls. As far as we know, no scientific studies of this fruit have been conducted.

Aframomum meleguetta K. Schum. (Ginger)

Gun: *Ara;* Fon: *Atakun;* Gèn: *Taku;* Yoruba: *Atanre;* French: *Maniguette.*

The fruit, once dried, has the same multiple properties as Xylopia aethiopica, and plays an important role in magical practice. It is used in decoctions made to cure coughs, asthma, headaches, dysentery and gastric illnesses. The seed has a peppery taste and can be used as a spice. A powder made from it is an ingredient in the manufacture of a black vegetable soap for the treatment of rheumatism. It is also used in the preparation of suppositories for treating constipation and haemorrhoids. In traditional practice, suppositories and vaginal capsules are generally prepared by mixing a soft, malleable excipient with some medicinal powder, normally in the form of ashes. The mixture is then shaped into a cone with the fingers. The most popular excipient is shea butter. Black vegetable soap is also used, but it has the disadvantage of hardening in the cool, dry harmattan season. Some pharmaceutical practitioners prefer to use the sap that flows from palm buds during the tapping of palm wine.

The maniguette clove is used in all magical prescriptions, its role being to boost the effectiveness of incantations. The healer, known as the Bokonon, chews up a piece of the plant, then sprays the resulting spittle on the other ingredients, reciting ritual incantations all the while. The plant reinforces his words with power.

Chemical analyses have revealed a yellowish, aromatic essence that makes up 0.30% of the seed by weight, along with a bitter essence, paradol, which resembles gingerol, the essence of ginger (Kerharo 1974; Adam 1974). So far no pharmacological tests have been published. However, it is possible that this plant has properties similar to ginger, in the sense that it is a stimulant, carminative, causes swelling, and irritates mucous membranes.

Ananas comosus L. (Bromelias)

Gun: Agon; Fon: *Agonde;* Gèn: *Blafogbe;* Yoruba: *Okpe oribo;* French: Ananas.

The fruit of the pineapple is known in Benin as a powerful diuretic and slimming agent. The pulp is eaten, while decoctions from the skin are drunk together with grape fruit juice. Normal doses are about a litre per day. The same decoction, with the addition of the rhizome Imperata cylindrica, is used to treat dysmenorrhea (painful periods). When rubbed over the body, pineapple juice softens the skin. Young pineapple fruits, pounded together with twigs of Costus afar and a dash of salt, disinfect pimples produced by outbreaks of fever.

Scientific studies show that pineapple juice contains an enzyme, Bromelaine, effective against bacteria and as an antihelminthic (Oliver-Bever 1986).

Carica papaya L. (Carica)

Gun: *Gbekpetin;* Fon: *Kpetin;* Gèn: Adubati; Yoruba: *Igi bekpe;* French: Papaye.

Papaya is a vitamin-loaded fruit with a pleasant taste, eaten green or a ripe yellow. It is also reputed to possess medicinal virtues:

a) Slivers of green papaya are rubbed over the hardened nipples of nursing mothers. The white latex flowing from the papaya helps to soften them.

b) Ripe papaya fruit works as a laxative, and is effective in the treatment of icterus and haemorrhoids.

c) The papaya tube is considered effective in the treatment of worms. However, tests conducted at Cotonou Hospital do not support this reputation. Substantial scientific research has been done on the papaya plant.

d) Unripe papaya contains a proteolyptic enzyme, papane, which boosts digestive suction processes and can be used to treat dyspepsia. It is used, incidentally, in the food industry for making chewing gum. Papane also has proven abortifacient and anti-ovulating properties, giving it a probable role as a contraceptive.

e) The juice is an anticoagulant. It helps to slow down heartbeats and to lower arterial pressure.

f) Ripe papaya fruit is an effective antibiotic against Staphylococcus aureus, Bacillus cereus, Eicherichia coli, Pseudomonas Aeruginosa and Schigella flexneri (Oliver-Bever, BEP 1986).

g) Papaya seeds have numerous properties. They are antihelminthic, causing proteolysis in treatments of cases of intestinal worms, and are effective as an antibiotic against microbes infesting the intestines and the urinary tract. They are also effective fungicides in the treatment of skin rashes, tuberculosis and inflammations (Kerharo, Adam 1974).

Citrus spp (Citrus)

Citrus aurantium: Bitter orange or grape fruit. Fon: *Gbo;* Gun: *Zigbo;* Gèn: *Bodo n'tisi;* Yoruba: *Jaganyin.*

With their round shapes, citrus fruits are part of the feminine world, in the same way as calabashes, eggs and pots. Their roundness indicates the matrical quality of women, like the birth-giving womb-shape. Grape fruit is used in numerous medicinal infusions as a diuretic. That is why it is often used in potions administered to treat fevers. It is also used in the treatment of arterial hypertension, gout, rheumatism and stomach ulcers. Amorous men can use it to make charms for ensnaring desirable women. Angry men, on the other hand, may use it to render targeted women sterile. Its juice is used to oil the fingers, labia minora and clitorises of pubescent girls or young married women in the ritual massage known among the Gun as Yodindon. The ritual is part of traditional sex education, and results in the elongation of the vulva. The oversized clitoris is then called Anaganta (Brand 1985).

Citrus aurantifolia: lime

Fon: *Kle;* Gun: *Kle;* Gn: *N'tisiti;* Yoruba: *Osan orombo.*

Lime juice is often used to make medicinal powders palatable in much the same way as palm oil and palm kernel oil are used. By itself, it is an effective treatment for fever, dysentery, head sores, mouth ulcers, coughs, diabetes and other ailments.

Scientific studies have confirmed that citrus fruits have anti-inflammatory, anti-histamine and diuretic properties, that they help open up coronary arteries, improve the stanchness of vessels, and boost capillary resistance. Citrus fruit juices, in effect, are clearly useful in the prevention of such illnesses as heart attacks, varicose veins, haemorrhoids, oedema, cirrhosis, strokes and hypertension. In addition, they contain vitamin C, effective against scurvy (BEP 1986).

Cocos nucifera L.: Coconut

Gun: Agonk; *Fon: Agon; Gèn: Neti; Yoruba: Agbon.*

The coconut is a plant of many parts, viz.:

a) The pericarp or fibrous cover, known as 'bourre' or cor';

b) The endocarp or hard shell;

c) The copra or firm seed albumen;

d) The coconut juice, the liquid seed albumen.

When copra is grated and squeezed, it produces a white liquid known as coconut milk. The fibrous and hard inner shell together make an extremely smoky, low-quality fuel much used in the coastal regions as a substitute for wood in areas where tree cover has disappeared. Coconut juice is used to make suspensions of medicinal powders. It is also used for treating tuberculosis. Furthermore, it is one of the ingredients used for making a magical good-luck charm. The standard prescription calls for steeping the following components in coconut juice, the whole to be kept in one's room:

a) Seven parrot feathers, all red;

b) Seven feathers of the savanna touraco, basic red but with white spots;

c) One dried chameleon;

d) An aspersion of perfume.

Coconut milk and cassava starch are used to make small, sweetened, aniseed-scented biscuits. Scientific studies indicate that:

a) Coconut juice is a fungicide effective against lice, tribhophyton and epidermophyton (Oliver-Bever 1986).

b) It is effective against the tuberculous bacillus Mycobacterium tuberculosis (Oliver-Bever 1986);

c) During the Vietnam War, it was used in the intravenous treatment of soldiers on the danger list. It proved to be a perfectly antiseptic medium (Kerharo, Adam 1974);

d) Like egg yolk, it can be used as a host solution for sperm in artificial insemination.

e) It stimulates root growth in cultures for growing tissue in vitro;

f) The shell produces a porous type of coal with excellent gas absorption properties when used in the manufacture of gas masks (Kerharo, Adam 1974).

Cucumis metuliferus E. Mey ex Naud (Cucurbit)

Gun: *Agbowonon;* Fon: *Gbowunon*

This fruit is said to possess magico-medical properties effective in the treatment of outbreaks of inflammatory fever provoked by the Vodun Sakpata. A formula for the prevention of smallpox is as follows: peel the fruit and steep it in palm wine (sodabi) or lime juice. Drink moderate quantities every morning or whenever the slightest symptoms appear. As long as this is done, the Vodun Sakpata may loiter around your home, but will never enter to sicken the inhabitants.

The following is a prescription for the cure of inflammatory illnesses: peel the fruit and steep it as in the previous prescription. Rub the resulting solution over pimples appearing on the body. It would seem that the thorny appearance of the fruit is the aspect that suggests a similarity with pox caused by inflammatory fevers. There is no evidence of any scientific research on this fruit.

Cucurbita maxima Duch (Cucurbit)

Gun: *Okpe;* Fon: *Kpe, Ayikpen;* Yoruba: *Elegede;* French: Courge

The squash is a magico-medicinal fruit.

a) Its seed, roasted, then pounded and mixed with water, eases labour pains;
b) Taken fresh, the seed helps to expel worms;
c) The peduncle is used in the Ouidah area in child outdooring ceremonies. If the child is a boy, the peduncle is cut into nine pieces, seven pieces if it is a girl. The pieces are dipped in black soap and given to the mother to consume.
d) After consultations of superanatural forces, squash figures among the sacrificial offerings given to invoke their help in the struggle against evil forces.

Musa paradisiaca L. (Plantains and bananas)

Gun: *Kokwe sozu;* Fon: *Kokwe sozu;* Gèn: *Amandan;* Yoruba: *Ogede Agbàgba;* French: *Banane plantain.*

Plantains and bananas are vitamin-rich food crops of the feculent variety. Normally, bananas are eaten raw, but plantains are cooked first. From a medical point of view, bananas act as intestinal astringents. When consumed in excess, they cause constipation. They are recommended as a treatment for diarrhoea.

In symbolic terms, bananas and plantains represent the circumcized phallus. The banana or plantain tree is the male plant par excellence. Women in Benin never harvest bunches of bananas or plantains. When they need leaves from the plant to wrap up their produce, they first ask a man's permission before cutting them. Women who deliver babies out in the bush place their new-born children on banana leaves warmed over a fire. The leaves represent the father receiving the child. The fruit and the tree both represent the fecundating potency of men as much as their physical power (Brand 1985).

From a pharmacological viewpoint, researchers have demonstrated that the ripe fruit tends to constrict blood vessels, thus contributing to hypertension. The flowers are hypoglycaemic: experiments on rats indicated that they provoked a 15 to 24 mg. drop in levels of blood glucose (Oliver-Bever 1986).

Schrebera arborea A. Chev. (Oleacea)

Gun: *Avinikpa, Akple, Gumaga;* Fon: *Vinikpa Agumoga;* Yoruba: *Okpele.* Pods of the plant are used in Fa divination sessions, when the oracle is consulted. A concoction made from the fruit is said to cure diabetes. We know of no chemical or pharmacological tests on the plant.

Tetrapleursa tetraptera (Schum et Thonn). Taub. (Mimosa)

Fon: *Lenja;* Gun: *Lenja;* Yoruba: *Ayidam.* This is a four-winged pod. In Benin it is used for apparently contradictory purposes as a stimulant and as a tranquillizer.

As a stimulant, the two non-ligneous wings of the pod are said to strengthen the resistance of children who drink and wash with concoctions made from them. The same wings are among the ingredients used in preparing a stimulating drink taken by persons about to enter into ritual possession trances. The following is the formula: candidates for possession are first brought into a dazed state by drinking a decoction made of roots of Rauvolfia vomitoria, shoots of Sabicea calycina, the bark of Erythrina indica and leaves of Datura stramonium. All these four plants have tranquillizing effects. Candidates then imbibe a stimulant brewed from pods of Tetrapleura tetraptera, Cola nitida and Cola acuminata, plus the Garcinia cola seed. This sends them into a trance (Brand 1985).

As a tranquillizer, the pod as a whole is used in numerous prescriptions for the treatment of stress, hypertension, insomnia, coughing, whooping cough, tuberculosis, rheumatic pains and stomach troubles. The following is a prescription for treating belly ache making children cry at night:

Make a decoction with seeds of Xylopia aethiopica, Monodora myristica, the pod of Tetrapleura tetraptera and the seed of Entada gigas. Administer one teaspoonful per day orally to expel intestinal gas. Higher doses may cause dizziness.

From a scientific viewpoint, pharmacological experiments have shown that liquid extracts from the pod act as tranquillizers, and cause body temperatures of rats to drop. An extract of the plant, dissolved in alcohol and given to a rat previously given a peritoneal injection of a convulsive drug, kept the animal from convulsive seizures normally associated with that drug.

Extracts from the plant have a steadying effect on heartbeats, and they are an effective treatment for constrictions of the bronchial tubes. It is thought that the plant contains an active principle, a saponoside that makes it an effective insecticide. (Oliver-Bever 1986).

Xykoplu aethiopica (Dunal) A. Rich. (Annonacea)

Gun: *Kpejele;* Fon: *Kpejelekun;* Gèn: *Eso;* Yoruba: *Eru, Eunje;* French: Poivre de Guine

This is a plant of many virtues, used in the preparation of numerous medicines, often simply to make them more palatable. It is said to be an effective remedy for coughs, gynaecological afflictions like metritus, skin diseases, rheumatism, mental illness, stomach ulcers and epilepsy. The skin, emptied of seeds, is used to treat liver ailments, but the seeds turn people's eyes yellow. Chemical analyses indicate that the plant contains xylopic acid, alcohol and oily essences. It is thought that the active principle responsible for the plant's effectiveness against Sarcinia lutea, Mycpacterium phlei, Staphylococcus aureus, Bacillus subtillis, Pseudomonas aeruginosa and Candida albicans is xylopic acid.

Seeds

Abrus precatorius L. (Papillonodea)

Gun: *Vivina Azetonuken;* Fon: *Vivina Azetonuken;* Gèn: *Jenjenklenjen;* Yoruba: *Ojuologbo;* French: *Jequirity, liane reglisse.*

In times past, this tiny red seed was used as a gold weight by the Ashanti of Ghana. The seed is poisonous to humans and animals. A single one can kill a person who chews it. Swallowed whole, it has no poisonous effect, because its thick skin keeps in the plant poison known as Abrine, of which 0.5 gm is sufficient to kill a human being. In Benin the plant is best known as a magical plant, with power to ensure the success of projects. The prescription for ensuring success is as follows: take seven Abrus seeds, the skull of a cat and steep in palm oil in some secluded corner of your house. Rub your face and hands therewith at the start of the day, or before embarking on any enterprise.

Censuplinia bonduc (L.) Roxb. (Cesalpinodea)

Fon: *Ajikwin;* Gun: *Ajikun;* Yoruba: *She ayo.*

The plant has a grey, spherical seed, commonly used in Benin for the game of Aji, in which seeds are dropped into sets of holes carved in a wooden base. The seed is used in divination. Persons consulting the oracle make their requests while holding the seed in front of their mouths. They then deposit it in the left corner of the diviner's plate. The plant is also part of the range of masculine sex symbols. It represents the testicles in general, and sperm in particular (Visin in the Gun language) which men deposit in the vaginas of women (Brand 1985). From a scientific point of view, the medicinal properties of the seed identified indicate its effectiveness as an antibiotic, diuretic, a treatment for fever and an anti-estrogen. The latter property makes it potentially useful as a contraceptive (Oliver-Bever 1986).

Cola nitida (Vent). Schott and Endl (Stercullacea)

Fon: *Goro;* Gèn: *Goro;* Gun: *Gbanja;* Yoruba: *Gbanja.* Cola acuminata (P. Beauv.) Schott and Endl (Stercullacea). Gun: *Avi;* Fon: *Vi;* Gèn: *Evi;* Yoruba: *Awedi;* French: *kola.*

The astounding virtues of the kola plant have long been known on the African continent. sixteenth and seventeenth century European travellers mentioned it as one of the fabulous products encountered on their travels. The name Goro is a derivative form of the Bambara name, Woro.

Throughout Africa, people chew the kola nut as an antidote to thirst. René Caillé reports that in 1830, in Guinea, kola formed part of the dowry young men paid for brides. The bride's father would take the kola nuts and throw them in the air, interpreting the pattern they made as they fell to find out what the future had in store for the new couple. In northern Ivory Coast, kola nuts used to be exported across the Sahara along caravan trails. Currency used in this trade consisted of salt bars, each three fingers long, called kikotta. From 200 to 600 kola nuts were exchanged for a kokotta (L. Ake Assi, «Les surprenantes vertus de la Kola», *Balafon Maagazine*).

Traditional priests have taken great care to keep alive the belief that kola nuts are a gift of the gods. Islam, in turn, has not only maintained the religious role of the plant, but has also recognized its uses as a stimulant and tonic. In Benin, cola nitida, a red or yellow nut with two lobes, is chewed fresh as a stimulant, or to quench thirst. There is a local cult around it, originating from Ghana, known as Goro-Vodun. In shrines dedicated to this Vodun, offerings invariably include kola nuts. Sometimes they pile up into little mounds, and some even begin germinating.

Cola acuminata is a red or yellow nut with four or five lobes. It is chewed much the same way as cola nitida, but it is supposed to have extra powers useful in geomantic divinatory rites. Shells from the follicle of the kola plant make a stimulating potion with aphrodisiac properties. Furthermore, they are supposed to be effective charms for attracting women's love.

Scientific studies have confirmed the efficacity of the kola plant as a stimulant and an analeptic pick-up. Taken in excess, it can even provoke convulsions. It contains caffeine and theobroma, which raise blood pressure and accelerate the heart beat. Kola can be used to make tonic and stimulating drinks conducive to intellectual performance (BEP 1986).

Dioclea reflexa Hook. f. (Papilionodea)

Fon: *V*; Gun: *V*; Gèn: *Ov*; Yoruba: *Agbanrin, ege, ishe.*

This almond, roasted and pounded, is said to stop hiccupping. Mixed with palm oil, it calms colic and is rubbed on muscles undergoing convalescence and rehabilitation, rheumatic joints and scars left by scabies. It also cures angina. The same mixture added to the pounded fruit of Aframonium meleguetta is licked as a treatment for pneumonia. It is supposed to have magical effects on anal sores. Hollowed almonds strung on a waist band are tied around the waist. Through gradual friction, the almonds lose their outer cover, by which time the sore has disappeared.

No findings based on scientific chemical analysis or pharmeceutical studies on the plant have so far been published.

Elaeis guineensis Jacq. (Arecacea)

Gun: *Datin*; Fon: *Datin*; Gèn: *Deti*; Yoruba: *Igi okpe*; French: Palmier à huile.

The variety known scientifically as idolatrica is called Fade, meaning: 'the palm tree of the Fa oracle'. The appelation 'Elaeis' means 'olive'. The nut comprises the following: a fibrous pericarp, red in colour, loaded with a pigmented carotinoid oil; a woody endocarp; a white, oily seed or almond.

To manufacture palm oil, fruits of the oil palm are boiled on a wood fire, generally in recycled oil drums. As soon as they reach the requisite degree of softness, they are mashed in holes dug in the ground. The decorticated plant is then immersed in water to separate the three components, each useful in its own right: oil, fibre and shell. Top quality oil, known as Zomi, is reserved for human consumption. Inferior grade oil is used for making soap. The fibre and shell make extremely good fuel.

To manufacture palm kernel oil, fresh palm kernels taken from cracked seed are ground and squeezed out. The resulting oil, Adin mi, is a sweet liquid of light brown colour. It is much in demand for frying bean cake known as ata, and for cooking in general. It can also be mixed with medicinal powders to make them easier to swallow. It is used in making soap.

Roasted palm kernel is ground, then heated to extract oil called Tchotcho. This process never takes place at home, since it is supposed to attract misfortune in the form of Sakpata, the smallpox Vodun, the most effective hex that an enemy can invoke. This kind of oil is therefore invariably processed in the bush, always at night. Tchotcho oil is a much prized ingredient in pharmaceutical practice in Benin. Medicinal and medico-magical powders are mixed with it to make them easier to swallow without irritating the throat. Certain families are allergic to it, however, and therefore cannot consume it. Its uses include the following:

a) it is rubbed in sores and ulcers;

b) it is used in cooking, most often for bean cake;

c) it is used for making a black soap, sometimes mixed with medicinal powders.

The Idolatrica type of palm nut is used in geomantic practice during Ifa divination sessions. The nut must be produced by cracking fresh fruit, not after cooking or roasting it, for Fa means "sweetness and gentleness". Other interpretations, however, derive the word Fa from Ifa or Ife, the Nigerian city from which the oracle originates. In any case, fire would abrogate the nuts' geomantic properties.

Twin palm nuts, smaller than ordinary nuts, are used in Ouidah as a rough and ready method of measuring the salt content of water used to dissolve ground salt in the salt manufacturing process. The nuts float when salt content is high. When it is low (near level 1), they sink to the bottom. The soil-dousing procedure is then halted.

Entado gigas (l.) Fawcett and Rendle (Mimosodea)

Gun: *Gblagbla;* Gèn: *Gblagbla;* Fon: *Gbagba, didi;* Yoruba: *Agbaa.*

Crushed pulp from the kernel is said to alleviate coughing. Mixed with Curculigopilosa or Monodora myristica and Xylopha aethiopica, it calms stomach aches of various origins, both intestinal and gynaecological.

Monodora myristica (Gaertn.) Dundi (Annonaca)

Gun: *Sasagbakun;* Fon: *Sasalinun;* Gèn: *Asioti, Asisanti;* Yoruba: *Shashagbakan, Ariwo.*

These seeds, like the fruit of Aframomum meleguetta, are used chiefly to spice up the taste of medicinal preparations. They are also reputed to cure stomach ulcers, digestive ailments and gynaecological infections (prescription quoted for Curculigo). They are used in the manufacture of pommades smeared on hernias or cutaneous inflammations. They are also supposed to be effective in the treatment of asthma. There are no published scientific studies on the plant.

Raphia Hookeri Mann. and Wendl. (Arecacea)

Gun: *Gba;* Fon: *Badekwin;* Gèn: *Bade;* Yoruba: *Iko, Igi ogoro.*

The part most in use is the seed of the scaly fruit, made up of an embryo covered by a hardened and mottled sheath. Ground and mixed with palm oil, it can be rubbed on the heads of babies with late-closing fontanelles.

Bulbs and Rhizomes

Allium cepa L. (Liliacea)

Gun: *Ajubasa;* Fon: *Ayoma;* Gèn: *Sabulvi;* Yoruba: *Alubosa;* French: Onion blanc.

This tiny white onion is mainly used in magical rituals. One prescription is as follows: take a small quantity of ash from the previous night's fire. Mix it with crushed onion, tie it up in a piece of cloth to make a protective talisman for warding off evil spirits.

The following is another top secret prescription: to acquire prophetic powers, eat these small white onions with dried fish for 40 days. There are charlatans who go about throwing cowries, claiming to be visionaries. But their cowries are only props for show. In fact, they use this prescription. Any individual following this prescription acquires foreknowledge of future events, and is therefore clairvoyant.

Curculigo pilosa (Schum. and Thom.) Engl. (Hypoxidacea)

Gun: *Yoglen;* Fon: *Ayote;* Yoruba: *Ekpakun.*

The rhizome of this savanna plant is used in many prescriptions for treating belly aches, genital infections, constipation, diseases of the spleen, icterus and prostate glands. It is used in a decoction together with the pod of Pentaclethra macrophylla, seeds of Monodora myristica and one kernel of Entada gigas. No scientific analysis or pharmaceutical findings on this rhizome have so far been published.

Zinziber officinale Rose (Zingiberacea)

Gun: *Dote;* Fon: *Dote;* Gèn: *Dote;* Yoruba: *Atale, Ataile;* French: *Gingembre.*

This rhizome is a popular spice, used fresh and whole or powdered and sold in jars. Steeped in palm wine (sodabi), it is said to work wonders as an aphrodisiac. Chewed fresh with a bite of sugar, it sedates coughing and alleviates sore throat. Mixed with other plants in potions, it cures headaches and anaemia. Black soap mixed with powdered ginger is used by rheumatics to wash, and it is rubbed on testicles afflicted with hernia. Chemical analysis shows that the plant contains an active principle, gingerol, with stimulating, carminative and stomach-settling properties. On the other hand, it causes swellings and irritates mucous membranes (Kerharo and Adam 1974).

Cowries and Shells

Cowries

Gun: *Akweo;* Fon: *Akwekwin;* Yoruba: *Owo eyo.*

Cowries are seashells of the genus Cypraea. It is thought that the word cowrie is derived from a seashell known as Cypraea carita. The cowries used in Benin are Cypraea moneta and Cypraea annulus. According to traditional African beliefs, they came from certain inland marshes. It is known, however, that cowries are usually collected on the Indian Ocean seaboard, in the Maldive Islands, on the Island of Zanzibar, and in the Philippines. Cowries are warm ocean shells found mainly in the Indo-Pacific regions. In Benin they are survivals from an ancient monetary system. They are often found buried or on display on market stalls where traditional medicines are sold. In the eighteenth century cowries were used for buying slaves. When washed and strung like beads, they were the equivalent of a bundle of modern bank notes. In the nineteenth and twentieth centuries when guinea coins and textiles became the going currency, the use of cowries as currency was stopped. (Rivallain and Iroko 1986).

In South Benin, cowries are used in divinatory practices because they have two faces, one open, the other closed. A cowry is always placed on the diviner's table. Cowries represent the female element, while kernels of Caesalpina bonduc represent the male (Brand 1985). Traditional healers use powdered cowries as a treatment for running sores, and give the powder to patients with mouth sores to lick. Like other seashells, they are used as a treatment for calcium deficiencies. Lime juice mixed with cowry powder, used as an eyewash, helps remove foreign bodies from eyes. The suspension, mixed with ground Boerhavia erecta root, is a cure for cataract.

Mineral Substances

Alum

Gun: *Sunmi;* Fon: *Sindaken;* Gèn: *Jesra;* Yoruba: *Alomu.*

Alum is available in the markets of Benin. It is a crystallized bisulphate of aluminium and sodium, in appearance much like a piece of white stone. Women washing their laundry with muddy creek water dissolve bits of alum in their wash basins. The alum causes the precipitation of colloidal matter, thus clearing the water. Powdered alum sprayed on sores helps the formation of scar tissue and healing. Alum is also used to treat diarrhoea, hiccups and asthma. It has abortifacient properties. Mixed with powdered sulphur, it is used during childbirth. Solutions of alum are used as eyewash as well as to wash sores, to clean the mouths of nursing babies, and to treat mouth sores. Women use alum to keep their private parts fresh.

White Clay

All languages of South Benin: *We.*

White clay, rolled into balls, cut into chunks or shaped into sticks, is used to whiten the bodies of Vodun priestesses during ceremonies, to set off their ritual beads. Sticks of white clay dipped in water are used to decorate busts and arms with white spots.

Grey Clay

All languages of South Benin: *Kalaba.*

Grey clay comes in the form of rough, irregular spheres, moulded and fired to give it a brown sheen when its iron content gets oxydized. Made in Ghana and brought to Benin by the Mina people, it bears its original name, Kalaba. It is used in various medicinal prescriptions intended to treat diarrhoea and dizziness among pregnant women. It is used as a dressing for running sores, as well as a stomach lining for patients with stomach ulcers. Young women are advised not to use it, since they risk becoming sterile if they eat it.

Incense

Fon: *Za.*

The incense used here is made from the sap of the savanna tree Daniellia iliveri, or from the forest tree Daniellia ogea. Incense placed on live coals burns, releasing an aromatic smoke used for ritual purification. In some psychopathological cases where patients are said to be possessed by evil spirits, the smoke is supposed to exorcise demons. The potency of incense reportedly increases when pods of xylopia aethiopica and powdered sulphur are added to it. Incense is burned in tiny ritual brasiers made of clay.

Iron

Iron occurs in two forms here: iron filings or pig iron from the smithy. The names are as follows:

Filings: Gun: *Ayami;* Fon: *Aliande;* Yoruba: *Kpekpe agbede.*

Pig iron: Gun: *Ahaya;* Fon: *Awlomi;* Gèn: *Sokpe;* Yoruba: *Idaro.*

To regain lost youth and banish all disease, the recommendation is to keep a piece of iron permanently in one's bath water. Healers always place some iron at the bottoms of jars used to store medicinal infusions made from herbs. Iron is said to have curative effects in cases of heart disease, asthma and anaemia. It is a treatment for the illness known as Chakatu, in which needles and assorted small stones are mysteriously projected into the body of an individual by an enemy. Iron filings steeped in bathwater cause the dissolution and evacuation of such hostile foreign bodies.

Author's comment: In African pharmaceutical practice, there is no plant with sufficient quantities of iron to make it as effective against anaemia as spinach is in Europe. Grey clay and iron may supply this deficiency.

Potash

Gun: *Akango;* Fon: *Akanmu;* Gèn: *Akan.*

What is known as potash in Benin is in reality a collection of salts with high potassium content. These salts are obtained after the evaporation of solutions of ash obtained after the burning of male inflorescences of Elaeis guineensis and Amaranthus spinosus. The two plants are particularly rich in potassium. Potash is much appreciated by cooks because it speeds up the cooking of okra, vegetables and herbs of all sorts. It also helps them keep their appetizing green colour. An infusion of Ocimum gratissimum prepared with a pinch of potash alleviates coughing. Potash mixed with palm oil is applied to boils to hasten their maturation.

Gunpowder

Fon: *Du;* Gun: *Adu;* Gèn: *Adu.*

This black powder is obtained from commercially available cartridges for hunting rifles. When lit with a match, it produces an extremely bright fireball. To honour dead dignitaries, gunpowder wrapped in paper is set on fire and thrown up in the air. At funerals of hunters among the Fon people of Ouidah, there is a ceremony called Doso in which gunpowder poured into small tubes is set alight, producing explosions representing illustrious exploits of the deceased.

Gunpowder also has medicinal uses. It is used as a treatment for inflammatory fevers. The powder is put into a bowl with leaves of Vermonia amygdalina and set afire. The ashes are then smeared on the skin of the patient, who might also drink a solution thereof. Normally, this remedy is prepared at home, though crossroads are a preferable venue. There are reports of home-made abortifacients, produced by mixing gunpowder, blue laundry powder and aspirin, causing death.

Black Soap

Gun: *Adiyu;* Fon: *Adiwi;* Gèn: *Akoto;* Yoruba: *Oshe dudu.*

Black soap is a wholly vegetable-based soap produced by heating oil from the cabbage tree and potash made from plant ash. A number of plants are well known for their high potassium salt content. They include Elaesis guineensis, Amaranthus spinosus, Anogeissus leiocarpus. Blighia sapida seeds have similar properties. Ashes obtained from burning these plants are steeped in water and left to settle. Water from the upper layers contains salts in solution. It is emulsified to obtain soap. Roasted cabbage produces a deep black soap credited with numerous medico-magical uses, depending on the powders mixed with it:

a) mixed with the powdered fruit of Aframonium meleguetta, it is used to treat rheumatism;

b) those who wash with black soap are generally protected against all sorts of ailments. Evil spirits are driven off, incantations are given greater power, and the most intimate wishes come true;

c) gargling with a solution of black soap cures angina;

d) black soap can also be shaped into suppositories. It is hazardous, however, to use such suppositories in the dry harmattan season, when black soap hardens as temperatures drop.

Sulphur

All languages of South Benin: *Hwemi*.

In Benin, sulphur is obtained at stations where it is loaded and offloaded on its way to Arlit in Niger, where it is used to make sulphuric acid used in enriching uranium ore. Sulphur has been adopted in pharmaceutical practice in Benin to cure skin diseases. Mixtures containing sulphur are used in numerous medico-magical formulae.

Among natural substances used in traditional medical practice in Benin, many are yet to be subjected to scientific studies capable of confirming or refuting the claims made for them. In other words, there is good work awaiting chemists and pharmacologists.

Discussion

The following is a transcript of the discussion which took place after the presentation of this chapter at the National University of Benin, research seminar (see introduction for details).

Servais Smith: Some magico-medical prescriptions include animal blood. What role does this ingredient play? Are traditional healers born or trained?

Simone de Souza: Some prescriptions require ceremonial invocations of the divinity supposedly responsible for the illness in question. The shedding of animal blood is a symbolic gesture designed to placate and please the Vodun.

No one is predestined or born to the profession of traditional healer. It simply requires outstanding qualities. The secrets of magic and traditional medicine are handed down only to children showing signs of a serious vocation. Under normal circumstances, children and grandchildren of healers, provided they show some aptitude, are in the best position to succeed. They gain experience through helping to prepare prescriptions, gathering herbs and plants, burning and pounding them, and learning to make the necessary mixtures.

Victoire Nombime: Modern pharmaceutical drugs sometimes cause illness. Do plant remedies also have a negative effect at times? And do naturopaths have a system of plant classification?

Simone de Souza: Modern medicines can provoke allergies, stomach ulcers, dizziness, heart problems, circulatory ailments, etc. The same is true of plant remedies, which are made up of complex ingredients. Take the root of the Madagascan periwinkle, which contains over 40 alkaloids. One of them is an effective treatment for leukemia. We know that some alkaloids, taken in moderate doses, have medicinal effects, but are poisonous when taken in excess. That is why in modern medical practice, the active principle used as a specific treatment for a particular disease gets isolated and purified. Traditional plant-based medicine, in other words, has its share of risks.

None of the traditional healers I interviewed in Benin gave me the impression of using a system of classification for medicinal plants. Specialized scientific documents arrange plants according to their therapeutic uses. For example, there are hypoglycaemic plants, antibiotic plants, stimulants and cardiotonic plants.

Epiphane Houngnon: In Africa, where intravenous injections are not practiced, scarification is used instead. In her research, has Ms de Souza come across prescriptions in which fruits, seeds and various ingredients might be used for scarification?

Simone de Souza: The proper analogy for scarification is not an intravenous injection but a sub-cutaneous injection. In my opinion, the moderate pain resulting from the incision produces a psychological shock that catalyzes the healing process. My research, however, is limited to an ethnological survey. It does not cover the constitution of formulae.

Satchon: In the colonial period, Catholic priests and their Christian followers were forbidden to use traditional herbal medicines or to participate in associated magical rites. The reason given then was that such practices were against religious precepts. Today, however, we see foreign and African priests paying a great deal of attention to traditional medicine. What does Ms de Souza think of this situation?

Simone de Souza: Ideas change with time. The issue involved has been settled. Today there is no confusion between curative plants, on the one hand, and associated pagan ceremonies, often merely mystificatory, on the other. In Europe, our grandmothers used herbs to cure diseases. For their pains, some got called witches. In the mid-twentieth century, modern medicine developed at an extremely rapid pace. At the same time, there was a series of discoveries revealing causes of diseases. This progress tended to push traditional medicine, based mainly on empirical practice, into obscurity. Today, however, plants have also become better known, and there is a trend back to the use of "subtle medicines" which work slowly at moderate doses.

All individuals, religious or lay, should be free to try this option. But naturally, one can hardly expect a monotheistic priest to make sacrifices to a Vodun even if, according to the diviner diagnosing the ailment, such offerings are necessary.

Paulin Hountondji: There are reports about the effectiveness of the Acacia nilotica pod as a treatment for coughs, even though the plant has not yet been tested scientifically. There are many other examples of plants, fruits, seeds and other ingredients which are said to be similarly efficacious. All this lends support to your conclusion: there is a need for further research.

Some plants are said to have magical properties; others are credited with strictly medicinal qualities. What criteria are used to distinguish between the two types of properties? An example is the Dioclea plant, seeds of which work as a cure for anal sores when they are strung around the waist. Should scholars be content merely to observe and note such an effect? Or should they try to arrive at a rational explanation? If so, what methods should they use?

I have another question related to the secrecy surrounding the knowledge traditional healers guard so jealously. Much of their information is esoteric. In the course of your research, did you come up against obstacles and problems? Do you feel you are betraying secrets when you publish information obtained from traditional sources? Incidentally, the issue of esotericism in our societies should not be treated as if it were an isolated aspect, a peculiarity of our societies alone. Even in Western societies there is what is known as the scientific secret. We do not, for instance, have access to all data generated by atomic research. These are nothing less than state secrets carefully protected by a range of police, military and other security arrangements.

In our own societies, then, it seems clear enough that beliefs in witchcraft, as well as the range of threats levelled against individuals suspected of revealing secrets, might all be considered as measures designed to protect intellectual property. Still, endogenous knowledge should be updated and revitalized, so that we can make the best use of it within a scientific, technological context, by linking it with the knowledge and know-how we inherited from the West.

Simone de Souza: We say a plant has a magical effect when, intellectually, we have no idea precisely how it achieves that effect. For example, the fruit of the Adenopus plant, suspended in a corner of a house, is said to protect members of the family from smallpox and other inflammatory fevers. There is no visible or tangible connection from cause to effect. In the current state of our knowledge, there is no scientific proof of what happens. Might there be some connection with wave theory, still only partially explored by science? It is the work of pharmacologists to test plants on cultures of microbes, or on animals, in an effort to identify their properties with precision.

We say a plant is medicinal when, on being applied externally or being ingested, it produces a cure in the patient, under circumstances that can be reproduced under laboratory conditions. For example, leaves of the goosefoot plant, reportedly an effective treatment for worms, contain a chemical known as ascaridole which kills ascaris worms. The process can be checked with experimental equipment. Similarly, the root of the Fagara plant lowers blood tension. It contains reserpine, which, when injected into mice, produces that effect, proving the plant's effectiveness.

In situations where part of the effect is scientifically observable while part of it remains occult, we speak of a plant with medico-magical effects.

Regarding the issue of secrecy, and the specific matter of the formulae I have described to you, I have no feeling of having violated any trust or revealed secrets. My information was freely given, by open-minded traditional healers. Government agencies have mobilized healers. Now that they are motivated, the healers wish to co-operate with researchers to help advance the cause of traditional medicine in Benin. There are many hospital nurses who are conversant with modern medicine, and also use traditional pharmaceutical substances. Sometimes they leave out the incantations supposed to go along with the treatment. Their argument is that the only effective element is the plant. I have the impression, however, that Africans in general and the people of Benin in particular need rhetoric as seasoning for herbal remedies. Their minds need that conditioning. Sick people need to be convinced that they are going to get well. Where the psychic condition of the patient is negative, cures are difficult.

Ben Johnson: Is there any justification in the supposition that natural substances used in our traditional prescriptions are more dangerous than chemical substances? Plants have their positive and negative aspects. It is the way they are mixed that balances them. An example is the Tetrapleura pod. Depending on the particular dosage, it can act as an upper or a downer.

Geoffroy Botoyiye: Why are traditional prescriptions supposed to lose their power once they come into contact with the ground?

Simone de Souza: People of a modern scientific mindset, if they accidentally spill medicine on the ground, will not use it. The reason is that it is contaminated by microbes. In traditional medical practice, the tendency is to think that potions spilled on the ground lose their effectiveness on account of beliefs about supernatural powers. The earth is a divinity, with supernatural influences.

Victoire Elegbe: Some plants have scientifically proven qualities, others do not. To what extent are traditional and modern medicine compatible?

Simone de Souza: Traditional and modern medicine are perfectly compatible. They coexist in all countries in the world. All Westerners are familiar with sedative herbal infusions which help to overcome insomnia.

Moukadam Bourama: Are those plants whose chemical composition and properties are known and tested not similar to the products sold in our modern pharmacies? As far as pharmaceutical practice is concerned, could these plant remedies not be substituted for the marketed commodities, which cost an arm and a leg?

Simone de Souza: With regard to certain plants, you are perfectly correct. Here in Benin, for example, there is the Cassia alata plant which contains chrysophanic acid, a substance with well-known decongestant properties. Pommade containing chrysophanic acid, sold in pharmacies, is extremely expensive. Well informed healers could advise patients to buy Cassia alata leaves inexpensively on herbal stalls in the market.

Mama Katchon: Modern medicine is never taken to the accompaniment of incantations. In our traditional societies, however, incantations are a matter of prime importance. Are they indispensable? Are they not used to mystify us?

Simone de Souza: The West has become rationalist in the manner of Descartes. People there mainly believe only what can be proved, even if the proof transcends a particular person's educational level. Doctors there do not administer medicine with any spiritual ritual. Rhetoric plays no part. Still, psychological factors also have a role to play in the recovery of patients. Rapid remissions from cancer have been observed where patients had a strong belief that they would get well. African man is much more mystical than Cartesian man. He believes in natural forces with which one has to come to terms if one is to regain one's health. Incantations are not mystificatory. They are intended to ready the mind, to reassure patients and convince them that in the search for a cure, no stone has been left unturned.

Epiphane Houngnon: According to your presentation, iron-rich grey clay is eaten by pregnant women, but it can make girls sterile. When then is it advisable to consume it?

Simone de Souza: It is not known why young girls who eat grey clay become sterile. Is it a contraceptive? Is the belief itself a myth? What is known is that this mineral ingredient may be consumed to make an intestinal lining in cases of gastric ulcers. It can also be a source of iron in cases of anaemia.

Ben Johnson: What is it about these traditional prescriptions that interests you?

Simone de Souza: My purpose is to help in the advancement and development of pharmaceutical resources in Benin, in collaboration with you, students at the University of Benin. All of us have untold riches within our reach. My concern is to find out how to use them for the benefit of all.

Servais Smith: How is it that animals do not eat deadly plants? Second, traditional healers ask to be paid large sums to make their remedies effective. Is this belief credible?

Simone de Souza: Deadly plants have a smell that repels animals. There are traditional healers who travel great distances to collect the plants they use. And they buy prescriptions from colleagues. The payment they ask for should cover these costs. However, those who demand exorbitant amounts are cheating. In any case, the cost of a remedy is no guarantee of its success.

Note

1. This chapter is the full version of an article published under the title 'Fruits, Seeds and Other Medicinal Ingredients on Sale at the Market', in *Medecine traditionnelle et pharmacope*, 1988, the French Cultural and Technical Cooperation Newsletter, Volume 3, Paris.

8

Traditional Models of Mental Health and Illness in Benin

Gualbert R. Ahyi

In health matters we tend too often to focus exclusively on the biomedical aspect. In so doing we give priority to bodily concerns, to the detriment of life's social and psychological dimensions. As medical doctors, we have sometimes been forced to recognize our weaknesses, and to try and reach a corrective balance through the interplay of the humanities, the social sciences and medicine. In truth, though, such efforts are by force of circumstance few and far between. By ourselves, after all, there is little we can do to change institutional curricula and personal habits. That is all the more reason why I appreciate the opportunity of the seminar to establish working contacts with other students. I hope our collaboration will be fruitful and long-lasting. I trust, in addition, that it will facilitate future collaboration between us in the examination of a number of common issues.

These days it is particularly difficult for any individual to specialize, simultaneously and with the same degree of thoroughness, in both Western and traditional psychiatry. Hence the humble prudence with which I venture onto this duplex field, knowing that with your store of acquired knowledge and personal experience in the field, you probably know as much as I, and possibly more.

We should note, to begin with, that the model of mental health followed in Benin is not entirely different from that of other African countries, given the powerful impact of culture on issues of mental health. The examples we give here might therefore be applicable to a substantial proportion of Africa's population.

If we define a model as a representation of reality, then when we speak of traditional models of mental health and illness, we include the following dimensions:

a) A description of ways in which mental health and illness are understood and explained in the cultural environment of Benin. Here the focus is on African culture;
b) an assessment of the adequacy of the models under discussion. By this we mean an evaluation of their capacity to enhance therapeutic, preventive and predictive action;
c) a comparison, within the field of psychiatry, of African models with those foreign models we are most conversant with, i.e., Western models.

At this point it might seem that our objectives are clearly defined. However, there are numerous problems on the path to their attainment, some of them formidable indeed. Let us look at three of them.

First, we ourselves start from a given position, that of representatives of a specific model, in this case the Western one. This confers on us the established position of people endowed not with a particular brand of knowledge, but of the quintessence of knowledge, period. In that capacity we function, unconsciously, as allies of a lopsided system in which on the one hand there is a conscious protagonist, the colonizer, and on the other hand a creature with a peculiar mentality, the colonized. Under these circumstances, it is legitimate for us to wonder if we are indeed the kind of individuals qualified to give due recognition to African psychiatry, that is to say, a psychiatric system tailored to the cultural realities of Africa.

Our circumstances, however, are not altogether negative. We have the good fortune to practice within an African environment. In that milieu, a number of traditional healers have built up a record of successful therapy. We are therefore bound to adopt less overbearing attitudes, and to dissociate ourselves from the position of the Western expert as teacher of ignorant Africans, a position that was such a central part of our colonial history. We have therefore been able to reach an assessment of African models, to make enquiries about the knowledge of traditional healers, to study their methods and concepts, and to assess the effectiveness of their techniques. Western psychiatrists have begun to pay attention to African traditions and healers. They have given up the position of teacher to adopt the pupil's attitudes. Their purpose now is to find out about ethno-psychiatry, no longer defined merely as a comparative study of different illnesses in different cultures, but as the way in which 'societies produce madness and make use of it or protect themselves from it by stretching or shrinking the gap between sanity and insanity'. The contemporary challenge, in other words, is to decode and understand current practice in every culture.

The second problem is related to our position as practitioners committed to a biological emphasis. That emphasis has found its rationale in, and been reinforced by, advances in research on pharmacological resources, biological factors and the physiology of the brain. In these areas our traditional healers are notoriously weak. It has been pointed out that 'the esoteric, sacred and religious aspect of traditional therapy constitutes a block in the path of foreign psychiatrists'. Indeed, it also inhibits African psychiatrists trained in Western universities. The rejection of this aspect is connected to the following factors:

a) a reluctance to rush into an area of mental illness in which therapists are confronted with evil forces, with neither preparation nor protection;
b) the dangerous aura of a sacralized environment;
c) the inhibition associated with queries on the fundamental beliefs and myths of individuals and their social organizations.

Western-trained psychiatrists avoid such confrontations for fear of getting shaken, or having to face challenges to ideational systems painstakingly adopted and internalized.

The third problem is again a function of our position: that of researchers bent on understanding African models from external viewpoints, starting from a basis of Western models and concepts. Under such circumstances, we run a high risk of distorting and misunderstanding the information we process.

Still, it seems inevitable that faced with the reality of African science, we should have to analyze traditional knowledge using Western concepts such as the healer's profession and tradition. Human beings are products of their culture, which is itself a way of life, of sensing and perceiving the social and human organization of the world. The question is whether it is possible to perceive and experience connections between human beings and their culture without first stepping out of our own culture. It is against a backdrop of such formidable problems that we shall here attempt to discuss models of mental illness in Benin, in Africa, and in the world at large.

Models of Mental Health and Illness

We arrive at an understanding of ways in which a given society construes and explains mental health and illness by examining specific factors identified or blamed, in that society, as causes of illness. From a descriptive standpoint, in Benin as in most African societies, two main explanations are given for mental illness. It is considered to be the work of living persons; alternatively, it is attributed to the influence of spirits. Where the putative instigator is a living person, mental illness may be caused by a direct or an indirect attack.

In instances of direct attack, one individual, using no intermediary, directly attacks another individual, using methods of human-devouring witchcraft. The aim is to kill the victim. In almost all areas of Central and Southern Benin, this phenomenon is known as 'Aze'.

In cases of indirect attack, an individual attacks another individual indirectly, using the services of an intermediary to do so. The intermediary may be an initiate in an esoteric cult, a Muslim marabout, or a magician, supposedly capable of mobilizing and controlling the forces intended to act on the victim according to the wishes of the aggressor requesting the service. This is the kind of esoteric, magical operation known in other French-speaking countries as «maraboutage». In Benin it is called 'Bodome'.

Mental illness caused by spirits is traced back to spirits of traditional, ancestral religions or those of imported religions such as Islam, the Judaeo-Christian sects, and local syncretistic religious movements. Each category of illness has a corresponding method of attack and an associated syndrome, that is to say, a set of symptoms. Each category of illness also requires an appropriate therapy.

Healers normally do not focus much on symptoms, the clinical signs of disease. Instead, they are primarily interested in pointers leading to a diagnosis. Their primary aim, in other words, is to find out who the instigator of the illness, the aggressor, might be. Pointers may come from discussions with members of the patient's family. They may also emerge from an assessment of the patients' own talk, visions and dreams, all products of their experience, whether they are conscious of them or not. Other indications may come from an understanding of relations between the individual and the group. This method of explaining what happens to sick individuals, or individuals regarded by close ones as ill, situates psychiatric realities outside the specific field of mental illness. The problem is not in the victim's body or personality. It originates in an act of aggression.

The Suitability of Models

Our purpose here is to determine what really is at the root of these models. We intend to assess their therapeutic efficacy. In other words, we want to see whether they facilitate predictive, preventive and operative therapy. Acts of aggression, whether they originate from human beings or from spirits, refer to levels of comprehension other than those expressed in the statements of patients, their families or the healer. The entire set of models refers back to sources of illness. In specific terms, these are situations of conflict which human beings are bound to experience, in their capacity as social beings interacting with other social beings and with the law.

Beyond what is articulated within the system itself, there are further levels of explanation. In effect, it would seem that what is overtly identified as a cause obscures and serves as a cover for other aspects about which nothing is overtly said. For that reason, we decided to begin with an analysis of the initial system that posits an act of aggression by a given individual, who may be the sorcerer himself, or an expert acting on behalf of a third person. The act of aggression imputed to the sorcerer refers back to something basic and original: a conflict in inter-personal relationships. Conflict being an inescapable aspect of all human life, people have to learn to cope with it. As social beings, we cannot deny the reality of conflict with significant others.

Of such significant others, the first is one's own mother, the one with whom we develop our first relationship. From conception to birth, the dual relationship linking foetus to mother is bound to leave a conflictual imprint which will surface in all subsequent relationships. In later life, this relationship is experienced in the oral mode, in the form of a peculiar tendency towards aggression. And oral orientations, coupled with aggressive stances, might refer back to some basic principle of attack, a tendency to devour.

It is, I think, this conflictual relationship with the other which is given recognizable form in the system of human-eating witchcraft and the 'bewitching' process I referred to earlier. It is quite possible, if my hypothesis is right, that the initiate or expert functions only as a transmission belt for the act of aggression. And if this hypothesis is right, then the primary system, in which there is the supposition of an act of aggression committed by an individual, raises issues involving the patient, the sorcerer and the healer.

From the information given us, sorcerers are like other persons, except that they are supposed to possess certain skills, know-how and powers. In some cases these powers are innate; in others they are acquired, handed down to the sorcerer in question. Using these powers, sorcerers are presumably able to strike directly at long range, in multiple locations. We do not intend to enter into a detailed discussion of these suppositions at this point, since they raise a number of problems we shall be analyzing when we come to a comparative analysis of the two models, traditional and Western. For the moment, let us focus on the assertion that the aggressive sorcerer is a human being like any other. This brings us back to my statement about the primary relationship within the mother/child duality.

Sick people, in describing and formulating their symptoms, express specific personalities. They make declarative statements, claim they have been attacked, and project onto the other, the accused, a number of desires and actions defining their guilt. Healers, as their self-appointed advocates will tell you, are also like sorcerers. The difference is that they do not kill people. Still, they have the power to hurt. Healers, then, are sorcerers who 'do not eat people', and part of whose vocation it is to keep sorcerers from devouring people.

What we have, then, is a system made up of a triad in which two principals at least are sorcerers. One eats people, the other does not, claiming instead to protect people. Look at the triad a little more closely, and it becomes clear that both sorcerers are entitled to use their powers of aggression. There is the patient, who claims he is being eaten, points to the putative man-eating sorcerer, and accuses him. Within the system, the sorcerer is endowed with a form of aggressive power. But the person who hunts down and destroys the sorcerer also deploys a kind of aggressive power.

The situation changes when we come to the system of attacks by ancestral spirits or by spirits brought in by imported religions. In such circumstances we no longer have a dual relationship between two individuals. What we have instead is a relationship pitting an individual against an established law, that of the ancestors. The relationship in this case is with a tradition, with a set of taboos.

It is through deliberate effort that human beings become social beings. We are not born that way. This means we each pay a price for our socialization. Individuals, suppressing their impulses in this process, project their animal aspects outwards. When people talk of attacks by spirits, they often say the purpose is to renew some past alliance, that we have forgotten our dead, that we have forgotten our relatives, including the living, that we have become alienated from others, and that we have adopted lifestyles no longer really compatible with our culture. Possession by spirits, or repossession by them, is a way of reminding us of our obligations. It recalls the possessed to forgotten duties towards members of the family.

For the family of the patient, an attack by spirits might signify that errors have been committed, and that something anomalous has been happening within the dynamics of the family or social group. The first system, in sum, is based on individual, personal relationships. The second is based on relationships with laws and traditions.

The two systems outlined above are well understood by patients, relatives and family members, as articulated by the healer. The systems refer back immediately to rituals and other therapeutic modalities familiar to all and accepted by them. The healer is simply an individual who knows something others do not know. But everyone is capable of understanding, explaining, identifying and naming illnesses and their causes, and discussing them in a common language.

Models: African and Western

We shall now move on to a comparison of our African models with Western models, in an attempt to put the meaning and performance of each in perspective. The ultimate aim is to assess how such performance can benefit society in general, and patients in particular. First, we shall discuss African models.

Assessments of African models fall generally into two schools of thought. The first is that of the humble "pupil" seeking knowledge from traditional sources, willing to obtain it at the feet of past masters, keepers of traditional lore. From this viewpoint, when healers say such and such is the cause of a given illness, their statements are not mere words with interpretative connections to reality. Let me clarify the point. Consider some of the most obscure statements heard in this field. When someone says a sorcerer is eating someone; that an expert healer can weaken a rival wife or cause the dismissal of a government official; that our ancestors have spirits capable of causing us to fall ill if we offend or neglect them, members of this school of thought would argue that the person is only speaking the truth, and that the actions and forces referred to really exist. And they would urge us to study and try to understand the phenomena invoked. As in all research, it is possible, starting from this viewpoint, to reach positive or negative conclusions, to the extent that research confirms or disproves the existence of these supposed realities.

Unfortunately for us, so far, knowledge of the phenomena in question, shrouded in mists of esoteric mystery, is not universally available. Since the condition for acquiring the knowledge in question is that one should get committed to this particular school of thought, we have no clear idea as to what must be done before these esoteric teachings can be incorporated in a general system of knowledge on the same level as all modern, scientific knowledge. Let us put the question another way: what sort of discipline would provide an appropriate framework for parapsychological phenomena? Is it thinkable that beside our own realm of being, there is something para-normal that would enable us to act on things and persons at long range, to speak to each other and give commands at long range, to conduct experiments and experience new realities, to leave our bodies and be incarnated in other bodies, to be here and elsewhere all in the same moment? Here we face an obvious conundrum, and only laboratory studies and research can give us answers. It is much too easy to dismiss such possibilities out of hand, to adopt the arrogant stance of the Westernized master and to say with no proof whatsoever: 'it is all hogwash'.

This is my criticism of certain colleagues who, simply because they see no proof of such realities, dismiss them. At the moment I am engaged in research designed to help me understand these African realities. I am working with selected healers, on a professional basis, in a sense. I have to be able to communicate frankly and seriously with them, because if the phenomena they speak of really exist, their contribution could be of immense value. And it would be a pity if in the end their esoteric lore turned out to be mere hogwash after all. For in that case, Africa, once again and in yet another domain, would have been proved to have made no contribution to the world at large. So much for the viewpoint I described as the first school of thought earlier.

The second school of thought treats the issue of para-normal phenomena and the healers' use thereof as 'a grand practical joke'. From this point of view, what is involved is a lie, but a lie that produces effective results in some areas of life. If this viewpoint is valid, it would indicate that Africans have understood that there are some realities they cannot discuss openly, since naming names would produce no positive results, and would only shatter families.

Suppose, for example, that a mentally disturbed person feels an irresistible urge to make love to his own mother, or that a male twin impregnates his female twin. Nothing would be changed by calling a spade a spade in such a case. The real problem is to determine whether the revelation of such realities would heal any wounds. The fact that a mad son sleeps with his father's fifth wife, or that a child murders his mother, or that some man commits suicide, merely presents us with a raw slice of life. Such facts can be identified and named. But they are facts in a crisis, and the germane question is: to what extent does discussing them openly help resolve the crisis?

In the present state of our knowledge there are a number of facts which, even if we understand them, we are impotent to explain. Let me cite a case related to sexuality. A fellow was able to marry a woman much desired by his bosses and several other rival suitors. On the wedding night his relatives waited for him to consummate the marriage, but he found himself impotent. Nonplussed, he asked his best friend for advice. They hit on a cock-eyed plan: to let the best friend stand in for his impotent friend under cover of darkness. But before daybreak, the groom imagined he heard the radio blaring his secret to the universe. Mortified, he begged his wife's pardon, then went around asking neighbours if they too had heard the news.

This young man's case was hard to treat at the hospital. The African healing system, on the other hand, understood that there were truths better left unsaid, facts better passed under silence because to discuss them openly would only rub pepper into open wounds.

Within this model, then, it is possible to transform the situation, going beyond the simple matter of naming names into a more complex area where the anomaly, without being openly named, is projected elsewhere. The psychological work of healing is then transposed to intentions supposed to exist elsewhere. Some of the available testimony is quite revealing as to what happens in such cases. It might be said, for instance, that 'It was not really my intention to commit suicide. How on earth should I want to kill myself simply because of a failed romance? It is my colleague at the office who cast a "soukpa" hex on me to try and kill me'. This reasoning completely absolves the patient of blame, and the cause of the illness is then located elsewhere than within his person.

A similar explanation might be given for the child who kills his mother: 'He is not the one who committed this weird crime. The fact that a child broke traditional taboos in this way is a sign that a spirit came to disturb his mind, and that is because we neglected such and such a sacrifice'. The child, who previously risked being the accused, becomes instead the victim, carrier of a spiritual message for the community as a whole. Instead of being accused, he is cared for, even honoured. He might actually become a ritual priest, since the spirits have chosen him to bear their message.

There are realities we may feel confusedly, but do not articulate. In certain situations, what happens is a covering up of potentially harmful traces. We can get a good idea of this process of rehabilitative cover-up by considering what happens at family meetings. Elders selected to settle family disputes sometimes find it hard after a meeting, to recapitulate accurately what exactly was said, who was right, who was wrong. Often, the meeting remains wrapped up in a cocoon of confusion conducive to consensus. The guilty party is also wrapped up in this consensus and protected by it, in the interests of general agreement. He knows, though, that he is guilty, and that the cover-up is an encouragement for him to mend his ways. Blameless parties come from such meetings knowing they are right. But they resist the temptation to make too much noise about it, knowing that everyone else wants the affair buried under silence.

In short, the basic concept behind our traditional models seems to be the idea of a cover-up: they are there to mask other realities. And if the system works, the reason is possibly because the truths thus hidden are not broadcast elsewhere. For if every truth were revealed, some day people would be confronted with truths they could no longer live with. The advantage of the model is that it casts guilt on no one - neither the individual nor the family.

Statements made by the traditional healer, the family and the patient fit into a consensus that facilitates cooperation within the group as a whole. At certain family ceremonies each member is asked to bring a small contribution. These are family collections of money, designed to fund ritual observances, etc. Even after conflict, then, willingly or not, all members are called upon to adopt flexible positions and modify their inter-personal relationships, to make possible the emergence of a new world, a new relationship.

A further characteristic of traditional models is that their operative thrust is not focused on the patient or victim. A man may be mad, but only because someone or something has attacked him. Therapy therefore means combating the source of aggression, not focusing on the patient. The one to neutralize may be the expert medicine man or sorcerer who caused the disease. If the instigators are spirits, they must be pacified. And if they happen to be mischievous, evil spirits, genies of a particular location, efforts will be made to placate them, shift them, or drive them out. The operative field of therapy, in other words, is located in some other being, some other environment, within the social group, or in the imaginary world.

Let us turn now to an examination of Western models. Of these the first is the medical, purely biological variant. According to this model, human beings become sick because inside their heads or bodies, something breaks down. The solution is to look for the defective part within the body, then to repair it by injecting it with medical substances, or by operating on it. Within this Western model, patients are alone in their misfortune. The illness, after all, is located within their bodies. They are the ones directly involved in diagnosis and therapy. Therapeutic resources are designed for them. By its very nature, then, the model subjects patients to a certain degree of rejection.

There is a second, psychological model, which we might here take the liberty of calling the psychoanalytical model. According to this model, illness results from behaviour patterns, socialization problems, breakdowns in relationships. The trouble is that psychotherapy, especially in its psychoanalytical variant, operates with and on the individual in need of healing. The patient is alienated; yet therapy is focused on him, not on the reality he needs to be integrated into.

The last Western model is the sociological model. It says no one gets mad by accident. Madness signifies that society has failed to solve its problems. The individual madman is not to blame. In the sociological model, society is a factory that does not want to recognize and take responsibility for its waste products. Not everyone can make it safely through the usual socialization routines. To produce fewer mad persons, society would have to solve its problems. It is an observable fact, after all, that in a given society, when contradictions abound, the number of suicides, behavioural disorders and mental illnesses etc. also rises.

This is admittedly a novel way of looking at the problem. However, it does little to help the mentally disturbed. In short order, they tend to be isolated by society and showered with guilt. Therapists, advocates for the mentally ill, if they belong to the sociological school, also find themselves in a minority. Society creates, educates and trains us, not to criticize it, but to help it make adjustments pinpointed by its effective critics. The sociological movement in the medical profession is also sometimes called the anti-psychiatric movement. It has not been able to make the mentally ill feel better. It has instead contributed to their isolation, widening the gap between the mentally ill and the mentally well-adjusted.

Here we come to a problem, a confusion of methods. It has become fashionable to talk of a complementary relationship between Western and African psychiatry. In reality, however, the tendency is to neglect African models and to concentrate on scientific Western models with their background of laboratory analysis and testing. The problem is that the Western and African models do not use the same methods; neither do they have a common goal.

The traditional model operates in an esoteric mode, assuming the existence of paranormal powers in us, and locating the focus of activity outside the diseased person. Within the traditional model, the phenomena threatening the mentally ill are extraordinarily dangerous, and they exist for all persons. Their invocation does not isolate the patient. Furthermore, the model demands of everyone that together, they agree not to speak the whole truth but to cover up selected aspects of reality. The purpose is to use 'the minor lie' adopted by consensus to ensure group cohesion, the power and dominance of group interests.

This indicates that one of the models does accept responsibility for madness. The mad person is taken over, reintegrated into the traditional milieu, brought back into the social fold. He lives together with others. His statements are understood, experienced, accepted. Where necessary, purification rituals are performed.

The other model leaves the mad person on his own. He is accused, subjected to treatment. This may be because he has had hereditary problems from birth, a likely scenario. Or he may have acquired handicaps due to his upbringing. Or he may suffer from emotional and other inadequacies. In some cases, people get ill because society fails to provide them with employment.

The case for considering the African and Western models as complementary is not particularly clear. An African psychiatrist confronted with a specific case might need to decide which model to operate on. Should he favour the 'objective', modern, Western model? Or should he opt for the traditional African model, with its emphasis on esoteric forces and the power of the group? The trend today, unfortunately, is towards the wholesale adoption of the Western model. This is not true only of the modern medical profession. Traditional and esoteric modes are being consigned to the dustbin. What, under these circumstances, are we to do?

Would it not be a good idea to maintain the tradition of 'the salutary lie'? Is it not preferable, if we can, to recognize our powers, instead of denying them? On the other hand, what sense does it make to reject or deny scientific knowledge on the grounds that the educational system dispensing it is imported? How could anyone neglect or reject this entire heritage? Such is the situation these days: psychiatrists practice on the horns of a dilemma.

To conclude this presentation, let me tell you an anecdote to put matters in perspective. I hope it will also move you to contribute to our discussions, and to offer fruitful advice: A young man, having obtained his high school certificate, entered the university as a first year undergraduate. His studies went badly, so he decided to quit the university and go to work outside. He got a job as an accountant with the Carder-Mono establishment, where he chalked up a record as a serious, sober, diligent worker. One day his boss asked him to give him a travel allowance from the firm's interest. He gave over the money, but forgot to get his boss to sign a receipt. When the boss returned, he asked him to sign the receipt, but the boss refused, deaf to all the accountant's entreaties.

Angered by the matter, the young accountant complained to the District Commissioner, who promised to settle it. He summoned the two and tried to persuade the boss to be reasonable, but the boss got angry. Shortly thereafter, the accountant hastily requested leave and left his job. Leaving a suitcase with his elder sister, he said he was heading for Parakou. Next, he was found in Niger, where he remained for four years.

What had happened? Had he abandoned his job and run away to Niger? He came back entirely penniless, wearing a tattered shirt and ranting gibberish all day long. He was ill. His high school certificate and accountant's diploma had become useless. He felt unseen forces attacking him. He said they were behind the house. Once, hearing more of them coming to get him, he threw a stone in their direction. It broke the windshield of a car parked behind the house. Its owners grabbed him, tied him up, took him first to the Police Station and then to the Local Area Commissioner, before finally taking him to the psychiatric ward.

I had a chance to see the patient. He was young, slender in a rangy sort of way. He showed signs of hallucination, smiling and laughing without visible cause. These were symptoms of a psychotic state, a case of schizophrenia, a serious illness. That was the situation when the patient's sister told us the story I've just told you. She ended with a declaration that at first everything was fine. The only trouble was that her brother did not want to be corrupted. She said the boss had been dismissed for his misconduct, but had threatened the accountant in the following words: 'You want me to lose my post. You can't keep yours either'. We asked the sister what she had been able to do since then. Her answer was: 'I'm a Roman Catholic. All I do is pray'.

There's the story. See what you think of it. For our part, we arrived at a diagnosis, which turned out to be correct. We shall now try and get him to settle down and go quietly about his business. But he will not forget this other dimension, real or imaginary, which hounds him because an interpersonal relationship was not smoothed over to make things happen more harmoniously. Here we have a sister who suggests to us the possible source of the problem. But she is a Catholic, and Catholics only pray.

What, we may wonder, does she really want to communicate to us? Does she really believe there are things hounding her brother? If that were the case, we psychiatrists would have nothing left to do. The patient would have to go elsewhere to get cured. If, on the other hand, the problem had a different cause, then we would have to go to work on the particular case, to try and make out the chain of events leading from the patient's conception and birth through childhood to the day he lost his mind. The incident on the job might then turn out to be no more than a tiny spark that set alight material already in a combustible state, perhaps rendered volatile by some hereditary defect. And we are still left with our dilemma: how to harmonize the African and Western viewpoints?

Discussion

The following is a transcription of a discussion which took place after the presentation of this chapter at the National University of Benin seminar (see introduction chapter for details).

Paulin Hountondji: I find the theory of the effective lie put forward as an explanation for the therapeutic effectiveness of mythical aetiologies particularly stimulating. The thinking behind such aetiologies appears at first sight to be completely deranged, yet it sometimes produces perfectly tangible results.

Bouraïma Moukadam: First, I wonder whether the two approaches to mental illness do not put you, as a specialist, in the problematic position of having to restructure an established classification of illnesses in the Western style, and beyond that, having to face a comprehensive challenge to the scientific tradition in which you have been trained. Second, I would like your ideas on ways in which Christian and syncretistic religions might be a source of mental illness.

Gualbert Ahyi: You have put your finger precisely on the conundrum confronting me. As I said, the choice is a difficult one. I've pointed out that the Western and African models do not really complement each other. To go back to the example I gave at the end of my talk, if the African model, properly understood, turned out to be true, then as modern psychiatrists we would simply have to close shop. Clearly, the model is a challenge to our practice. Occasionally, we come up against real cases which raise exactly this kind of problem. Where we have hesitated, or where our therapeutic efforts have failed, relatives of patients have sometimes quietly asked us to let them go and try their luck elsewhere. In some cases we went along with that idea. They tried suggested models and methods, and achieved prompt results. When I said just now that we sometimes had doubts, I meant there were cases in which we did not apply esoteric methods ourselves, yet understood that it might have been better to hand the patients over to traditional healers, even if all they got was some communal rhetoric. Sometimes, problems get solved in unexpected ways.

Unfortunately, though, we have had cases where the traditional, rhetorical methods have been applied, with no positive result. On the other hand, in my experience as a psychiatrist, I have often 'exorcised sorcerers' using medical pills. Patients have taken them and been cured. They were sick people supposedly 'attacked by witches'. Now I know nothing about witchcraft; yet my diagnoses, based on the patients' behaviour and my own information, turned out to be right. I administered the medicine, and it worked.

In some respects, I wonder whether the thing to do is not to gradually unravel the knots of interpretation and observation, separating fact from fiction. I have started doing research into sorcery. To minimize the risk of error, I began by identifying fake witchcraft. That already assumes there might be genuine witchcraft, but I confess I have yet to come across it personally. I hope it really exists. In my practice, I have dealt successfully with some cases of witchcraft, but I call them fake cases, and my concern is to understand the dynamics behind them. It is those cases that have baffled me that I suppose, possibly, might be genuine instances of witchcraft.

There was a question as to how the syncretistic religions could be held accountable for the increase in mental illnesses. Take the example of Islam. Muslim teachings can drive some individuals mad. As you know, Muslims believe in two types of spirits: devils and genies, identified as forces of evil and good. The mentality of believers interprets all events as results of the actions of specific spirits. These spirits have to be exorcised by ceremonial rituals. Within the religious context, then, that explanatory model is valid, in the sense that it is based on beliefs that determine mental attitudes and inform behaviour. Roman Catholics are in a similar situation. And Protestants, Pentecostals and members of other Christian sects all agree that there are evil spirits which drive people mad. And there are cases in which we identify the source of illness as a conflict between two parties at the office or elsewhere.

It is quite common for psychiatrists to learn, after some Christian patient stops coming to the clinic or hospital for consultations, that it is because the parish priest has taken over the case, and is busy exorcising some demon possessing the patient. Such demons do exist, and there are priests appointed by the bishop or archbishop to exorcise them. You know, of course, that among Catholics and Protestants alike, services and masses are sometimes held during which the congregation waits for demons to come out of possessed victims, freeing them from physical or mental illnesses.

Ignace Djenontin: There are frequent cases of mental breakdown in academic institutions, ordinarily described as madness. There is the example of a high school certificate candidate who, after a hard night's swotting on the eve of the final examination, woke up only to be told the time: 'twelve midday'. From that moment, he began to mutter over and over again the single word: 'midday'. What is the explanation for frequent cases of this kind? In such cases, can we talk of witchcraft or society as causes of mental illness?

A second question: you said some traditional healers were able to heal patients. Did you mean they achieved definitive cures? Or was it more a case of temporary remissions, after which in most cases the diseased persons relapsed, and were thus obliged to remain permanently with the healer?

Edouard Wallace: The speaker's dilemma is real. Western therapy is different from traditional therapy. I think, nevertheless, that these days it has become imperative to reconcile the two methods.

Albert Gbodogbe: I would like the speaker to give us a general description of mental illness, types of mental illness, and the difference between symptoms of mental illnesses caused by external factors and those not traceable to such factors. Lastly, what are the speaker's opinions about sociological causes of mental illness?

Gualbert Ahyi: Let us start with madness in the academic environment. There too, unfortunately, there are two schools of thought. As a psychiatrist, I would say that any emotional shock, pleasant or disagreeable, can cause illness. You cited the case of a student who overslept and woke up to find his future shattered. From our point of view, powerful emotions can cause mental illness, whether they are pleasant or unpleasant.

There are people who go mad because their children get married. Some people have been known to fall ill right after winning a lottery jackpot. Others fall ill because they lose. The modern explanation focuses on the strength of the emotional shock received. It is a plausible explanation. Traditional explanations, on the other hand, make no room for simple chance. On stepping out of my house, I stub my left big toe against a stone. Why the left and not the right? I must consult the diviner, because I have to get to the root of the incident. The factual truth or falsehood of the supposed 'root' of the problem is beside the point.

An individual's failure may be attributed to the machinations of a jealous colleague, or the evil wishes of a stepmother. The individual in question thus invents an aggressor, because it is hard to admit one's own fault in oversleeping, as in the case of the tardy student. It is just as hard to take the responsibility for missing classes, the real cause of failure. In this situation, the student gets absolved of all blame, because the cause of failure is some other person.

The trouble with this approach is that it can cause disturbances in other areas that should normally be left intact. Intelligent healers can shift the supposed 'root cause' into another dimension, thus opening up new operative perspectives and opportunities. For example, they might conclude that failure is the result of neglect of the ancestors, the omission of a libation for twins, etc. That removes the factor of blame. The libation gets poured at last, facilitating reconciliation and raising fallen hopes of future success. The optimism thus engendered holds out a promise of success.

In the modern system, however, we acknowledge that the individual overslept, and that the mistake was his. We prescribe an anti-depressant to help him cheer up and make the best of the situation. In that way we prevent him from collapsing into mental illness.

Methods used by the two models differ. One holds that nothing happens by accident, and that in all cases we must look for hidden causes. The other asserts that the problem is the result of the individual's own mistakes, and that he must make the effort to bear the consequences, with the help of drugs prescribed by the doctor.

Someone asked whether traditional healers heal their patients for good. I cannot say the cure is definitive in all cases. The reason is that most of our patients come to us after having consulted traditional healers and performed a number of ceremonial rites in the hope of a definitive cure. The last ritual was the shaving of the patients' heads. But they later relapsed into illness. Still, we have to admit that some traditional healers really do produce definitive cures, provided connections between factors involved in the disturbance are clearly established. In other words, the anomaly identified as the cause of illness must first be corrected.

Let us take an example: We know of a case in which a son unjustifiably cursed by his father left his home village and for ten years did not communicate with his father. One day he returned home with a son he had fathered during his exile. That same night he fell ill. Called to treat him, I discovered that the hidden cause of his illness was the paternal curse uttered ten years previously. According to his relatives, it had been heard and ratified by ancestral spirits. So certain ceremonies had to be organized to heal psychological wounds and ensure a more efficient management of past realities. From that time on there was never another crisis between father and son.

There are other situations in which we modern psychiatrists operate like removers not of causes but of symptoms. It is in such cases that traditional healers sometimes out-perform us. When you remove a symptom, the individual withdraws into himself. You give him stimulants and he may begin to move around, but soon he retreats into his shell again, because he still feels surrounded with permanently threatening presences. Drugs, in other words, alleviate disease only to a limited extent. When they are eliminated to enable the therapeutic process to focus on 'relationships', the patient stands a pretty good chance of getting definitively cured. In effect, traditional healers who succeed in re-establishing shattered relationships achieve definitive cures. Psychiatrists can achieve the same results, but in their case, instances of success are rare.

Psychiatrists also go to work on patients' bodies. During psychoanalytical sessions, psychiatrists target inhibitions, encourage patients to rediscover their potential, to take closer stock of their psychic bases in the interests of their own happiness. They may go some way towards admitting their shortcomings, but in that process they are all alone, since the responsibility falls entirely on their own shoulders. Those unable to tote that burden may commit suicide. There have been cases of patients leaving the psychiatrist's clinic to go drown themselves. Others come out all smiles, because they have been given fresh insights into their lives, and have at least tried to solve their problems, or at any rate to take charge of their own lives.

The basic difference between traditional healers and us, modern doctors, is that they heal relationships, we heal bodies. It is hard for us to heal relationships where we work, inside hospitals. There, patients are on their own. So what kind of relationship is it possible to create? We are reduced to giving our patients drugs and keeping them quiet. These days we have begun imitating traditional healers by hospitalizing patients with selected members of their families. This gives a sliver of hope. We watch what happens between patient and relative, then ask the latter questions. Where necessary, we call in the family to enable them to see the patient's progress or regression, and to help in his treatment. But at certain points, when we try to identify the problem with utter clarity, the situation slithers out of our control. The reason is that when we name the problem, we bring the truth out into the open, and the open truth is hard to admit, to accept responsibility for. In sum, we modern psychiatrists have yet to hit on that small lie which makes it possible to establish group consensus and heal the sick through the power of relationships.

There was a question about religions. It is true that religious bodies have their share of taboos. But if there is a rise in the incidence of illness, and religious groups are helping to deal with them, the reason is that the medical system is in some respects a fiasco. For the medical system should be so designed as to care for human beings in their wholeness, not for their bodies only. The solution is to accept responsibility for humans, wholly and completely. This modern medicine has failed to do. The mentally ill need human relationships, certain kinds of social security. African families provided such security in the past, but increasingly these days, they can no longer cope. Now it does not matter what drugs we give our patients; there comes a time, inevitably, when they feel all alone. There are certain communities and religious groups that have grown hugely successful, with multitude of adepts. Such a community may decide, for instance, that on Sundays their mass or religious service will last not a mere hour but the entire day. The faithful go there even to wash their laundry, and remain there to see it dry. They seize every opportunity for living together, eating together, because in this way they build up and enjoy a certain sense of security.

Concurrently, such religious groups try to dig into the traditional model, hoping to find resources absent in modern life. Many of these religions are now attempting to focus public anguish on witchcraft. From the traditional to the syncretistic religious vision, all members talk about is sorcery. Individuals joining them adopt a number of common group practices. But as a rule, the reason why so many people turn to these religious groups and communities is that they offer an atmosphere of family life. For that reason, I think we psychiatrists need to revise our working methods.

We now come to the crucial issue of definitive cures and temporary alleviation punctuated by relapses. After some thought, I concluded that if I could form a sort of 'community' with my former patients, relapses would no longer be experienced as collapses into illness. Let me give an example. Not far from where I live, there is a community belonging to a cult called 'Tigari', originally from Ghana. The intriguing thing is that while we interpret fresh hysterical crises as relapses into illness, members of this cult interpret them as new visitations from the spirit world. Individuals experiencing hysterical crises are thus accepted and socialized. Their identity is no longer that of sick people; instead, they are regarded as spokespersons for God or some particular spirit. Patients then become cult members. This gives them the time they need to fashion a new life, without having to change their status in all respects.

Now it is possible to give such patients a new vision in life without having to isolate or discourage them.. As far as they are concerned, they experienced such and such a vision or faced such and such a problem because someone attacked them. If there are fresh attacks, new interpretative visions can be found for them. Patients are not certified inmates in a concentration camp for failures. Instead, they remain part of a continuing process, based on a type of group thinking with its own logic.

By contrast, all the modern system offers is a bleak scenario of cure-and-relapse, the only basis of judgement being the general environment. It is in this respect that, in my opinion, traditional healers go us one better. We do maintain friendly relationships with our patients, of course. But there are unfortunate time limitations on our practice. After their brief sojourn with us, we give former patients medical chits declaring them cured, or convalescent; then we send them back to work. When we do this, we botch the solution to problems of interpersonal and group relationships, as well as our own relationships with patients. We have to keep seeing them, but under what circumstances might we see them again? Often, we assume no responsibility for creating, between ourselves and the patients we suppose cure, special social bonds that last, and which both parties want to maintain. In this department I think we have a lot to learn from traditional healers. They could prove of tremendous help in the creation of new African models.

To give a general description of mental illness, types of mental illness, and the difference between symptoms of mental illnesses caused by some external factor and those not traceable to such factors, I would have to summarize the entire field of psychiatry. That would take some time. But I can give a brief classification, along the following lines:

a) *Neurotics*: are people who have problems relating to others and creating an independent personality. On account of problems encountered in their infancy, they are permanently in conflict with others.

b) *Psychotics*: are noisy, agitated people, who experienced deficiencies extremely early in life.

c) *Psychopaths*: are antisocial people, prone to violence, destruction, rape, etc.

d) *Mentally retarded people*: have poorly developed brains. The kind of people we know here as *yèyinon*, that is to say, idiots.

In between the different categories come psychosomatic illnesses. In such cases, lasting emotional shocks end up affecting the body. Students sometimes contract such illnesses as exam time draws near, with scholarship stipends still unpaid. Fear of poor exam grades sends their glands into overdrive, and they come down with ulcers. Psychosomatic illnesses are makeshift expediencies that in the end leave basic psychological problems unsolved.

On the difference between externally instigated illnesses and natural illnesses, speaking as a psychiatrist I would say that mental illnesses cannot be externally provoked. But from the viewpoint of traditional healers, it has been observed that sometimes illnesses presenting the same signs may be natural or externally provoked, depending on how long they last. Natural illnesses can be cured quickly because they are simple, assuming they are not terminal. Illnesses that worsen over time, on the other hand, are sometimes construed as having external causes. For instance, a patient may contract an illness that starts out as something,but the traditional healer may find human factors associated and accordingly go to work to deal with it. The point is that it is not a consideration of symptoms alone that enters into the decision. As we have pointed out, traditional healers are not primarily interested in symptoms. After all, some symptoms may provide indications, but others are not particularly useful. The traditional healer therefore proceeds on the basis of continuing developments, and on information from the diviner's board.

François de Meideros: I would like to say simply that Professor Ahyi's contribution has opened up vast vistas for lay persons unfamiliar with the field. I found a number of the points he raised striking. First, Dr. Ahyi's conclusion gave the impression of a gap between the traditional and Western models so deep as to make their reconciliation difficult. I think that conclusion rather pessimistic. The assumed dichotomy on which it is based is somewhat farfetched. After all, judging from his own words, in Dr. Ahyi's practice he is far from adhering to a single model. His report indicates considerable progress in the treatment of the type of illness he discussed.

The presentation raised a large number of interesting points. I for one would like some more discussion of the primary relationship between mother and child. I was most struck by the perception of African man that makes the mother, then the parents and relatives, the primary significant others. A background for subsequent conflicts is located there. I find this interpretative approach extremely fruitful. I think it would be worth following. It could prove beneficial. Supposing a Western model that makes no provision for this relationship leaves a major lacuna, this could prove to be a new interpretative approach.

On the subject of para-psychology, let me present an anecdote. Last year, in the course of a magical show, the magician proposed that a number of people recite certain formulae. When they did so, there were immediate results. For instance, formulae were used to make the hands of volunteers get stuck together. This would only be possible because the volunteers had been hypnotized. Assuming there was no trickery, what happened was certainly an example of words achieving an immediate effect. This kind of reality has yet to be thoroughly explored, and Western models do not take it into account.

I wonder if, in the final analysis, the path described by Dr. Ahyi is the only one likely to produce ruptures in relationships. The issue of ruptured social relationships reminds me of a different kind of report I read recently, this time dealing with the impact of legal systems on human relationships. The author was a theologian, and his subject was Law. Taking as an example the statement that gas chambers were reprehensible in point of law, he argued that such an assertion was utterly inadequate. In his opinion the real issue lay deeper. For if individuals were permitted by law to abuse others as 'dirty Jews', and if society considered such behaviour acceptable, then the highway to the gas chambers was already open. In other words, legal activity, to be effective, had to focus on opinion, that is to say, the media. I think what happens in mental behaviour is somewhat similar.

Victoire Elegbe: A moment ago the speaker explained that madness could be caused by either type of emotional shock, positive (as a result of marriage) or negative (as in the instance of the student who slept past exam time). From what I understand, it seems that in order to cure mental illness brought on by an emotional shock, an equally powerful emotional shock is needed to re-establish lost balance. I am reminded of the example of a woman travelling in a car with her husband. They get into a crash; the husband dies and the wife loses her memory. To help her regain her memory under the impact of a retrospective shock, attempts are made to reconstruct the accident. My question is: does such a phenomenon have a rational, objective explanation?

There have been cases of persons getting overstressed as a result of intense physical and mental exertion. They go into a depression, and are given medical treatment. But then it is observed that at certain times, often coinciding with the full moon, they relapse into illness. There are those who claim such relapses are caused by the lunar cycle. Are they right or wrong? And how might such a phenomenon be explained in medical terms?

Ignace Djenontin: I would like to know at what stage in the progress of mental illness the disease is still curable.

Gualbert Ahyi: I am a pessimist by nature. That , for me, might be a source of strength. I have said a lot remains to be done. But I have also said that we need to get to work. In my opinion, before a really close examination of traditional and Western models, it is easy to suppose that they could be nicely complementary. For a very long time in Dakar, a group of us psychiatrists believed we could cooperate with traditional healers. In time, and after terrible soul-searching, I came to understand that we had achieved nothing. All we had done was to conduct research into superficial details the traditional healers did not explain to us. This failure of open cooperation, which happens throughout Africa, is the real obstacle in the way of the complementarity of the two models. It makes me wonder if the goal is worth pursuing. There is a risk of a total metamorphosis in the long run. I say the obstacle is contrived, because if people really want to commit themselves to a complementary approach, it should be feasible.

The question, though, is whether we cam really be understood. After all, we are supposed to be the custodians of science with a capital S, and we come on affecting a particular status. Sometimes, among ourselves, there are statements we are unable to make at conferences, simply because not all experts agree on them. To utter such seriously controversial statements might lead to crises. In effect, a long road mined with problems lies ahead of us. I have had the experience of going to certain traditional healers to ask if we could work together. When they agreed, it was on a number of conditions. For one thing, they regarded the research group we thus formed as some sort of closed circle. Access to it was limited to a select few. The traditional healers would first of all have to submit each member of my research team to a loyalty test, based on divination, specifically designed to find out if they were likely to be traitors. Secondly, we had to limit our number to five. These precautions were related to taboos whose nature could not be made plain to just anyone.

The point is that some types of knowledge are double-edged swords. Within the traditional model, people do not become healers through simple selection processes like high school certificate examinations or competitive tests. The healers themselves identify certain qualities as indicating aptitude. It is only those who have them who can be entrusted with certain powers, knowledge and skills indispensable for learning and mastering the art of healing.

Western models clearly recognize the primary importance of the mother-child relationship. However, the relationship to one's mother, from the African perspective, is altogether special. Considering the permanent contact between mother and child, the lateness of the weaning period, and the range of physical manipulations children get subjected to by the group, mother-child relationships in Africa tend to constitute an extremely rich type of contact with strong psychological impact. This is important in our everyday behaviour.

I think it would be a good idea to have parapsychological laboratories. I tried a low-profile start, because when you move into such a field, you are not dealing with scientific realities alone. Para-psychological studies require the installation of laboratories and a substantial quantity of equipment for the conduct of analyses and tests. In some developed countries, para-psychology is already a university discipline. Here, paranormal phenomena of a crude sort are part of everyday life, according to reports, at any rate. But for now, no use is made of the information.

Once, I told an academic colleague that telepathy could have material foundations. His interest aroused, he immediately drew closer after I told him the following story: a couple, having quarrelled and fought, separated. So heavy were the insults they traded that it was inconceivable that they could ever again live together or even visit each other. One day, a family friend went to the separated wife and told her: 'I have a confession to make. At the time when you were living abroad and did not want to come and marry the man, I intervened to make you come and marry him. That was a mistake. I made it because he was my friend. Now I know him better, and I know he is worthless'. The woman replied that she did not believe a word he'd said. 'How on earth could you have made me come to Benin against my will? Can you prove you did that?' 'It is quite true', the friend answered. 'When you were out there, we had to go and consult a healer. He gave us a plant and told your husband to urinate on it, focusing all his thoughts on you and wishing your return. He said you would return. And sure enough, you did return'. To convince the woman, the two went in search of the particular healer. They asked him to repeat the experiment, targeted this time at the husband. The healer began by remarking that the husband had been ungrateful, then gave the same plant to the woman to urinate on, focusing her thoughts and wishing for her husband's return. The woman wanted him back that same day. She did as advised, and that same day her husband came to visit her. When asked why, he had no answer.

I think something other than simple juju is at work here, namely, certain truths not yet explained or experimentally tested, but which might be brought under control. If that is the case, we had better stop declaring such reports false without experimentation. These realities contain elements that call for research. Let me say that often enough, I have faced a number of problems that I wanted later to discuss with some colleagues here now. The reason was that these phenomena really happened, and I thought I could understand them within my rationalist mental framework. Yet people convinced me I was wrong.

One day, for instance, around 10 am, a woman came to my clinic and told me she was a witch. She came with one of my patients, and I was asked to sign a medical chit permitting him to take two months' sick leave. That would give him time to travel with the self-proclaimed witch to a venue where rituals would be conducted to counter the effects of spells cast on him by a community of sorcerers. I asked the woman why she was making such a statement. She said:

> This man knows very well why. He wanted to enter a seminary. We in the village were against the idea. So at a sorcerers' coven we decided to deal with him. Our aim was to dissuade him. But he had relatives in our coven. We decided not to kill him, but simply to cut him down to size. That is exactly what we did. Now he is out of the seminary; he did not become a priest. He is a teacher, but he is ill. He has been ill for almost 14 years. That is too long. We have to help him now. What kind of treatment have you been able to give him?

I gave her my diagnosis. She asked me if that was the only diagnosis he was getting treated for, and if I was the only doctor treating him. I informed her that another qualified professor was treating him for sinusitis while I treated him for a case of intellectual repression, each doctor treating him separately. She said that was not all; that the patient had said he was getting treated for hypertension as well, by a third doctor. In conclusion, the woman said we were all a bunch of ignorant idiots.

I must say I was somewhat displeased, but I took the insult in good spirit, mumbling that she could well be right. The woman then told me my patient had hidden something from me, another illness he was being treated for, or ought to be treated for: a permanent erection. At that point I took a close look at the patient. I had been treating him for over two years, but he had never told me about this ailment. He corroborated what the self-declared witch had said, whereupon the latter said; 'See, I told you so. Four of you have been treating him. Didn't I say you were idiots? Me, I know what we've done to him'.

> Listen. We put two types of hex on him. First, we asked a poor villager to go beg him for one of his old seminary gowns. He gave it up as alms, and we used it to hex him. He had left his mark on the garb, so even though he wasn't physically there, he was present. We decided to do two things with the gown. We tied a piece of it to a pigeon, recited an incantation over it and let it fly. Pigeons are thought to have good memories. The moment the pigeon flew off with a piece of his gown, our man could no longer become a seminarian. The reason was that his studies at the seminary were demanding, but he could no longer cope. He had a permanent headache. After handicapping him in this way, we had to point him in a different direction. We took the remainder of his garb and, after reciting an incantation, tied it to a ram. Since then, our seminarian has had a permanent erection, chasing women from dawn to dusk. Because he fears to disgrace himself, being a former seminarian, he spends all his time fighting the erection. So he has hypertension. You treat him for headaches, another tackles his cold, a third takes on his hypertension, and all the time the problem is much less complicated.

I gave the witch back the consultation fee, signed a chit giving the patient two months' sick leave, bade them goodbye and asked them to let me know what happened. The witch promised to come and see me next day at around 10 o'clock. My wife was worried for me and her children, who were disturbed at the mere presence of the witch. Before leaving, the witch said she was going the next 'Holy Saturday' on a 'trip' to the residence of a high ranking churchman where she and her colleagues had buried two stakes. The stakes had to be dug up as a first step in the treatment. On Easter Sunday she returned to show me two stakes, one worm-eaten, the other new.

Like any good rationalist, I pointed out that it was impossible for a stake to have remained spanking new after being buried for fourteen years while another, buried under the same conditions for the same length of time, had turned worm-eaten. The witch retorted that I was silly, and that people like me saw only the external aspect of realities. She said it was possible to hollow out a yam without physically touching it, and that the remains of objects could be used to restore them completely.

Thanking her, I told her I did not believe she could succeed, adding that I too knew something of the ways of traditional healers. I thought it incorrect of her to try on her own to change a group decision, if such a decision had indeed been taken. On that point she agreed with me, but argued that an issue of rank was involved. According to her, some members of the witches' coven were like simple lamps, some like hurricane lanterns and the highest like electric lights. I said I'd understood, wished her good luck, and to said good bye.

When she had pulled up the stakes, she had washed them to make an infusion with which she treated the patient's sinus condition. That was her first achievement. But 15 days after she left, I saw my patient, and he was sicker than before. Upon investigation, I heard that when the witch had gone back to the Mono area, where incidentally the patient also lived, she heard even before she got home that her two grandchildren were in a coma. Apparently, the village witches were upset at her attempts to cure the man they had hexed. Deciding therefore to abandon the patient to his fate, she picked up her grandchildren and took them to Northern Togo, where she had done her apprenticeship in sorcery. She needed to protect herself and her offspring. So once more I went to work on my patient. He is still a sick man. I gave him a medical certificate which helped him get a transfer to an administrative post, since he could not be expected to teach pupils in his condition.

I decided to write a report designed to stimulate greater interest in this aspect of traditional medicine. I gave it the title: 'Towards a Reorientation of Research in Traditional Medicine'. The point of the title is to underline the fact that so far, physiologists, bio-chemists, botanists and pharmacists have focused solely on the pharmacological aspect of traditional medicine. I think we should try and explore the paranormal aspects as well. I think in the esoteric domain, there is a lot of information we have yet to discover, about phenomena we do not understand. My intention, in short, is to urge researchers not to focus exclusively on aspects considered important in Europe. Our hopes of achieving significant breakthroughs are greater in such new sectors than, say, in the discovery of new molecules.

9

Foreign Objects in Human Bodies: A Surgeon's Report

Henry-Valère T. Kiniffo

A foreign object in a human body, as a coroner's report might define it, is any article that normally does not constitute part of said human body. The pencil before me now, for instance, is a foreign object as far as my body is concerned, because it does not belong within it. In my practice as a surgeon, I have occasionally come across unusual objects incorporated, in some strange manner, into the bodies of some of my patients. There is a wide range of possible explanations as to how they got there in the first place.

Types of Foreign Objects Found in Human Bodies

Foreign objects get into human bodies in a variety of ways. There are cases of children sticking pencils in their ears and breaking the graphite tips in there. Others push marbles up their nostrils, swallow coins or shirt buttons. Foreign objects, in other words, may get into human bodies by accident, through ignorance, or simply by mistake. On occasion, they might be introduced into human bodies with self-destructive intent, that is to say, in a suicidal bid. In such cases, individuals bent on killing themselves may swallow sharp objects such as razor blades or pins, which then get stuck in their throats.

Normally, the extraction of such objects is a straightforward matter. It takes only a pair of forceps to pull out objects stuck inside ears or noses. Accidents of this sort are of course spectacular, and doctors have to keep patients from panicking. This is easy enough, especially when the objects in question are not particularly sharp. If they are lodged in the alimentary canal, they follow the normal route from oesophagus to anus. For this to happen, care must be taken to sheathe them prior to their evacuation, to avoid the risk of their getting embedded in body tissue. The patient's relatives are advised to give the child fibrous food such as carrots, strings beans, or any other foodstuff that can insulate the object. Even cotton might be swallowed for the purpose. Once so covered, the object is likely to be evacuated in the patient's stool within a couple of days. An x-ray photograph is necessary at the start to locate the foreign object. Three days later, a second x-ray photo should help determine whether the object has in fact been evacuated. It is advisable, indeed, to have the patient use a chamber pot for defecation. This makes it possible to confirm the exit.

Other foreign objects might get into human bodies by more violent means. Well known examples include stray bullets or buckshot fired from hunting guns. Hunters sometimes get a shotgun blast right in the face. X-rays can track the precise locations of the pellets. Some pellets can be pulled out. Others, located in parts of the body where they can do no harm, are left alone. There are cases of ex-servicemen who got shot in the head, the bullets settling under the brain without actually touching it. There are similar cases of persons at the receiving end of salvos of gunfire ending up with pellets imbedded next to their backbones. Sometimes the natural motion of the bullets pushes them against the spine.

Where their extraction seems too dangerous, they are left in the body, but physicians keep track of their locations. When it is clear that they have to be removed, this is done through a surgical operation. First, the precise openings through which they entered the body are identified. The next step is to trace the trajectory of the bullet from the point of entry to its final location, using ballistic techniques. After that it is time to go after the bullets. Sometimes all such pellets and bullets are found. In other cases only some are extracted, because the remainder have already made their exit after transiting through the body. In such situations the surgeon examines both the entry and exit holes. Where the numbers of the two sets of holes match, there is no problem: all bullets shot into the body came out. When there is a mismatch, for example with 12 entry holes and only eight exit holes, it becomes necessary to look for the remainder, four bullets in this example. The procedure involved is a basic part of forensic medical practice, and there are trained specialists in the field.

We have looked at two ways — one peaceful, the other violent — in which foreign objects can get into human bodies. Foreign objects can get into human bodies in other ways, some of them curious indeed.

The exhibits at the Medical Museum in Paris include a series of amazing objects that people at some time pushed into their bodies. For example, certain persons are known to have pushed wooden phalluses up their you-know whats, where they got stuck, necessitating retrieval. Other exhibits show crosses retrieved from young girls' bladders. You can imagine how they got up there: boarding school girls masturbating with crucifixes turned into dildos. Doctors got to know of such cases because the presence of such foreign objects, detected by X-rays, caused ailments such as urinary infections.

Incidentally, there is another category of foreign objects such as gallstones that get formed inside bladders or bile ducts. These are not normal bodily components. They cause ailments, and have to be extracted too.

In the world of deviant behaviour, there are spectacular cases of foreign objects getting into human bodies. For instance, whole containers of yoghurt have been found in the large intestines of homosexuals who inserted them in the anus and then lost them as they got sucked upwards. Since the container blocked the intestinal tract, making normal evacuation impossible, illness ensued. In such cases also, surgical work was necessary. If the container was not too far up the intestines, the patient was simply made to lie down, the passage was dilated, and the object removed either manually or with the aid of forceps. In my courses on forensic medicine for magistrates and judges, I often cite this type of case when dealing with the subject of sexual deviance and social mores.

To conclude this survey of ways in which foreign objects get into human bodies by accident, we should mention cases resulting from technical errors committed by surgeons or other health workers. The problem might be caused by hypodermic needles breaking inside the body. As you are probably aware, needles tend to travel in the body. A needle might enter a body through the buttocks but end up in the knee. In lucky cases they get embedded in body tissue and can easily be removed.

It is possible for quite a number of other objects to get stuck by mishap in patients' bodies after surgical operations: compresses, scissors, forceps, etc. Just a year ago I actually came across a surgeon's lancet inside the body of a patient I had to operate on. An abscess had grown around the buttock where the lancet had been sewn in, and for years the patient had walked around with it floating in a small pool of pus under his skin.

Apart from foreign objects introduced into human bodies through surgical malpractice, oversight or the firing of projectiles, there are others which get into people's bodies by less clearly defined means. For the moment, let us simply call these means 'mysterious'. Let me recount an anecdote on this head. Thirty-two years ago, when I was a young student in Dijon, I went to hear a lecture given by a white priest. His topic: 'Mysteries of Africa'. He told a series of weird stories like those I am about to narrate here. At the end of his lecture I told him: 'Father, I'd like to express my appreciation to you. I'm glad you took the initiative of saying all this. I'm in a position to support what you've said. If I had delivered this lecture myself, the audience would have responded with sarcastic smiles and thought I was just another young African telling tales. But you are a priest, a man of God, and you have reported what you saw. As an African who knows these things, I bear witness to their truth'.

A moment ago I described a broken bit of a needle that stayed stuck in the right buttock of a man for eight years before we pulled it out. A needle like that might enter a human body neither by accident nor by deliberate insertion, but in much more mysterious ways. To give you a better understanding of my drift, let me tell you another story: As you are no doubt aware, in our country, inheritance disputes give rise to problems galore. Now there was a catechist whose father died young. The dispute about the inheritance caused a rift between him and the rest of the family. One day, standing at his window, he felt a searing pain in his left forearm. Right then there was no other development, but two weeks later the forearm swelled up, and the catechist saw he had an abscess on his hands. He was taken to the local clinic, where a nurse incised the abscess to drain the pus. But in addition to the pus, a needle came out. The catechist masked his astonishment at the time, but a week later the forearm swelled up again. Back to the clinic for another incision. Result: more pus, then another needle. At this point the nurse, with admirable presence of mind, asked the catechist to undergo an x-ray test. The resulting photo (see Figure 1) showed a number of other needles imbedded in the forearm. The conundrum was: how did all these needles get into the catechist's forearm?

Figure 1: X-ray of a Man's Left Forearm*

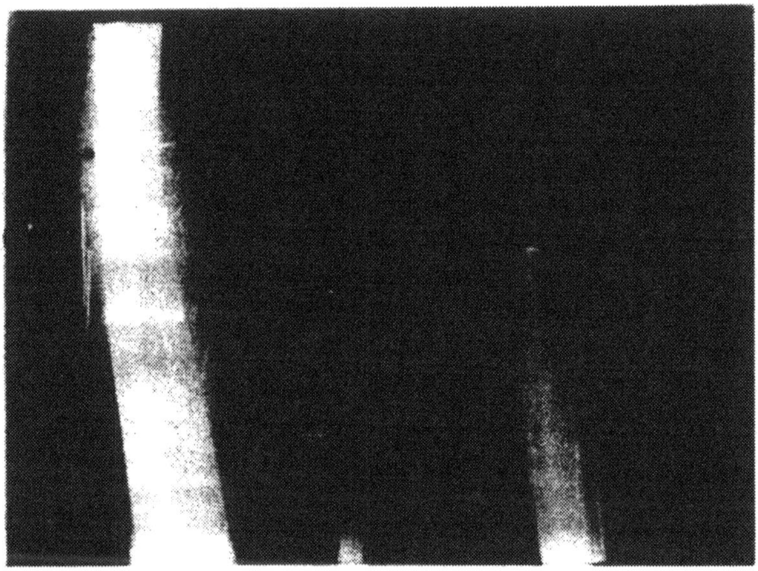

* Note Mysteriously Inserted Needles

Now the catechist was not a little boy. He was quite unlikely to have fallen on a bunch of needles. He told me as much, then reported the matter to his bishop. The bishop, a local man, understood immediately what had happened. He asked a traditional healer to draw out the needles, using a method that might be called a magnetic laying on of hands (this involves a motion or sign made by the healer over some parts of the body to draw out foreign objects imbedded there). The healer claimed he could not do as requested, because two incisions had already been made over the 'psychic area' he would have had to work on. The area, in other words, had been desecrated. The bishop then brought the catechist to me, told me the story, and asked what I could do about extracting the remaining needles. I told him: 'All I have to work with is my lancet'. I located the needles, operated on the patient, and drew them all out.

The needles were undeniably there. The x-ray photo confirmed their presence, and I actually drew them out by surgical means.

A little over two months ago, around the time when Professor Hountondji asked me to deliver this talk, a woman came to my surgery complaining that she felt sharp objects pricking her, and that she felt generally unwell. I told her: 'This is a case of chakatu. You have to try and do something about it'. (Chakatu is the name given to a discharge from an invisible gun that hurls miscellaneous projectiles into the human body). She therefore went to a traditional healer, who extracted from her body numerous objects including fishing hooks, shards from broken bottles, bones, needles, cowries and snapped-off tips of scissors (see Figure 2).

Figure 2: Foreign Objects Found in a Human Body

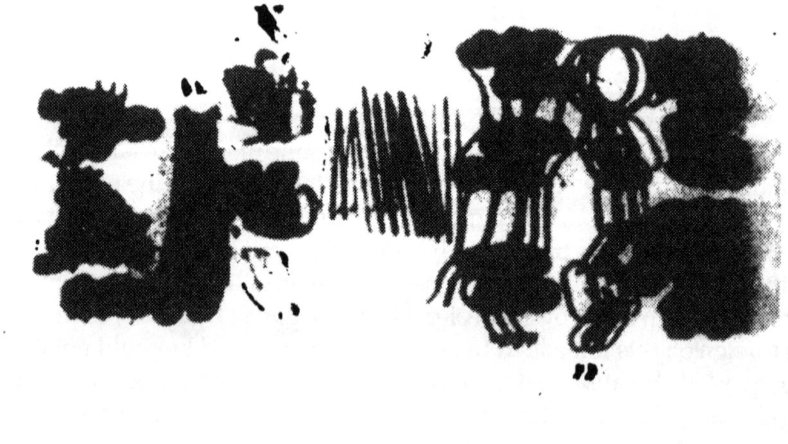

Then there is the story of a high-ranking seminarian at Ouidah (Benin). His mother brought me a number of foreign objects said to have been extracted from his body. Both of us wondered how they had got there. Another of the same woman's children had had cat meat with the hairy hide attached extracted from his body. It is possible for people to consult traditional healers who can extract such objects, using the technique of the 'magnetic laying-on of hands'. I have had the following direct experience of this sort of thing: some years ago, a well known politician, now no longer with us, sent for me one night. 'Doctor', he said, 'I feel strange objects inside me, needle-pricks in my joints'. One day he sent for one of his uncles from Bassila, who prepared some root potion for him, laced it with rum and told him to drink a tot (the measure we know here as 'talokpy') morning, noon and night for eight days. On the eighth day the uncle returned and performed a series of sucking operations all over the patient's body. Out came an impressive array of objects: rattles, broken glass, thorns, pins, stones, needles.

The phenomenon has a name: chakatu. It is a process whereby objects are injected into human bodies in a fashion altogether foreign to rationalist logic. No one sees them get in. It is possible for broken glass to enter human bodies during accidents, when windshields are shattered and pieces projected into body tissue. In such cases some are taken out, others overlooked, to wait for two or three years in some cases before they get extracted. That is perfectly understandable.

What is not so easy to understand is the kind of situation I have described above. I have had direct experience of this sort of thing. Some 10 years ago, I knew a 14-year-old girl who grew as thin as a skeleton, except that her belly kept growing. On touching her belly, one felt something strange and hard lining the abdomen walls. X-ray photos revealed nothing comprehensible. Something ill-defined was located, and that was all. But every time I planned to operate on her, something cropped up to block the operation. Finally, one day I decided to go ahead with the operation no matter what the obstacles. The girl was laid out in the operating theatre, surrounded by my staff. On cutting into her abdomen, I found the stomach pushed out by an object that had taken its shape. I tried to determine if it was outside the stomach by slipping my hand behind the stomach, but failed. That told me the object was definitely inside the stomach. I therefore opened the stomach and extracted this object. At the time it looked like a small 'aguti'. It was a ball of hairdressers' string (see Figure 3) broken in two. A French colleague shown the object concluded: 'The girl ate some hairdressers' string'. Later, in her mother's presence, I asked the girl: 'Agatha, you must have been hungry, with nothing to eat. You were sitting beside a hairdresser, and you ate these bits of string'. 'But Papa', she protested, 'I did not eat any string'.

Figure 3: Ball of Hairdressers' String Found in the Stomach of a 14-year-old Girl

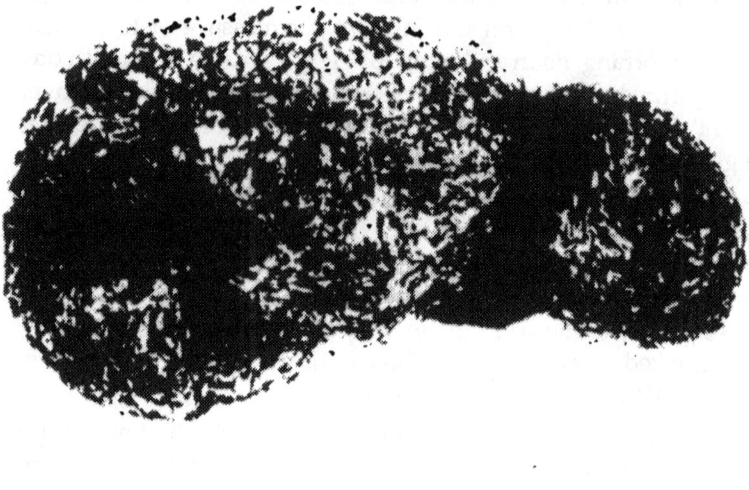

I bought some of this thread and tried to swallow a piece of it. After all, in every situation we have to maintain an experimental attitude. I confess I could not. It felt awfully scratchy in my throat. Furthermore, the strings in the ball swallowed by the girl were woven into a tight tissue of black, green and red thread. How did they get into Agatha's stomach? And once in there, how did they manage to get woven into sometimes intricate patterns of red and green thread? What I have described is a fact. I have shown you the evidence: this ball of thread which I have kept for ten years. On the day of the operation, we invited all medical students, trainee nurses and midwives to watch. Even relatives of the girl who had heard what was going on came in their numbers to the hospital.

Since then I have used the ball of thread in several lectures. I remember in particular one lecture I gave at the Health Development School with Professor Collon, a French psychiatrist based in Dakar (Senegal), who had done some research into African techniques. I presented the exhibit as an oddity. Among the audience there were some traditional healers, and they asked me to let them examine the object. After checking it out, they informed me that the ball of thread had not been swallowed but projected into the girl's body from outside. This had been accomplished one night, when the girl was asleep with nothing covering her belly. The healers said the people responsible came from the family of the girl's father. Next time I saw the girl's mother, she confirmed that there was indeed bad blood between her and her in-laws.

At that time the girl had yet to reach puberty. Today she is a married woman, with three children, I think. So here we have a set of strange objects that can be extracted from human bodies either through the traditional technique of 'the magnetic laying on of hands' or by standard surgical means. You have seen the exhibits with your own eyes, and some of you have felt them with your own hands. I am told that certain Nigerian colleagues have had to extract from their patients' bellies nothing less than calabashes. I personally have not had to perform any such operation, but then perhaps it is only a matter of time.

We have now reviewed various foreign objects found in human bodies: broken glass, rattles, needles, broken teeth, bones, cat flesh, soap and what have you. These objects got into the patients' bodies in invisible ways. At any rate the patients had no idea how they got there. They became aware of their presence only because of the illnesses they provoked. How, then, do we interpret these realities?

An Interpretive Approach: The Need to Encourage Traditional Medicine

To start with, factual data requires supporting evidence. As the philosophical dictum goes: 'Every statement must be supported by clear proof'. Here we have provided the requisite proof. We have foreign objects extracted from human bodies. You have felt them yourselves. So even if I happen to be a scholar, a surgical doctor and a member of

European learned associations, I have to admit that these objects exist. It was I myself who extracted them, after all, and I still have them with me. There is nothing imaginary about them. They are tangible. I vouch for them, and you who have also seen them can do likewise.

There are those who might suppose that the statements made about these objects come from minds prone to hallucination. But then these are real exhibits, and I carry them around with me as proof that Africa has its wonders. As I have said to my European colleagues, of course all this is not at all logical in the spirit of Descartes. In other words, it is unscientific. Still, it is a fact that these foreign objects spent some time inside human bodies. The question is: how did they get there?

In answer, we have to recognize that Africa has its share of mysteries. That brings us to the issue of the conception of traditional medicine, that is to say, of medicine approached from traditional perspectives. It is clear, to start with, that traditional medicine looks at illness from a perspective that combines theological, metaphysical and mystical factors. In other words, God, the mysteries and mysticism are all simultaneously involved. In the near future, we shall be prescribing traditional medicines for ordinary illnesses. For a cough, for instance, decoctions from a particular leaf might be indicated. There are similar prescriptions for diarrhoea, like those available at the paediatric clinic run by Doctor Dan at the National University Hospital Centre in Cotonou (Benin). The National Horticultural and Nutritional Centre at Guando (Benin) has come up with formulae for baby powder. These are all examples of ways in which local pharmaceutical resources can be put to rational, scientific use.

The mystical aspect comes in when there is reason to think that the ailment has given rise to complications. The environment is thought to have been violated in such cases, making it necessary to conduct reparations so as to restore its lost balance and wholeness. The reparations in question entail sacrifices of animals such as sheep and pigeons, along with rituals like the treatment of bodies with herbs, to oil and purify them. Incidentally, purification rituals are not an African peculiarity. Remember the use of hyssop for the same purpose in the Christian Bible. In effect, Christianity and Judaism are just as familiar with the concept of purification. African purification ceremonies are similar in nature, except that in Africa, there is clearly an additional element. This is a viewpoint from which rites are necessary. But care must be taken to distinguish genuine ritual from hocus pocus.

The same Professor Collon to whom I referred earlier on made a film on possession entitled *Le N'Deup*. At the time, he was taking courses with a group of traditional healers, and to make the film he collaborated with some of them. The subject of the film was the possession of individuals by various spirits. In such cases, atonement was needed to exorcise evil spirits. To start with, consultations were held to find out which evil spirits were involved. Next, the patient was washed with blood from sacrificial chickens, with a prayer that the situation return to normal. To conclude the ritual, there was a procession.

The point is that there are realities that are difficult to deny. In the first place, it is absurd simply to treat traditional and official (Western) medicine as if they were polar opposites, as a particular Minister of Health here in Benin did. Such an attitude is futile. The way I look at it, there is no opposition between the two. I think, rather, that each type of medicine has a role to play, as well as its own limitations. For instance, I think there are excellent traditional prescriptions for treating diarrhoea, coughing and, to some extent, asthma. I work together with traditional healers with a scientific approach. These were trained agricultural engineers and hospital nurses who at some stage began to conduct research into medicinal plants.

We have, for instance, numerous medicinal plants capable of curing diabetes, hypertension, etc. It should be remembered, moreover, that many important drugs produced by the Western pharmaceutical industries are based on plants from Africa or Madagascar. Certain drugs used in the treatment of hypertension are a case in point.

Findings from other ongoing research so far seem inconclusive. There are persons who claim to be able to heal or treat cancer. Some have been given cancer patients to treat, but have failed to produce a cure. I think, in other words, that there are areas in which healers do effective work, and others in which they cannot achieve much. For instance, there is little traditional healers can do to stop internal haemorrhaging or a ruptured liver. In these cases, the magnetic laying on of hands can hardly be expected to produce results. The best course is to ask a surgeon to operate, to stanch the bleeding and repair the rupture.

I think it is a mistake to treat traditional medicine and modern, Western-type medicine as diametrical opposites. They can complement each other. There are countries like Nigeria and Ghana in which a great deal of progress has been made in this domain. Here in the Republic of Benin, numerous meetings have been held in an attempt to get traditional healers organized in a federation. So far these attempts have failed, because the healers have the impression that they are going to be hustled out of the knowledge which gives them their livelihood, in return for nothing. Things are different in Nigeria, where traditional healers are given patents for their inventions and formulae. For instance, the inventor of a formula for whooping cough is awarded a patent. If the formula is mass-produced, he is paid royalties. Here we have done nothing of the sort for traditional healers, hence our failure. Stripping traditional healers of their knowledge only to abandon them without support is hardly the right way to go about encouraging them.

The situation in Ghana is similar to that in Nigeria. When we travelled to Ghana on missions with the Ministry of Health as part of the Benin-Ghana co-operation accords, we observed experiments there which gave us a clearer insight into the reasons for our own failure here in Benin. Our delegation contacted the Director of Traditional Medicine in the Ghanaian Ministry of Health, who arranged for us to visit a Centre for Traditional Medicine in the town of Mampong. That centre is run along 'scientific' lines.

The Director of the Centre, Professor Acheampong, holds the Chair of Pharmaceutical Resources at the Faculty of Medicine, University of Ghana, Accra. In Mampong, invitations were sent out to traditional healers. Those who responded came with their formulae and samples of their medicines. Together with Western-trained doctors, they held consultation sessions. If a plant was considered effective in the treatment of, say, diabetes, laboratory tests were conducted to determine the level of blood sugar registered by selected patients. The treatment was then administered, and at the end of it a new blood sugar reading was taken. The initial level might, for instance, have been 2g per litre. If after treatment it was seen to have gone down to a normal 0.9g, that was scientific proof of the effectiveness of the treatment. From that point on the Centre would help the innovative healer by conducting analyses of his formula, fixing the requisite concentration levels or isolating the active principle in order to ensure the long-term preservation of the medicine.

In Ghana, then, there is a system of co-operation involving traditional healers, chemical engineers, nurses, pharmacists and doctors. Furthermore, the operation is scrupulously free of hype: a signboard at the gate to the Mampong Centre announces: 'Here we cure thirteen diseases'. And the illnesses in question are individually named: hypertension, arthritis, dermatosis, asthma, etc. There is even room for laughs. The signboard concludes: 'For help with other diseases, please try elsewhere'. That, in my opinion, is what needs to be done. Traditional medicine reaches out to modern medicine, and the gesture is reciprocated. Together, the two techniques help in the advancement of science.

Regarding the issue of the magnetic laying on of hands, there is no way we can clear up the mystery just yet. The technique works. That is a proven fact. But for the moment, we can put forward no scientific explanation as to why it does. My point is that there is a science that is so far latent. I am reminded of a statement with which my high school physics teacher was in the habit of ending his lessons on electromagnetic waves: 'Human beings can see the range of the spectrum between ultra-violet and infra-red rays. Beyond that span, they see nothing. That means the range of human vision is infinitesimal. Everything outside it, from the tiniest to the most gigantic, lies beyond human perception'. In conclusion, the teacher used to say that human beings may not be blind, but that we are only a hair's breadth from that state.

Such a conclusion is no doubt astounding. After all, humans consider themselves lord of the universe. They make all sorts of intricate contraptions, from the miniaturized tape recorder to huge supersonic airliners like the Concorde, capable of flying from Paris to New York in under three hours. Remember, on 29 July 1969, the American Neil Armstrong took a moonstroll. Yet here we are concluding that man missed blindness by a hair. In other words, what we understand now is nothing compared to what we still do not understand. This is something great scientists and scholars have always known. The great physicist and mathematician, Albert Einstein, for instance, said of the French scientist Paul Langevin that he was very fond of him, because when the latter explained his own theories, he could begin to understand them.

Personally, every time I perform an operation, working to the best of my ability, I am still struck with wonder, to borrow the words of Ambroise Par, father of French surgery, to see the patient healed. I know it is by the grace of God, who created man so admirably, combining in him the circulatory and respiratory systems, blood vessels and lung cells, the interchange of oxygen and carbon dioxide in the blood stream, etc.

Humans are created beings, and philosophers now inform us that the date of their creation has been shifting farther and farther back, and that human beings first appeared scores of million years ago. Our ancestors included Australopithecus, the Javan Pithecanthropus, the Chinese Choukoutien man, Neanderthal man, Grimaldian man, Cro-Magnon man. And it was only in 1847 that the Englishman Harvey discovered the circulatory system. That knowledge had stayed occult for several million years.

There are, in effect, areas where scientific knowledge and control are possible, even imminent. But there are other domains of reality that are bound to remain unknown, areas of esoteric 'science' explored only by mysterious initiates. That kind of unusual knowledge is known as 'the occult sciences'. It is a way of looking at reality, and there is nothing simple about it.

Discussion

The following is a transcript of the discussion which took place at the National University of Benin research seminar, after the presentation of this chapter.

Paulin Hountondji: The speaker began on an extremely technical, positive note — I am tempted to say a down-to-earth note, in the sense that science tends invariably to be down-to-earth — before lifting off into more rarefied realms.

This lecture raises a number of thorny issues confronting those unfortunate thinkers trying to break out of metaphysical mindsets.

Ms Wiesermann: I found the lecture most interesting. It raised a host of stimulating points. I am not in the medical profession, but the phenomena the lecturer discussed are encountered in other areas of life as well. Let me start with this point. If I am not mistaken, you said these phenomena were peculiar to Africa. I beg to differ. I have witnessed very similar phenomena in South America, for example. And Europe too, if we step back in time, produced the same sort of events. So these things do not happen here only. Naturally, explanations for and attitudes towards them differ. There was a time when such things no longer happened in Europe, but there seems to be a resurgence these days. There are certainly non-scientific, spiritualist explanations for them. But my main point is that these phenomena are encountered in other areas of the world.

Toussaint Tchitchi: What role do words play in the magnetic laying on of hands? What is the status accorded words? Is it possible to draw parallels between Biblical practices and the magnetic laying on of hands?

Amoussou Yeye: I have two questions: one for Professor Kiniffo, the other addressed to Professor Hountondji. First, is Professor Kiniffo not a bit scared to get involved in these rather weird goings-on, to deal with these foreign objects imbedded in human bodies? Has he not been afraid of possible repercussions? If indeed he has been scared, does he not take measures to protect himself against these occult practices? As for me, the mere sight of these objects on exhibit here gave me the creeps. And yet he has worked with them, touching them, feeling them with an open mind. I think that is risky. We know you are a skilled surgeon with an international reputation. We would hate to have anything nasty happen to you.

Second, I think these discoveries make it necessary for us to adopt a fresh epistemological approach, a new way of looking at these phenomena. The world has seen the rise and fall of various schools of thought on this issue. First there was the pre-Hellenic worldview. The Greeks accomplished an epistemological revolution in the conception of reality by giving it two dimensions, one physical, the other metaphysical. Then Marx and Engels accomplished another epistemological revolution. Taking off from the scientific approach of their time, they arrived at a dialectical conception of reality. But right here and now we see events that call for a different conception of reality. For the situations Professor Kiniffo described involve human beings acting on reality in ways incomprehensible according to our orthodox yardsticks for measuring the human impact on reality — the principles of praxis according to Marx and Engels. I would like to propose that we begin work on a new theory, laying the groundwork for a third epistemological revolution.

Victor Nobime: From September to October, 1985, I was ill. I felt there was an invisible hand inside me, messing up my internal organs. Then I began vomiting blood. I was taken to the CNHU in Cotonou, where for a month I underwent treatment. On my discharge I was told that my illness was psychosomatic.

My second question is addressed to the lecturer, Professor Kiniffo. It concerns something I have observed in our hospitals. Doctors there are in the habit of driving off patients who complain, for example, that they feel pinpricks in their bodies. The doctors tell them it is all in their imagination, and that they are mystified. At the time I was admitted to the hospital, there was a patient who said he felt sharp internal pains. The doctors gave him an injection that put him to sleep. He dreamed his father, dead for 13 years, was asking him what on earth he was doing at the hospital. He answered he was ill. His father said his illness could not be treated in the hospital and that he should try and get out and go to a traditional healer for treatment. He explained that he could not get out without permission from those who had brought him to the hospital. His father then led him to the environs of the hospital morgue, where he showed him a plant I happen to know well. He told him to gather the plant, then asked him if he knew the uses of the root and leaves. The young man said no. The dead man said he would have to give him a herbal formula. He was to mash some leaves in water, add salt and drink the mixture while waiting to go and get treated elsewhere. On waking up, the patient wrote down on a piece of paper the entire dream conversation with his dead father. Then he went and looked for the plant, but without using it he went to bed again. Then he began feeling sharp pains again. At this point he drifted into a trance during which he spoke with someone. When he came to, we asked him what the matter was. He drew out the piece of paper and showed it to me. After reading it I asked him if he had got the plant. He showed it to me. So I told him to prepare the potion. He did so, added salt, and drank it. Five minutes later he vomited traditional protective rings. He took a second swig and out came some cola nuts, the kind known here as Ahowe (Garcinia cola). After a third swig he vomited cowries; after a fourth he threw up seven pins and some blood. When he woke up that night he was definitively cured. I saw all this with my own eyes. Since then, I have wondered whether the official medical establishment is not shirking its responsibilities when it so often dismisses patients with this type of illness.

Paulin Hountondji: Let me take the opportunity to answer the question raised by my colleague Amoussou, about the possibility of a new epistemological conception. I am not competent to advance a new theory in that field. Before we get to that point, I think it would be well for us to remember, as Ms. Wiesermann said a moment ago, that Africa is not unique in this respect, nor even as exceptional as we might suppose. It is perfectly possible that the phenomena we are discussing here are much more universal, though our limited experience does not enable us to see that clearly.

Henry-Valère Kiniffo: I agree entirely with Ms. Wiesermann on the point that the phenomena we have been discussing are not peculiar to Africa. But the historical fact is that on the older continents these things have been left to simmer on the back burner of human consciousness, while here at home, people still consider them very much a major preoccupation.

10

Links Between Psychosomatic Medicine and Sorcery

Clement T. Adjido

African medical practitioners, whether they dismiss the issue of sorcery out of hand, or consider it unsettling, are likely to find it a recurrent embarrassment. African doctors, after all, though trained according to rationalist norms, are born and raised in a home environment whose psychological landscape still bears the shaping imprint of ancient myths. Confronted with peculiarly difficult cases, practitioners might be tempted to dodge the issue by pointing fingers at 'the occult sciences', even if occasionally they suspect that consciously or unconsciously, sorcery operates along some of the same wave lengths used in psychosomatic medicine.

How, in such cases, might the psychosomatic profiles of victims of 'dark, nocturnal forces' be accurately described? Second, in our operative context, what impact might sorcery have on modern medical practice? Third, in what ways can it influence traditional medical practice? By sorcery, we mean the phenomenon described as an 'invisible iceberg', seen from the perspective of its operative mechanisms and its functional role in social life as well as in the individual psyche.

There certainly are links between psychosomatic medicine and sorcery. To get a clearer picture of these, it is a good idea to begin with a look at the state of the art in psychosomatic medicine today. The next step is to examine the essential content of sorcery, i.e., the structure of its operative mechanisms, its functional character, and its capacity to produce an impact. There would then be a simultaneous examination of the traditional concept of illness as related to sorcery, with special reference to the way it manipulates rhetoric and language, particularly through the use of incantations and magical formulae. One would also have to examine the issues at stake in the link between psychosomatic medicine and sorcery. This implies a study of traits rooted in the cultural environment, based on the exploitation of somatic referents in prevailing images of the body. Examples include the way the body as a whole is conceptualized within a given culture, mothering techniques, and so-called psychosomatic transferences.

We would also have to examine such psychoanalytical issues as aggressivity, sexuality, power and security within the context of individual competition, and the limitations imposed by all these problems. Concurrently, thought should be given to the sectorial aspect of medico-legal problems as related to magical and mythical mental attitudes which connect with the vast field of symbolic meaning so frequently encountered in our lives. Lastly, we would look into individual imagination and fantasy life, before examining collective modes of representation and fantasy as related to sorcery. That is the structural outline we intend to follow in our study of the topic.

Now what might psychosomatic medicine possibly have to do with one of the central mysteries of African life, sorcery? Africa is a land of many mysteries touching even on such domains as political, social and cultural life. Of these mysteries sorcery has a particularly powerful grip on the continent's population. As everyone knows, in medical terms epidemiology is a scientific discipline focused principally on the study of phenomena with a high impact on given populations.

Psychosomatic Medicine: An Overview

There are indications of an emerging consensus in the scientific literature on psychosomatic issues. Nowadays no intelligent, honest person denies the interaction of psychic and somatic processes. In general, psychosomatic medicine gives due recognition to psychic realities within the context of individual temperaments, social factors, problems of adjustment facing patients, their behaviour in the social context — in short, all internal and external factors responsible for the onset of psychosomatic disturbances.

Where such disturbances and imbalances lie at the root of an illness, effective treatment requires that we look beyond and ahead of the illness itself. In this process it is sometimes necessary to examine the unknowable in order to determine the conscious and unconscious paths and byways along which mental activity impacts on somatic processes.

Psychosomatic medicine is a medical approach that identifies aspects of general pathology related to psychic life in conscious and, especially, unconscious ways. There are different schools operative in psychosomatic research, but the leading groups today are the American school of Alesander, Dunbak, Weiss, English and colleagues, whose focus is on psychosomatic factors; the Soviet school led by Bykon, with its focus on the study of reflexes; and the German school of Schwartz, Krehl and Von Weizsacker, with its biological and philosophical focus.

Other schools have been conducting sporadic research in psycho-physiology, but it is the three schools cited above which have come out with complementary findings. On the basis of their experiments, it is henceforth permissible to speak of a psychosomatic approach, a trend which posits that the accurate understanding of a given situation begins with the conception of the organism as a whole.

From such a viewpoint, whenever the physiological experience of an illness coincides with its psychological manifestation in a pathological unit, the intersection point at which the two expressions of illness cross is the venue of what is called an elementary psychosomatic syndrome. In other words, at the crossing of the two manifestations, one physiological, the other psychological, we have a psychosomatic unit at an elementary level.

Another category embraces manifestations which are a peculiar and prevalent expression of a subject's reactions to his or her living conditions. Here the individual's syndrome is not simply a reaction to external stimuli, but may incorporate reactions to his or her own living conditions. In such cases, where living conditions give rise to psychological manifestations leading to disturbances, we are faced with instances of *pathological habitus* related to peculiar personality styles. Examples include asthma and arterial hypertension, both of which are pathological states in which psychosomatic factors are active components.

Like gastric and duodenal ulcers, asthma and arterial hypertension are psychosomatic illnesses. Psychosomatic medicine, by focusing centrally on deep-seated interconnections between the unconscious and our life processes, has been drawing closer to psychiatric methods, which require that the anthropological dimension be taken into account in medical practice. And this anthropological aspect brings us to an awareness of unconscious processes the subject might use in order to work out deep, unconscious conflicts in physical pathological forms.

Psychosomatic conceptions go farther. They embrace a constant questioning of established pathological aetiologies and a search for innovative solutions. It was such innovations that at one point stimulated reconsiderations of etiological factors in psychosomatic medicine. The question that arose was: if the approach works for a particular illness, might it help to treat some other illness? And that opened the way to the study of complementary causal relationships in the interaction of multiple fields.

The process involved is much like that implied by the use of the term 'field of tension' in modern physics. In the long run, this approach can help resolve fruitless contradictions between psychic causes and organic causes. It also reinstates comprehension of the relationship between external pathogenic agents and the environment in which they develop. Allergies and immunological studies provide enlightening examples.

In considering unconscious processes, then, it is important to emphasize ways in which ego dysfunctions can surface in psychosomatic ailments. People with psychosomatic illnesses have notoriously weak egos. In other words, an important part of the personality lacks adequate strength. This is a partial explanation for the occurrence of certain cases of psychosomatic regression. The reason seems to be an absence of mental integration. Authors like Cohen have indicated in their work on the origins of psychosomatic disturbances that as early as the intra-uterine stage, violent pressures from the mother's unconscious, along with conscious and unconscious rejection from the psychosocial environment all hamper the development of the life-force, inhibiting the organization of a psychological identity and biological immunity.

This provides evidence of the fact that as early as the intra-uterine stage, numerous factors connected to the experience of pregnancy are operative, quite without the subject's knowledge. Is the pregnant mother accepted or rejected within her psychosocial environment on account of the pregnancy? An Argentine psychoanalyst, Bleger (1981), has, in a book entitled *Symbiosis and Ambiguity*, drawn attention to the impact of early experiences in the development of psychosomatic ailments. In his opinion, such disturbances begin at a time when the nursing baby is overwhelmed by the pressure of incoming stimuli at a time when its capacity for psychic integration is severely limited, at a time when it has not yet learned to speak. Psychosomatic responses in later life, according to Bleger (1981), are due to the memory of such excessively intense stimuli, recorded in the most archaic area of the brain, the proprioceptive area.

Dolto (1984), in *L'image inconsciente du corps*, tells us that the way individuals understand any word depends on their corporeal scheme, their image of the body, and those live exchanges which in their experience were associated with the acquisition and integration of that word. In other words, the understanding of a word is not a simple process in which the symbol for the word is registered along with an accompanying image. The depth and power of comprehension depend on the conditions under which the word was learned. Certain emotional states affect the comprehension of the word thus learned. When we consider the kind of highly charged situations in which incantations are recited to produce a particularly profound effect on the subject, we are in a position to grasp the full meaning of this statement.

Tremendous advances have taken place in psychosomatic medical research. Findings from field research indicate that psychosomatic cases may be just one step away from psychosis. Some scholars think the concept of conversion would reward further study. The concept refers to somatization, a process whereby subjects express internal conflict or react to given situation by using body parts as a means of communication. An individual's image of the body might be considered as incorporating a structural outline of her or his emotional history. In that case the body might work unconsciously as the primary venue of self-expression. Explanatory psychodynamic studies have located the source of psychosomatic ailments in the earliest stages of life, in the very first relationships of the pre-objectal phase.

Gastro-duodenal ulcers as well as bleeding of the large intestines and rectum have been explained in this way. The reasoning is that the predisposition towards psychosomatic ailments results from failure to develop a positive defensive posture needed for nurturing the first set of objective relationships.

For his part, Von Weizsacker of the German school stresses the lack of mental integration as a cause of inadequate transfer mechanisms in psychosomatic subjects. According to him, inadequate transfer mechanisms can be traced back to inadequate fantasy lives. The root of psychosomatic illness might lie in a separation of the ego from the energy resource pool that should normally have been available to it. In psychotic cases this separation occurs within the ego itself, in the form of a dissociation, while psychosomatic cases involve a blockage of the ego's paths to those areas of being where it could otherwise tap into fresh energy pools of its own.

Research in the discipline has not been limited to a single field. It has stretched into psycho-neuro-physiological areas. In effect, intense emotional changes provoke gastric secretions. By what mechanism does this happen? To explain the process, we have to turn to psychopathology.

The workings of psychosomatic factors in a subject suffering from a gastric fistula has been demonstrated. Subsequently, there were many other assessments of physiological manifestations of emotional states, including muscular tension, sweating, the discharge of adrenalin or noradrenalin, and fibronylitic activity. In this latter condition, the blood vessels of persons with coronary troubles might produce perturbations in fibrin levels. Such coronary ailments work in spasms of the blood vessels. The spasms send pulses to the central nervous system and cause secretions of neural messengers, making it quite easy, through biochemical analysis, to trace the operative mechanism involved. Still, psychosomatic medicine kept raising further questions. Several problems had to be solved before the achievement of a more or less clearly structured model. Nowadays, the psychopathology of psychosomatic illnesses is an open book. In the medical field, it no longer presents any mystery.

The conclusions are as follows: first, illnesses are not caused by one factor alone. They are consequences of a confluence of various independent factors at a given moment. They are the resultant of a new power relationship that at least temporarily upsets the delicate balance of adaptive mechanisms on which our health depends.

Second, among these factors, psychological factors have a more or less important role to play. In some cases they can cause the pathogenic imbalance.

Third, the boundary between psychological and social factors is relatively artificial, or at any rate vague. The psychological realm is incorporated in the social. As far as our practice is concerned, we are interested in social factors to the extent that they provoke psychological reactions, our primary focus. In such cases the factors involved should be identified as psychosocial. By contrast, there is a case for establishing a real distinction between what might be called the psychic fragility of a subject and the environment within which victims of sorcery are selected and targeted.

Certain events in the lives of individual persons might play a significant role in the sense that they can lead to the eruption of an illness previously present in a latent state but kept in check by the individuals' normal defences. The triggering event happens when these defences are in a state of exhaustion. The correlation between emotional states and immunity levels, in any case, is now well established.

Links between psychosomatic states and the brain depend on the following cerebral structures: the hypothalamus, the limbic system, the reticular system and the neurocortex. Let us take a schematized look at what actually happens. The hypothalamus is a storehouse for a number of inborn automatic reflexes. It registers and integrates information on the body's condition, handles adjustments necessary for the immediate survival of the individual organism, and transmits the requisite information to higher structures of the brain.

The limbic system functions in close connection with internal events and sensations. It sifts through the environment for useful resources and elements indispensable to the organism. In other words, the limbic system operates like a modulator for reflexes regulated by the hypothalamus. In that role it is both pragmatic (in that it aims at maximum efficiency) and egotistical (in that it aims at maximizing pleasure).

Some specialists think the reticular system is a buffer between incoming information from the outside world and data from the neocortex. It regulates wakefulness and sleep, posture and motor activity, attentiveness, habitual patterns and conditioning, together with a range of vegetative patterns, through the mediation of the hypothalamo-hypophyseal complex. The main impact of its activity seems to be quantitative, qualitative and inhibitive. It is the neocortex, however, which, receiving information from the entire range of underlying structures, stores data, memorizes them, matches and compares elements and, working thus through abstraction, reacts both on the organism itself and on its environment, while its capacity to modulate underlying reflexes remains practically infinitesimal.

Under these conditions, psychosomatic reactions are clear enough. But abreaction from an instigating event, charged with power by overwrought emotions or an internal psychic conflict, provokes the range of reactions known as psychomotor and psychosomatic reactions. In cases where these reactions are not brought under control, they may overreach their purpose, leading initially to disturbances affecting the generality of vegetative and metabolic systems, more or less.

Let us not forget that in current usage, the term psychosomatic applies to all symptoms and syndromes of a 'functional' nature in which the doctor observes a pathological state involving both psychological and physiological manifestations in coherent form. However, the term is also used in a narrower, specialized sense, to describe various stages of affliction in specific instances of 'functional or lesion-related pathology'. In this usage, beginning with emotional reactions to stress, such as nausea and vomiting, we progress through such functional disturbances as diarrhoea, to syndromes involving lesions, such as gastric and duodenal ulcers and bleeding in the colon or rectum.

An analysis of theoretical research leads to the conclusion that according to the school of thought typified by Marby and Fain, psychosomatic personalities develop as 'lifestyle patterns'. That said, we still have to answer the question as to how the 'personality choice' involved gets made. And it is of particular interest to psychosomatic medicine to find out how individuals determine which organs they will 'use' to give somatic expression to their psychic states. That, in highly schematic outline, is the way psychosomatic medicine approaches these psychopathological mechanisms. We now turn to an explanation of the *modus operandi* at the mysterious hard core of sorcery.

Psychosomatic Medicine and Sorcery

I think it is important to point out that the historic longitudinal study on sorcery conducted with such masterly flair by Professor Leger (1982) of Limoges, France, provided definitive proof that in its evolution, sorcery as a 'system of magical beliefs' has undergone well known changes across time, and that each change reflected the state of society at that given period.

In our African societies, practices related to witchcraft involve sociological realities still hard to ignore. In treating the topic of sorcery, the first problem we usually encounter results from the hermetic nature of sorcerers' secret societies. The second problem is that the larger social group itself puts up a wall of resistance around the phenomenon of sorcery. Admittedly, it may not always be aware of doing this. But it seems in the process to consider sorcery a core value of African civilization in its representation of 'psychosocial reality', a role in which it helps to organize the individual subject's relation to the world at large.

Today we are asked to define the indefinable bases of our land and culture, within the framework of endogenous knowledge. We shall do our best, if not to define sorcery, at least to identify it. To do this we shall use an explanatory grid based on clinical observations and a series of relevant studies. Within this framework, it seems to us that sorcery is a socio-cultural system with the following characteristics:

a) It has proved its staying power over the ages;

b) It is based on traditional notions of mythical and sacred realities set in a given cultural matrix; and

c) It draws upon magical thinking and the human imagination in order to make strategic adjustments needed for its survival. When necessary, it links up with a traditional technology that gets increasingly sophisticated with the passage of time. In the process it exploits in varying combinations and permutations a number of factors including psychology, parapsychology, toxicology and geomancy.

From an examination of available reports on sorcery, it is clear that the most important process involving sorcerers is the 'congregation of spirits'. The spirits involved, practicing sorcerers, gather for a meal supposed to be the body of a victim, figuratively speaking. It is said that the spirit - the sorcerer's just as much as the victim's - takes leave of the body. Physical bodies, then, are absent from the sorcerers' meal. The proceedings take place entirely in the realm of symbolic imagery. It is the attack perpetrated against the victim's spirit which determines the seriousness of the resulting illness, the remedy to be applied, or the time left before death. All this, in turn, depends on the success or failure of various operations deployed by 'anti-witchcraft defence forces'.

We should point out, incidentally, that magical thinking does not dispute the reality of illness. But it conceives of illness as the result of operations mounted by a personalized instigator exercising some evil power over the patient. Illness therefore becomes the consequence of the aggressive actions of an enemy or spirit intent on mounting a premeditated attack, or wishing to remind the victim of some forgotten obligation. For example, cases of impotence, paresis or paralysis may be interpreted as the price paid for survival in a conflict in the course of which the surviving body failed to retrieve part of its inhabiting soul or 'double', or after which the double was left without due recompense.

Now Benin is the cradle of Vodun beliefs. Anyone growing up here is bound to be familiar with the famous legend of 'Toffa and the Thunderbolt'.

Once the supposedly external, malevolent source of an illness or disturbance is identified, exposed and hunted down by some other, supposedly superior force, the illness can be cured, the disturbance dealt with. Exorcism may take place through the rhetorical magic of incantations, contact or exchanges with the outside world, stress-reducing psychotherapeutic techniques, cathartic events or sacrificial ceremonies and performances. Anti-sorcerer healers, endowed with powers of sorcery themselves, deploy an irresistibly powerful arsenal of multiple-warhead anti-witchcraft missiles. The following is an inventory of this formidable arsenal:

a) The Missile of Divination: This geomantic weapon has such prestige that it sometimes draws seekers from various levels of the ruling bureaucracy.

b) The Missile of Magical Conjuration: This weapon supposedly has the power to cancel curses and a range of hexes. Within the rules of the sorcerers' code, however, those invoking it put their own lives at risk.

c) The Medicinal Missile: The use of this weapon involves symbolic images, philtres and ritual practices or confidence-inducing techniques associated with traditional pharmaceutical practice. Sorcerers are regarded as 'beings' invisible to the normal run of humans. They are supposed to be capable of appearing in various psychological and psychic guises, travelling over distances great and small, in purely immaterial forms or disguised as birds or strange, monstrous animals.

Sorcerers work within hierarchical social organizations regulated by draconian laws. The craft of sorcery itself can be summed up as a set of techniques with definite channels, none of which can ever be said to be the definitive procedural path. These combined channels are cultural, toxicological and psychological.

In cultural channels, the main factor is myth. The central myth of sorcery is a sacred, structural narrative in which the subject is immersed throughout the growth of his or her personality. The myth plays a role in the subject's self-identification as well as in his or her relationships with external objects and third parties. Simultaneously, these aspects of cultural life play an important part in the regulation of social interactions, with special reference to stress, major transgressions, and the handling of aggressive impulses related to jealousy.

In toxicological channels, the knowledge and use of toxic substances is a key instrument of attack. Initiates have developed it to peaks of tremendous perfection.

Third, the use of psychological channels involves the exploitation of the suggestibility of intended victims. The most effective striking moments are periods when 'the ego's defences are weak. At such times psychological manipulation can further weaken or destroy them altogether, reducing the ego to easy prey'. The point is that sorcerers choose their victims with great care. Preferred victims are children or adolescents, especially those with psychosomatic personalities.

The way witchcraft supposedly operates is that the shade of evil hovers in the atmosphere, moving from the putative initiate to the supposed target. Let me cite a clinical case to illustrate the scenario.

A 12-year-old boy was rushed from a village to Cotonou for emergency treatment. He had been whipped by his schoolmaster for persistently coming late after repeated warnings. He was admitted to the paediatric ward, but his treatment there produced no positive results. In spite of all the doctors' efforts, he complained of intense pains in his legs, and could not stand up. A physical examination showed a slight swelling on the right knee, plus a few bruises on the calf. A week later, the clinical chart showed that the boy's agony had worsened. Faced with negative findings from both the physical examination and x-ray photos, the boy's parents concluded that the illness was 'not the kind that could be treated at a regular hospital'. The case was therefore transferred to the psychiatric ward, and a report on developments at the paediatric unit sent along.

The boy, after a few psychotherapy sessions, eagerly explained how much his schoolmaster hated him, illustrating his argument with numerous examples. We in his audience were mesmerized by his account, especially when, in the heat of his diatribe, he moved both his feet and brought them firmly to the floor. Seeing our surprise, he immediately resumed a supine pose on the bed, and continued his complaints. By then we had understood the psychosomatic aspect of his illness and pain. This young man was giving somatic expression to a psychic state.

His polygamous father lived with his second wife. His supplanted mother was reacting to the rejection by withdrawing. On the rebound, she had developed a close relationship with the schoolmaster — too close for the boy, who still loved his father and missed him. A close relative of the younger, rival wife had been heard to mutter the ominous words: 'Everything has an end'. Since then numerous sacrifices had been made to protect the mother and her only child, but despite everything the child had fallen ill.

The boy's mother, unable to conceive a second child, accused her rival wife of having caused her sterility. Against this background, the boy hit on the option of communicating not verbally but through his body. Thanks to a combined regime of psychotherapy and, perhaps, magical rituals, the boy was able to pick up his favourite games again, playing football and hunting lizards, but only after going back to his father.

A Fon proverb says: *Mê wê non di bọ bô non di* (juju works only on believers). The corollary is also true: Belief in the reality of the healer's anti-witchcraft powers is a fundamental, indeed indispensable factor if ritual incantations are to liberate the victim from the malady.

In my opinion, then, one possible linkage between sorcery and psychosomatic illness is suggestibility. For a subject whose cultural background encourages the assumption that witchcraft is effective, suggestion can work along psychosomatic paths.

In that kind of cultural environment the psychosocial conviction underlying this sociological reality enables the sorcerer to commit aggression, strong in the belief that he indeed can do this through his focused influence and suggestive power. When the resulting tension is maintained over the long haul, the body of the prospective victim is caught up in the web of rhetoric and belief manipulated by the instigating party. The normal separation of psychic and somatic realms is thus abolished. The outcome is the psychosomatic unit.

It is our understanding that sorcery faces the issue of death on two different levels. On the first level we have the anthropophagic death of the supposed victim. On the second level we have the death of the alleged sorcerer. This could happen as a result of a physical attack mounted by the putative victim before the supposed sorcerer has a chance to strike, or in the wake of the victim's death, as an act of vengeance exacted by relatives. The latter situation raises attendant medical and legal problems.

Death through sorcery might happen of a sudden, through poisoning. Or it might be a long-term result of illness or some other agency yet unexplored, including psychosomatic transfer. Within this framework, psychosomatic transfers can be seen as part of the effort to destroy victims through exhaustion by shaking up their defence mechanisms, thus plunging them into a micro-environment of suggestion-induced insecurity, source of a lethal anguish.

In times of crisis, sorcery can operate as a stress reliever. When traditional conflict-resolution methods are lost, some people feel overwhelmed by the success of their peers. It is possible, however, for sorcery to worsen crisis-induced anguish, where the group's basic framework of rights, obligations and laws is shattered by socio-cultural changes, leaving people with no useable reference values.

In social terms, when social transformations are accompanied by a particularly harsh economic crisis, stakes in two-party conflicts or conflicts in community relationships rise steeply. This encourages the development of various beliefs and reinforces the sacred status of myth. In such situations the unconscious can help to give symptomatic form to psychosomatic phenomena, so that the Other in the equation is no longer simply part of the same body. The fact remains, therefore, that it is impossible to begin understanding psychosomatic realities without prior studies on the relationship of epistemological factors to bodily conditions.

Science, as we know, gives inadequate or unsatisfactory answers to questions confronting potential patients on such vital issues as happiness, money, pain and love. Into the aching void left by science in these areas, daydreams, magic and myth slide with consummate ease. Sorcery, with its arsenal of Kleinian weapons, camps securely in the heartland of the general territory of magic. For magic is the form taken by human initiative in a world dominated by the immanence of supernatural forces.

What this boils down to is that we have a lot of thinking ahead of us. Let me end this chapter with a pertinent quotation from Poincaré: 'Those who doubt all, as much as those who believe everything, abdicate the responsibility of thinking'.

Part Four

Forms of Transmission

11

Writing and Oral Tradition in the Transmission of Knowledge

François C. Dossou

Therapy as practiced by our traditional healers is a sophisticated, efficient skill. In other fields our ancestors possessed a stock of knowledge difficult to master. None of this information was recorded anywhere in writing. No school, in the formal sense in which we understand that term these days, taught such content in its syllabuses. How, then, did people manage to store all this knowledge from generation to generation, handing it down to the present with no loss of accuracy and no distortion? What makes oral traditions so resilient that they can withstand the ravages of time, remaining vital despite the powerful thrust of the art of writing and the potent impact of the modern school system?

We have a tendency, once we learn to read, to look down our noses at oral forms of communication. It is a received notion that education means literacy. The temptation to add 'and vice versa' is strong. Sometimes the view is held with extreme rigidity. In such cases there is a temptation to see illiterate persons not simply as human beings with no writing or reading skills, but as yokels who know nothing worth taking seriously. Research into oral forms of transmission might help restore a measure of balance into this skewed situation. But let us look, to start with, a bit more closely into definitions of the terms 'oral traditions' and 'writing'.

Definitions and Caveats

What do we mean when we say someone is literate or another person illiterate? Normally, people are called illiterate when they do not know how to read or write. The word 'illiterate' literally means 'unlettered'. In real life usage, however, the word is given much broader connotations. When you and I, talk of illiterate persons, we also imply, above all, that they are ignorant. For you and I went to school to learn the alphabet as a gateway to information, which in turn gave us access to knowledge. It follows then, no matter how modest we might wish to appear, that we suppose ourselves entitled to consider illiterate persons as somewhat more ignorant than we are.

It is this differential perception that Louis-Jean Calvet (1984:4) addresses when he writes that:

> In social usage the terms 'literate' and 'illiterate' as applied to persons (the latter defined in dictionaries as those who do not know how to read or write), are negative, disabling concepts. On the one hand they posit the existence of a type of knowledge (reading and writing skills); on the other hand there are persons (illiterate individuals) who do not have these skills. This negative vision gets blown up into a social phenomenon when we talk of illiteracy rates, so that we have societies with majorities which do not know how to read or write.

You noticed, no doubt, that the author thinks of reading and writing as skills. In this, his thinking is no different from ours in this society. An intellectual is known here as *akowé*, meaning someone who understands writing. Plainly, there is an established connection between the possession of the magic Western skills of reading and writing. This means that in this society writing is not merely a prerequisite for the acquisition of knowledge; writing is knowledge itself. That is observation number one.

Observation number two: from the evidence, modern societies place high hopes on the acquisition of writing. They spend huge sums on literacy campaigns and follow-up assessment programmes. Literacy has become a measure of development. Literacy rates are factored into the growth rates of societies. What all this tells us is that the current meanings given to literacy and illiteracy, literate and illiterate individuals, are far removed from the etymological meanings those words should normally have. Those words no longer mean what the dictionary says they mean. They have been given ideological, political, sociological and economic connotations far distant from purely etymological or epistemological considerations.

We turn now to a second concept, that of oral traditions. Here it is helpful to bear in mind the fact that orality does not mean simply the absence of writing. Such a supposition would be wrong. A contemporary linguist, Maurice Houis (1980:12), has presented a definition of the two terms, designed to obviate ambiguity. 'Orality', he says, 'is a characteristic of communication systems that emphasize aural perception. Scripturality, on the other hand, is communication with a visual bias'. For the most part, we shall be working with these two definitions. They will provide us with a starting point for examining the meanings we give the two terms and their concrete connotations.

To recapitulate, then, I think all societies based on oral traditions confront this core problem: how to preserve the memory of human experience, keeping alive in a given time and place the trace of realities no longer present, having passed out of common usage. How do learned and esoteric practices get transmitted? And how, in the process of transmission, does one ensure that their intellectual excellence is preserved, so that they are kept from degenerating into vulgar, profane lore? This is the normal meaning of problems encountered in the upkeep of libraries, archives, the preservation of knowledge. What is required to keep knowledge from withering and losing its content? Needless to say, the type of memory we are discussing here is not individual but social and historical. In this connection Calvet (1984:8) writes:

> This problem of social memory, partly solved by scribes and libraries in societies with written traditions before those forms of storage were superseded by computers, provides a good definition of the major foci of our presentation. It breaks down into a set of problems: what to preserve, how to preserve it, how to transmit it, and for whose benefit.

Now let us take the specific example of 'chakatu'[1] in Benin. The practice raises a number of questions. Is the knowledge involved worth preserving? If so, what form should such preservation take: sacred or profane, mystical or rational? Why and to what purpose? On this point we have to be clear. We preserve knowledge only with the intention of using it later. In other words, the preservation of knowledge necessarily implies its transmission. If the problem of transmission is not settled at the same time as the problem of preservation, the effort is useless, because future generations might find themselves in possession of stored-up knowledge incomprehensible to them, and therefore doomed to disappear. This also indicates that oral traditions do not preserve knowledge indiscriminately. Only those elements are preserved which meet the highest standards of the civilization in question, thus becoming a part of its tradition.

To conclude this series of definitions and caveats, let us say a few words about the emergence of writing itself. This happens to be a controversial matter. Was writing invented at a specific time, long after the spoken word? Or was it a natural practice refined over time to produce the alphabet? Linguists, anthropologists and ethnologists look at the issue from a very broad perspective. Drawings on a wall, pictographs, etc., are supposed to have been precursors to alphabetical writing. There does not seem to be any necessary connection between the writing forms known to us today and spontaneous thought processes that moved people (and still do) to make marks on walls or sticks as ways of jogging their memories. Let us turn once more to Louis-Jean Calvet to help us understand the state of discussion on the issue.

There are those who hold that writing originated among farming communities. Pierre Amiet, for instance, writes that 'in its origins, writing was linked to the need of agricultural and stock-herding communities in Mesopotamia and the vicinity of Iran to develop accounting systems'. Others, on the other hand, argue that writing originated in urban societies: 'On the whole, genuine writing systems developed only among urban populations. For the craft of writing implies highly complex manufacturing skills as well as sophisticated transportation facilities and social arrangements in general' (Marcel Cohen). For our present purposes it is a matter of little relevance whether writing originated in Sumer or China, among farmers or traders. We shall focus on the following facts, on which there seems to be general agreement:

a) Whatever its geographical origins might be, writing was 'invented' for such practical purposes as accounting and the drafting of contracts and legislation, not for literary ends.

b) Given both its origins and the processes of social evolution, writing belonged primarily to ruling social classes (Calvet 1984:102). We shall be returning to this point after discussing the question whether the motivating impetus behind the invention of writing was scientific and scholarly or political and administrative. Which makes the most efficient use of writing: science or political power? It is a key question, and we shall address it in our presentation. With the problem thus summarily outlined, let us move to a more detailed discussion.

Oral and Literary Biases

I have pointed out that those of us who know how to read and write, taken individually as well as collectively, suppose ourselves superior to those who do not. And in general, literate societies consider societies without writing as inferior. For instance, one of the standards historians use to distinguish history from prehistory is the presence of writing. For numerous reasons, justified or unjustified, they tend to be suspicious of oral traditions. The reasons advanced are sometimes unconvincing. Occasionally they are downright contradictory. The following is a sample:

a) Oral traditions dating back to remote periods are untrustworthy.

b) Oral texts often stray far from their source content.

c) No one knows how to sift genuine material from apocryphal additions.

Such suspicions are the basis for a bias towards writing which takes the form of a theoretical denigration of oral civilizations. Writing is taken to be a super-intelligent invention that transformed human destiny. Peoples without writing systems are considered simply to have remained at the level of primitive savages. As Claude Hagege (1985:70) points out: 'This prejudice was inevitably ratified by incompetent reports written by missionaries with no linguistic training, incapable of conceiving the learned complexity and historical continuity of numerous oral languages. In various forms these notions have been the dominant intellectual staple of the West since the Renaissance at least. The invention of the printing press certainly contributed decisively to it'.

Verbophilia: The Oral Bias

Let us look at the fresh, original position of a well known thinker, Jean Jacques Rousseau. For our purposes, the originality of Rousseau's ideas springs from the fact that they are imbued as much with literate biases as with oral preferences.

Rousseau's philosophical purposes and objectives are well known. He aimed to legitimize the myth of the noble savage by arguing that civilization exerted a corrupting influence on humans. In his view, humans were happy only in a state of nature. Civilization corrupted them. From this premise, Rousseau only had to prove that writing was a product of civilization to draw the conclusion that reading was to be avoided. Children had to be protected from books in order to preserve their innocence and sincerity, for books were liars, books presented falsehood as truth, even though adults and children had a tendency to assume that books were always right. Roseau described writing as an artificial process demeaning thought. In his view, libraries were repositories of intellectual poison.

In his *Essai sur l'origine des langues,* first published in 1817, Rousseau listed various types of writing according to categories. For him, the cruder a writing system, the closer it was to the state of nature. The more refined and scholarly, the closer it was to civilization. Scriptophilia, the love of writing, was at the latter extreme. Rousseau's three-part classification of writing systems was as follows: painting; the use of signs to represent words and statements; and the alphabet. Painting involved representations not of sounds but of ideas. He gave Aztec glyphs and Egyptian hieroglyphs as examples. What was involved here was 'the representation of words and statements by conventional characters. These three types of writing rather accurately reflect the three stages of human organization into nations. Representational painting is suitable for savage peoples; the use of signs to represent words and statements corresponds to the stage of barbary; alphabetical writing is the appropriate form for people organized in the polis'.

As might be expected, Rousseau was partial to savages, a preference reflected in his verbophilia. 'Languages', he said, 'were made to be spoken. Writing is useful only as an adjunct to speech'. The same book contained a series of famous aphorisms, a sampling of which I shall quote here: 'Children who read do not think'. 'The excessive use of books kills knowledge'. 'The key is not reading but seeing'. Rousseau's type of verbophilia had a tremendous impact on such ethnologists as Claude Levi-Strauss.

In *Tristes tropiques,* Levi-Strauss approaches the issue of writing from a Rousseauian point of view. 'Writing', he says, 'may not have worked adequately to consolidate knowledge. But it was probably indispensable to the strengthening of power structures. Let us take a look at realities closer to home. In the 19th century the European states worked steadily to promote compulsory schooling. That campaign went hand in hand with the extension of military service and the proletarianization of the population. Literacy campaigns were thus synonymous with the strengthening of government control over citizens. For all citizens had to be rendered literate before the State could say: 'No citizen has the right to be ignorant of the law'.

Later, Levi-Strauss (1956:344-5) practically repeats Rousseau's words: 'In gaining access to the learning piled up in libraries, the people open themselves up in increasing numbers to the lies propagated in printed documents'. Such is the undisguised face of verbophilia.

The renowned linguist Ferdinand de Saussure is also a verbophile. He argues, over several pages, that writing was imposed on us in illegitimate fashion. In his *Cours de linguistique générale,* he argues that 'language and writing are two distinct sign systems'. The sole rationale of the latter is to represent the former. The purpose of linguistics is not the study of the written and the spoken word. The spoken word alone is the proper study of linguistics. However, writing interferes so intimately with speech that it ends up usurping the leading role. Thus we find ourselves giving as much importance, indeed more, to representations of vocal signs than to the original signs themselves. We act as if we thought that in order to get to know someone, it were 'better to contemplate his photograph than to look him in the face'. He adds later:

> Language is independent of writing... Language, then, has an oral tradition independent of writing, with an entirely different system of standardization, which we cannot see because we are blinded by the prestige of writing'. Further: 'Literary language further boosts the undeserved importance given to writing. It has its paraphernalia of dictionaries and grammar books. The school system teaches us to use books, according to bookish standards. Language, it seems is regulated by a code. That code is a set of written rules with rigorous traditions of usage known as spelling. It is this which makes writing so primordially important. In the end, we forget that we learn to speak before learning to write. The natural sequence is reversed.... Writing thus acquires an importance to which it is not entitled.

Scriptophilia: The Bias Towards Writing

I need not expatiate as long on scriptophilia, since most of us here belong to that school. We are practically all mystified by writing, since in our time everything is set down in writing. To illustrate scriptophilia I have selected two examples of its votaries, Jacques Derrida and Paulin Hountondji. In his book *De la grammatologie*, Derrida mounts a sustained attack on Claude Levi-Strauss and Rousseau (the verbophile). Derrida argues, justly, it must be admitted, that Levi-Strauss confuses 'government' with 'oppression'. That criticism is borne out in the passage we quoted above. The reader will note that whenever Levi-Strauss mentions government, he immediately identifies the concept with oppression. The truth, however, is that power is not always political, nor is it necessarily oppressive, unless one espouses the anarchic supposition that makes all government anathema. Derrida (1967:191) writes in connection with *Tristes tropiques*: 'In this text Levi-Strauss establishes no difference whatsoever between hierarchy and domination, between political authority and exploitation. The dominant tone of his argument reveals an anarchic mindset that deliberately confuses law with oppression'. Derrida (1967:16) also presents a long critique of Jean-Jacques Rousseau. He takes care to point out, however, that 'to speak of writing as a primary form does not necessarily mean to say that in chronological reality writing came first'.

I turn now to Paulin Hountondji. This professor became a scriptophile quite early in his career. In his doctoral dissertation (1970), he was already advocating the following viewpoint:

> Writing seems to be the most refined form of language, the most suitable means for ensuring stabilization, communication across time, immortality, in a sense. Scientific knowledge, precarious as long as it remains individual, can only be preserved and transmitted as the permanent heritage of humanity (or at any rate of a given society) if it takes the form of written documents.

In other words, those ignorant of writing lack an essential human dimension. For among them, language does not fulfil its mission of 'stabilizing' thought. Presumably, the thoughts of such people go wandering where they may, and, like the muddle in the head of that poor fictional character Victor de l'Aveyron, are incapable of taking fixed form.

In 1973, Hountondji again wrote:

> It seems hard for me to imagine a scientific civilization which would not also be a literate civilization. It is equally difficult for me to conceive of a history of science, a scientific tradition in a society using

only oral methods for the transmission of knowledge. It seems therefore difficult to imagine African civilizations becoming an integral part of what we now call the world of scientific learning, which might more accurately be called the world of scientific practice and activity, unless African societies first accomplish the basic, prerequisite transformation from oral to literate civilizations. The point, I think, is clear enough to make further comments.

The Mystification of Writing

The question really facing us with regard to the transmission of knowledge is this: what role does writing play in the process, and what role do oral traditions play? We shall be speaking of the mystification of writing, the juju status, shall we say, conferred on the alphabet. But let us take care, from the start, to acknowledge the real power of writing. For we have come (and in using the inclusive we, I am speaking in all sincerity) to consider science and even history as forms of knowledge mainly transmitted in written form. As for oral traditions, we tend to think they are inadequate means for the transmission of knowledge. I think we make these assumptions spontaneously. And that makes us all unconscious scriptophiles. Because we already know how to write, we have a tendency to worship writing. I suppose that is merely normal. At any rate, the sociological context provides a perfectly logical explanation.

In our societies today, what is valued is basically individual merit, personal worth. In the bourgeois society we live in, all arrangements tend to facilitate the eclipse of the group, sometimes even the family, by the individual as achiever. Writing is precisely relevant in that it helps us affirm our individual worth. That is why we assume that thinking itself is a strictly individual activity, a personal affair, since writing enables those capable of handling it to create their own personal worlds (to borrow Max Stirner's words), and enables each of us to create our own heaven.

If I write something down, it is my property. Hence the well-known concept of copyright. And the moment I put my signature under a thought, it belongs to me. No one is entitled to take it away from me. If someone says the same thing without quoting me, he is an ignoramus. He should have read my work before talking. In extreme cases he will be pilloried. It has therefore become hard for us to imagine thinking as a collective activity, the kind of process encountered in oral societies: collective, anonymous ideas.

Such ideas are not treated seriously as ideas, and they have scant chance of being recognized as philosophy. And then how is it possible to imagine human groups with no individual thinkers, people whose work it is to think, and who have a particular style of thinking? In other words, how can we imagine thoughts without thinkers, ideas without owners? Scriptural civilization has brought us to the realization that only the alphabet makes the objective manipulation of thought possible. Such objective manipulation of ideas covers not simply my thoughts, not merely those of the living, but the ideas of the dead as well.

It is equally true that writing has become an indispensable instrument, so indispensable, in fact, that today we are hardly aware of it as a tool. Those who possess writing are deemed simply to possess knowledge. So writing has become a kind of juju. It ratifies and lends credibility to all forms of speculative thinking. Partisans of the written word have gone so far as to assert that what is unwritten is untaught.

The social order is equally permeated with writing. If there were no writing, we would have no administration, no bureaucracy, no department heads, no secretaries, nothing. The modern world is practically built on writing. Whatever is officially valid can invariably be found written somewhere. Speech is dangerous from the point of view of administrative systems. For that reason, in the world today, illiterate people are in a strict sense social invalids, absolute invalids, condemned to live as if they could not walk, see or hear. Illiterate persons are an underclass. If you have ever bumped into illiterate individuals in the tunnels of a European subway, you will understand what I am talking about. You cannot find your way about a modern city unless you can read. We are all forced, therefore, to learn to read and write. Personally, incidentally, I'm quite glad to be literate.

From a literate viewpoint, then, there clearly were no administrative systems in our traditional societies. By administrative systems I mean bureaucracies of the type we have today, with all their red tape, circulars, forms, receipts, identity cards, chits and sundry licences, certificates, affidavits and degrees. Writing has produced nothing less than what might appropriately be called a paper civilization. 'Officially', no one knows who you are unless you can produce a piece of paper saying you are X or Y. It does not matter how deeply you believe you are who you are. Without papers you cannot prove your identity. This has given rise to numerous cases of false pretences, a phenomenon against which numerous states have been waging a losing war.

In the past, facial scars and 'natural' forms of initiation into social groups were the equivalent to our modern identity papers. They were proof against fraud. Administration was a simple, practical affair, 'automatic' if you will, for no one could survive unless they were integrated into a community. One reason was that the division of labour was then not as intensive or sophisticated as it is now. That is the proof that writing originated not to meet the need for knowledge but to satisfy the demands of power structures. Society, faced with the tremendous development of the production system, of forces of production and the division of labour, could no longer be managed as before. Science had nothing to do with it.

If science and scholarship managed to take advantage of writing and got transformed in the process, the reason is that there was already a scholarly corpus in existence long before writing. Let me repeat: writing was no prerequisite for the development of knowledge.

Democratic systems are impossible without writing. Democracy as currently practiced in major urban societies is principally based on writing. On this point I agree wholeheartedly with Levi-Strauss. The axiom: 'Ignorance is no excuse before the law' means nothing unless all citizens are literate. In societies with high illiteracy rates, the implementation of such an axiom would be unutterably complicated. There is, in other words, an ideological function of writing controlled by the powers that be. In order for governments to function normally, citizens have to be literate. That is the reason behind free and compulsory schooling. Democratic governments force all citizens to go to school up to a certain level, not through kindness, generosity or Christian charity. The reason is to teach them to read and write, to make them more amenable to control, so that they can get integrated into the dissemination system propagating the dominant ideology. If the governed do not know how to read or write, the dominant ideology can only reach them in distorted echoes. That does not suit political rulers.

Lastly, literate societies give an impression of being extremely pluralistic. With individuals writing whatever they please, the sense is strong that everyone enjoys freedom of thought, and is free to come up with the most original ideas. Such is the power of the written word.

Orality seems, by contrast, like a weakness synonymous with illiteracy and ignorance. Extreme partisans of literacy go so far as to suppose it a sign of primitive status. Fortunately, however, linguists these days have begun to react against such views, so they are dated. Still, I maintain there is a need to tread carefully. What really goes on in societies based on oral traditions? How did thought processes begin? How did people begin disseminating stories or proverbs, getting them popularized and used throughout the community? One thing is certain. The process was much more complicated than simple mouth-to-ear transmission.

In this connection, Papa Massène Sène (1985:6-7) writes:

> Western society has accustomed us to the concept of authorship. Here, however, the term is no longer entirely suitable; it needs to be redefined. In effect... authors here are recognized as individuals. The concept of authorship in oral literature embraces both the transmitter and the receiver of literary rhetoric. In addition, there are many other participants scattered throughout the society.... In other words, at the inception of every literary work there certainly might be an individual creator, but his work acquires the status of a literary piece only when it is assessed by the collectivity according to its aesthetic and ethical criteria, accepted, then ratified for dissemination.

Needless to say, we accept such statements with a great deal of caution. Research in oral traditions is in the teething stages. We know little, so far, about the precise ways and means by which ideas circulated in societies based on oral traditions without degenerating into mere rumours. We can only speculate for the moment. But I am optimistic, judging by research findings from various sources, that all these interesting ideas can soon be subjected to experimental demonstration. Meanwhile, the idea is that oral societies operate on a consensus synonymous neither with unanimity nor a determination to achieve unanimity.

All members of the community express their individual thoughts, but only some thoughts earn social approval. Our contemporary societies may seem on the surface to operate differently; at bottom they work the same way. I may write a book, but that does not mean everyone will read it. By force of circumstance it will have to undergo a selective process, first among my contemporaries, then in the hands of posterity. In the upshot it may be left to gather dust, or become a treasured part of the human heritage. The difference between oral and written traditions is that the latter is preserved.

On now to the specific question: which is the better choice: scriptophilia or verbophilia? In my opinion the two are aspects of a single coin. As I have said, I am perfectly happy that I can read and write. We all share that position. The problem is that these days it is hard to defend oral tradition, or, to be precise, to advocate the rehabilitation of oral traditions. It is some time now since Paulin Hountondji sparked the debate, and its terms are well known. We are all scared of being stigmatized as 'ethno-philosophers'. Yet the debate on orality is radically different from that on African philosophy. The way I look at it, it is possible to take Hountondji's position in an extremely dangerous, obscurantist way. I would add that certain aspects of that position need to be transcended.

Is it feasible to advocate verbophilia in this day and age? Let us put the question this way: supposing you want to study animals whose normal lives are entirely nocturnal. You will have to illuminate their habitats. In so doing you modify their behaviour patterns, studying them in an environment alien to them. Yet we do not conclude from this circumstance that there is no point studying nocturnal animals. What we have to do is to take all necessary precautions, the better to be able to study them under conditions as close as possible to their normal situation. That, in sum, is my approach to the problem of scriptophilia and verbophilia.

Is it impossible, today, for us to profit from the study of oral traditions? Shall we limit ourselves to the study of knowledge contained in books, as required in school curricula? The question is germane, since we are in the grip of a powerful classroom education that fills our heads exclusively with information from books, written information. It is this mesmeric power that keeps us repeating, with Professor Kiniffo, ideas such as that the practice of *chakatu* belongs to a realm alien to Cartesian logic. Why do we say a particular practice is outside the scope of Cartesian logic? What do we mean by that? That it is irrational? What is the status of rationality?

Is it what is known or what is understandable? Or is it simply what has been rendered rational? Is any event rational a priori? Is any crude fact rational? Is it not up to us to make practical investments of time and energy to render it rational?

To conclude, this topic is not exclusively epistemological. It has an ideological aspect that deserves equal treatment.

Discussion

The following is a transcript of the discussion which took place after the presentation of this chapter at the National University of Benin seminar (see introduction chapter).

Paulin Hountondji: I would like to express my gratitude to the speaker. In suggesting that he address this topic, I had no intention whatsoever of forcing it on him. Neither did I imagine that the issue was simply ideological and political. I was naive enough to suppose that it was also a scientific, scholarly issue.

Edouard Wallace: I do not wish to deny that writing has a clear importance in contemporary society. However, the speaker's presentation raised numerous questions in my mind. It seems to me that when we speak of orality, there is nothing that necessarily indicates weaknesses in the practical uses of oral methods. Traditional societies, after all, had numerous representational systems that enabled them to memorize and store what was called rhetoric. More than we do, such societies relied heavily on memory, developing it to prodigious levels.

In this respect, I would say that the calculators we find all over the place these days are among the evils of scriptophilia, because they are products of the emphasis on literacy. These days it has been observed that many people are unable to do even basic arithmetic without leaning on such gadgets. People in oral society did not have such machines, yet they were able to handle complicated problems. The quotation you gave us from Professor Hountondji's article gave me the impression that knowledge could not be scientific unless it was set down in writing. For me that raises a question: is our endogenous knowledge, purely oral and African as it is, not scientific?

You also said there could be no administration without writing. On that score my question is this: in precolonial times, was there not a form of administration? If there was, was it necessarily based on writing?

François Dossou: There is indeed a problem of memory. Let me say that societies dependent on oral tradition used a series of mnemonic techniques to help them remember texts. Oral texts do not have the same structural scaffolding as written texts. They contain a whole range of techniques imbedded in the story or fable. They are designed to help the teller to remember the tale, as well as to enable the audience to follow and understand it.

Oral texts fall into different categories. There are exoteric texts for the uninitiated; there are texts targeted at people with a certain degree of training and status within the social structure. The two types of text do not have identical content. Knowledge is hierarchically structured for purposes of communication.

It is true that in our time we are losing our powers of memory. A contemporary linguist goes so far as to assert that these days even the most gifted among us can barely remember the names of all our friends. Everything these days conspires to erode the faculty of memory. On this particular point, with permission from Professor Hountondji, I would like to ask Ms Midiohouan, a specialist in oral traditions, to supplement what I have just said.

Thécla Midiohouan: As Professor Dossou said, research and studies on oral traditions are still in their infancy. The reason is precisely that having no written documents to inform us of the exact nature of past processes, we have been trying to reconstruct those realities from available evidence. What we know for certain, though, is that orality was not a crude matter of mouth-to-ear transmission, as you pointed out. Societies based on oral traditions have their training systems and schools, or at least had them in the past. Incidentally, when discussing oral societies, we shall have to speak in the past tense.

They had schools. They had techniques for developing the power of memory. There were candidates who concentrated solely on expanding their mnemonic capacities. Those who failed were dismissed, no argument about it. There was a whole series of techniques, not necessarily literary, involving repetition, key words etc. Their purpose was to develop memory to the point of absolute fidelity. Furthermore, adepts used 'magical potions' to expand mnemonic capacities to prodigious levels.

Thécla Midiohouan: We should add that writing did not necessarily bring about a scientific renaissance. Just because ideas and cultural realities are transmitted orally does not mean they are valueless, and that we have to start from scratch. As the proverb says, writing is yarn linking us to the past. Today, writing is a must. The modern world cannot exist without writing, even if the only activity that is absolutely dependent on writing is speculation. This is true in arithmetic as well as in speculative philosophy.

You quoted a statement from Louis-Jean Calvet to the effect that 'Writing was invented to facilitate accounting and legislation ... and not specifically for literature or scholarship'. That is a key fact. It means that knowledge does not necessarily have to be transmitted by writing. As you demonstrated, writing appeared when societies needed it. Some societies needed it at a particular point in their development, and they invented it.

Orality functions quite differently. By the way, no society, oral or literate, remembers all its history. That is impossible. And oral traditions select only a strict minimum for retention. What is preserved is what is needed for the survival of future generations. As for your analogy about nocturnal animals on whom it is necessary to shed light, we think it may be rather far-fetched. On the whole, however, it may be a useful comparison. Even now, when we want to study oral traditions, we have to set the information down on paper in order to analyze it. Writing certainly facilitates speculation and analysis. But that does not make it an indispensable standard.

Paulin Hountondji: On the basis of what Ms Midiohouan has just said, I would like to ask the Professor Dossou a question: is she a scriptophile or a verbophile?

François Dossou: Using the opportunity offered by Ms Midiohouan's contribution, I would like to answer a question likely to arise in any case. I had left it out, thinking it was going to come up as soon as we got into the discussion period. Now I have to bring it up myself. Writing is not necessarily the avenue to knowledge. I separated writing from the printing press on purpose. We have to take care to distinguish the dissemination of writing from writing itself. No doubt about it, when published by the printing press, the written word enhances the proliferation, popularization, secularization and preservation of knowledge.

As a form of expression, writing has not always served to disseminate knowledge. Sometimes it has done the opposite. In the past, writing was used to keep scientific discoveries secret. In the 15th and 16th centuries, many scholars and scientists learned to write in reverse order so as to hide their discoveries from colleagues and friends. Writing is extremely conducive to confidentiality. When we talk of writing and dissemination, we normally only think in terms of the wide distribution capacity of the written word. What we forget is that it is also capable of hiding information. For example, the famous scientist Leonardo da Vinci kept his findings in secret notebooks in a protectively reversed script, because he was dead set against others finding out about his research. Another scholar, Tartaglia, refused to show Cardan his method for solving third degree equations. The method was written down in his notebooks, but it was a secret, kept under conditions of high 'security'.

This is why we say that the best way to keep an idea secret is to write it down. All that remains after that is to hide the document. Spoken words are hard to hide, unless several people conspire to create a secret language like the jargon used by vodun votaries, who are called vodunsi (disciple of vodun cult).

Paulin Hountondji: I would like to discuss the points raised by the speaker, by pointing out that the examples he gave do not in any way prove that writing has an accessory, unessential, superfluous role in the effective establishment of modern scientific knowledge. What the example of Leonardo da Vinci proves is simply that we need to distinguish between the preservation and dissemination of knowledge. Both are functions of writing, but they are distinct. Now I would like to go even farther, and turn into the devil's advocate. I think that writing does not merely guarantee improved preservation of knowledge. Nowadays it is an essential factor in the very production and institutionalization of knowledge.

How is research on oral traditions conducted? It is conducted by linguists and anthropologists toting notebooks and pencils. They may write purple prose about the good old times of orality. They may write long articles to say writing is unnecessary. But they do it all in writing. In the process they do not simply transcribe thoughts ready formed in their heads. They outline and develop their ideas, articulating them at the moment of putting down their written texts. That is definite proof that writing is now inexorably integrated into scholarship. Today, scholars studying oral traditions are not only equipped with notebooks and pencils. They also lug recorders for taping sounds. Once again, this proves that in the process of research on oral traditions, we are deeply immersed in writing and reading.

We might find this state of affairs delightful or deplorable, but that is hardly the point. The point is to take a clear-headed look at the way practical research, live research on dynamic scientific topics, gets conducted today. From the perspective of such dynamic, scientific research, writing is a prerequisite, and illiteracy does not mean idiocy. I do not know a single serious author who claims the opposite. Perhaps the speaker could mention names of serious authors who have asserted or at least thought that illiteracy meant idiocy. It seems to me rather foolhardy to make a long speech just to argue that illiteracy is not idiocy. It is a case of barging aggressively into wide open gates.

I also had questions of detail in mind. To start with, I would appreciate a clarification from the speaker concerning the concept of verbophilia. Did you coin or borrow it?

François Dossou: I thought this was clear enough, since the term is widely known. Of course I did not invent it. It comes from Louis-Jean Calvet, and it means precisely what it says.

Paulin Hountondji: Now what is the relationship between this concept of verbophilia and that of logocentrism which, to be precise, lies at the core of Jacques Derrida's critique. That critique indicates that in the long run, beyond the opposition between scriptophilia and verbophilia, etc., the whole of Western thought has been basically logocentric and somocentric; that in other words, since Plato — and only since that thinker — it has invariably considered the living word as the highest instance of language, and that furthermore, whenever attempts have been made to reinstate writing to a status of importance, the effort to conceive of writing as an original form in relation to speech has never really succeeded. The tendency has always been to think of writing as a secondary transcription of a primary reality, speech.

What contemporary thinking enables us to identify with increasing clarity is in the first place the enormous expansion of the concept of writing, which goes beyond alphabetical forms, and secondly, the fact that writing has become an operative factor in our very thought processes. There is a book by an excellent anthropologist who incidentally lived for a long time in Ghana, Jack Goody, entitled *La raison graphique*. Its subtitle indicates that it is about 'the domestication of savage thought'. A more recent book by the same author is entitled The Logic of Writing. In the latter book he tries to analyze the transition from an oral to a written civilization.

Needless to say, the creation, preservation and eventual dissemination of knowledge are not , generally speaking, the primary function of writing. And of course, this strictly theoretical function of writing derives from political and religious functions. Incidentally, we have overlooked the religious function of writing. In the great revealed religions, from Christianity and Islam all the way to Buddhism, the word of God is a series of texts in written form, the Holy Scripture. Religious, political, administrative, social and other functions of writing obviously antedated its strictly theoretical function, a derivative function. But the moment we begin to investigate the real modalities of scientific practice today, we are bound to acknowledge that the relationship between writing and science is not at all extrinsic but intrinsic, intimate, in fact.

If I gave you O level questions in mathematics to answer, you could knock yourself out trying to answer them, but unless you wrote them down, set the equations down on paper, as students say, I'm sorry, but you would never go beyond the level of mental arithmetic. My point is that modern mathematics is a written science. It would be impossible to develop it outside a literate framework. Admitting this is not tantamount to feeling contempt for 'illiterates'. Neither does it imply that illiteracy is synonymous with stupidity. It is a simple recognition of a real situation. It is a simple requirement of honesty with ourselves. It simply indicates a willingness to face up to the effective practice of scholarship today.

Now I would like to ask the speaker a single question. But as a prelude, since the issue is extremely ambiguous, let me ask the speaker whether his real focus was on the mystification of writing or on the power of writing. He used both expressions. It is therefore not very clear whether he acknowledges that writing has real, objective power impossible to ignore, or thinks instead that people endow writing with some illusory power. That is my question: is the power of writing, in the speaker's opinion, objectively perceivable or an illusion resulting from mystificatory manipulation? I admit it could be more precisely phrased, but it is still rather vague in my mind, and I would appreciate some clarification from the speaker, beyond asserting that illiteracy is not idiocy. We all agree on that. No one ever said or thought otherwise. Now on to my final question: what are we to do, here and now? What do you propose beyond all the ideological polemics on the relative value of writing and oral tradition? In any case I think the argument is rather dated. The real issue is what to do here and now.

Ms Midiohouan: The question is very precisely put, and extremely interesting. But before the speaker answers it, permit me to raise a point I have not heard discussed this evening. The speaker quoted a linguist, de Saussure, to the effect that speech precedes writing. I consider the point well taken. As far as Europeans are concerned it is perfectly true, since Europeans invariably learn to talk before learning to write. But the situation in Africa is different. Children here have to learn to read and write in a language they do not speak. I wonder to what degree this situation affects our entire attitude, our approach. The situation we experience in childhood provides an entirely different base for Africans and Europeans. Now I wonder to what extent it has a mystification impact if the language I write is my mother tongue, or let us say a language I understand perfectly, because I speak it naturally. Matters become more complicated when the language I write is revealed to me in the very process of my learning to write it.

François Dossou: What you just said is tremendously important. I myself had not thought of it before. It explains why Africans are in general such scriptophiles. In effect, we acquired knowledge after acquiring writing. We are therefore overly impressed with the power of writing. Now this enables us to answer Mr Hountondji. Let me state simply that writing has real power. I think I said as much before. I also said I was quite happy to be literate. I went even farther, saying that illiterate people in our society were handicapped in an absolute sense. That much I think is clear.

So where does mystification set in? It begins, I think, with the assertion that it is in the process of writing that we think; that it is when we put pen to paper that our ideas take shape and get structured. That is the precise onset of mystification. I am happy that Paulin Hountondji, in front of this audience, has repeated what he has always written, that is to say, that unless we write we can only have messy thought processes, and that we cannot structure our ideas. I hope I'm not misrepresenting his ideas.

Paulin Hountondji: But you are — absolutely. You have crudely misinterpreted my words. What I said was that anyone who cannot write cannot answer an O level mathematics exam question.

François Dossou: That example was a booby trap. I refuse to fall into it. In the first place, the mathematics you talk of was designed within and for a literate context. This is another attempt at mystification: to select a discipline that originated only after writing, and then to challenge us to confront it as if writing did not exist.

As I have already told you, I am quite pleased that I can read and write. So I can handle mathematics. There are mental exercises in the school system which require writing. On that we all agree. What I disagree with, and on this point I think lots of people are with me, because the notion flies in the face of common sense, is the supposition that my thoughts get structured only while I am writing. That is hype, and should be exposed as such.

There is an ideological approach to writing, and I think that is what we are confronted with today. Otherwise we would not be having this argument. Let me repeat my point. I agree that writing has stimulated a lot of work, academic work included. Writing was at the origin of scholarly disciplines. It is a fact that I cannot handle mathematics without writing, as Kepler well knew. All these disciplines were literally invented within a literate framework. In an oral context, they would be meaningless. We all agree on that, I think.

But my being illiterate does not necessarily mean I am incapable of reasoning and reflection. If I were illiterate, that would not mean I was necessarily incapable of achieving supposedly scientific levels of thinking. Emphasize the word 'modern' as you will; it makes no difference. My position is this: writing does have real, objective power, on the one hand. And then on the other hand, there is a subjective, mystificatory power conferred on writing. The proof, needless to say, is plain for all to see.

Paulin Hountondji: I confess I do not know of a single author who ever claimed that as long as one cannot write, one cannot think; that those who cannot write cannot reason. People who emphasize the fact that writing is an indispensable medium for the practice and development of scientific thought are not talking of thinking in a general sense. Neither are they referring to reflection and reasoning as general processes. Their focus is on the precise area of scientific and scholarly activity, scholarly reasoning, scientific reasoning. Of course there are constituted bodies of knowledge in oral societies. Had we not recognized their existence and their extraordinary importance, we would not have organized this seminar. There are divisions of knowledge passed down from generation to generation in oral tradition. Incidentally, let me correct a statement made by the speaker. It is untrue to claim that only literate civilizations manifest pluralism, while oral civilizations know only collective thought.

François Dossou: I did not say that. My statement was a qualified one.

Paulin Hountondji: I wanted to highlight the numerous research findings and publications which for decades now have been refuting the ethnographic prejudice according to which oral societies were ignorant of individual theoretical contributions. Intellectual and ideological pluralism are by no means a monopoly of literate civilizations. Now the question is: what is the comparative value, the comparative efficiency of constituted bodies of knowledge handed down from generation to generation, on the one hand through oral tradition, on the other hand through writing? My question is the following: What do we do here and now? Do we fall back on bodies of knowledge inherited from our ancestors? That is the only question: yes or no? For these bodies of knowledge do exist. That is the sole question I, for my part, would claim to address when I say that the transition from an oral to a literate civilization is today inevitable. People who accuse me of worshipping writing as if it were some form of juju attack me unjustly.[2] Writing against the worship of writing, in truth, is beating a dead horse. Obviously, scientific discussions take place in the oral mode, like all debates. Our symposium here is an oral process. We use spoken, live words. So even in the domain of scientific research there is a level at which oral transmission is absolutely essential. That is clear. But that is not the issue. The issue is to determine if the dynamic process of research can be satisfied with oral discussions, or if it must inevitably develop in a literate framework. I think, for my part, that my question is pitched at a much more specific and precise level, a much more technical level, than the fuzzy ideological plane on which some people would prefer to keep it.

François Dossou: I think there are a number of points on which all of us here in this hall agree. But just a while ago, Mr Hountondji, speaking about specialists in oral traditions, used exactly these words: 'It is in the very process of writing that their ideas get organized'. I think we all heard these words, and I assumed they were supposed to mean something.

Paulin Hountondji: I was saying that the logical structure of these specialists' articles was the structure of written texts, that was all. I said some of their articles were organized and structured like written texts. By that I did not imply that their ideas would have been chaotic if they had not set them down in writing. I meant they would have been structured differently, and differently organized. Written words come in a particular order quite different from the order of speech.

François Dossou: I have said it was extremely hard for people trained within a literate system, people who already know how to write, to combat scriptophilia. We can write and we can think. But we only speculate well when we write. I think the contribution Ms Midiohouan made just now fits into this framework, and it should help Professor Hountondji and myself reconcile our viewpoints. We learned to write before learning to speak French. That circumstance has affected our attitude towards writing. I think we should understand such realities.

Beyond that, there is an issue we need to clarify: the matter of Holy Scripture. Biblical texts were initially oral. Only later were they put down in writing. People talk of Holy Scripture because those texts represent the word of God. In technical terms, this issue was settled long ago. Obviously, it is possible, on that basis, to suppose that all writing is sacred, and to expect everyone to adopt a reverent attitude.

Now on to the question: what must we do here and now? In all honesty, I think the list of Mr Hountondji's publications is something to be proud of. For our part, we think he has done a good job. At the same time, and again in all honesty, we reserve the right to express opinions and proffer arguments that might not please him entirely. That is also good, in my opinion, and it should be encouraging for everyone.

Moukadam Bourama: This question is for both the speaker and Ms Midiohouan, who has now and then stepped in to help him out on specific issues. Four years ago, when we were first year undergraduates, Professor Midiohouan informed us she was going to give us a course in oral traditions. I do not know if she remembers this, but I asked her if she would translate the information after collection, and into what language. She said French. I then asked if she did not think the original ideas would not be distorted, indeed betrayed, in the process. I think it would be profitable now to address this issue in answering the question raised by Professor Hountondji: what is to be done here and now? I trust the lecturer has some enlightening insights here.

Jean-Baptiste Baimey: I would like to address this question to both the speaker and Professor Hountondji. Their argument reminded me of a debate that took place a few years ago in the Ivory Coast. It was between two researchers, the sociologist Professor Niangoran Bouah and Professor Bernard Zadi, who has a PhD in Literature. At the time, Professor Niangoran Bouah was doing pioneering studies in a discipline he called drumology or the study of drum language. The literary Professor Bernard Zadi saw drumology as the grotesque mask of a dying science. As far as he was concerned, it was impossible to think of a discipline consisting simply of the study of drumbeats used for transmitting information. Now drumology is an integral part of oral traditions. My question is: can it really be conceived of as a science? The controversy notwithstanding, Professor Niangoran Bouah continued his research into what has come to be called the science of sounds. The term is accepted now. Is it a science, or is it merely endogenous knowledge? I think there is a difference between the two.

My second question is for the speaker. In my opinion, writing has an economic aspect. I think there is more to writing than mystification. I think, for instance, that writing is an energy-saving invention. Once a text is written, there is no further need to repeat it whenever one needs to communicate its message. One no longer has to travel just to go and speak to someone. In traditional Africa, for example, people had to travel hundreds of kilometres to have conversations. As a matter of fact, the fact that right now we talk so much instead of writing means we waste energy. If we simply wrote down what we had to say, we would save that much energy.

As for the origins of words and writing, let me remind you that the Bible begins with the following words from the Old Testament: 'In the beginning was the Word, and the Word was with God, and the Word was God'. I think the proof of the fact that, after all is said and done, speech is superior to writing, even though writing is necessarily and more economical, is that words have a certain power. For instance, when diviners give you an incantation, they often refuse to let you write it down in a notebook. According to them, once you write down these incantations, they lose their power. That shows that within a mystico-religious context, words have power.

Mama Katchon: My question comes from simple curiosity. We know of Socrates as someone who was happy to philosophize without ever writing his thoughts down anywhere. I would like to take this opportunity to ask our professors why he felt it was all right simply to communicate his philosophy without ever setting his ideas down on paper.

Geoffroy Botoyiye: A moment ago, Professor Midiohouan summarized the speaker's position, accurately, I think, by saying that writing is not necessarily the vehicle of knowledge. Now what I'd like to know is your own position. Should one be a scriptophile or a verbophile? You have stated your position from a political and ideological point of view. Now from a scholarly, scientific viewpoint, what is your position? In other words, what is the heuristic value of oral texts? Is our stock of traditional knowledge growing or levelling off? If it is growing, by what means? I ask because these days, more than ever, we know that the only way the various disciplines progress is through constructive work. So what, in your opinion, is the status of our endogenous knowledge?

Albert Gbodogbe: My question is intended mainly for Professor Hountondji. I would appreciate his telling me, or enumerating for me, the criteria of scientific discourse. I have no idea whether, in order to qualify as scientific, a statement has to be written or oral. Can oral discourse be scientific? If so, to what extent?

François Dossou: I think writing is an admirably practical skill. Yes, it does save us a lot of energy. I do not want to go into details, since it would take too much time to exhaust the virtues of writing. Writing is practical, energy-saving. It enables us to communicate in style ideas we cannot put into spoken words, since speech, once uttered, is forever gone. Written words, unlike speech, can be retrieved, revised, reshaped. That is a great help in the attempt to couch our ideas in practical statements. It may be said that writing is so seductive that we want to go down on our knees before it, assuming it is the source of modern science. I have said all that.

Now on to 'drumology'. I have read a few articles by Mr Niangoran Bouah. I have drawn no special conclusions concerning them.

Oral traditions do have heuristic capabilities, as proven by actual practice. Why do I say this? Traditional knowledge was a form of power. Not everyone had access to it, and initiation was a highly selective process. Those selected as repositories of traditional knowledge, then, knew perfectly well what to do to preserve it, how to disseminate it among appropriate audiences, so to speak. Needless to say, that knowledge was not popularized in the way writing now is. Preservation techniques were therefore extremely selective. It was not the entire stock of ambient knowledge that got preserved. A lot has been written on the subject, and I have cited a few titles. Those interested can get the necessary background information from them.

Regarding criteria for determining whether a particular discourse is scientific or not, I think that is the crux of the problem we have been discussing today. I am rather skeptical about the criteria proffered by Mr. Hountondji. Honestly, I think the scientific nature of a statement is defined according to explicit methods, never implicit ones. In our work on oral traditions here, we have to deal with real practices. It is impossible to say of any practice, a priori, that it is or is not scientific. Professor Kiniffo, in his presentation, spoke of practices unaccompanied by theoretical work. He raised some questions concerning such practices. His questions were scientific, because they followed a scientific approach that led him to the conclusion that the objects he discussed were foreign bodies. His methodology was entirely correct, scientific.

Careful observation had revealed that foreign objects found in the bodies of certain patients had not got there along any previously known paths. From that point on, the only rational hypothesis left was that these foreign objects had penetrated the human bodies in question along 'mysterious' paths so far unknown to us. If the time comes when the researcher no longer finds these paths mysterious, he can prove his new knowledge by repeating, under experimental conditions, what happened to the patients. At that point, what we shall demand from him is that he be able to explain the process, ending all the mystery. For now, however, someone, the professor or some other researcher, still has to discover the key to the conundrum.

It should be possible to find it, and it must be found. The practice known as chakatu, after all, has been going on for centuries. It exists, and it works. We should therefore be able to answer the question. The day when we find out how it is done, we shall have invented a new surgical technique. We will know then how to project foreign objects into human bodies, without operations or scalpels, and at long range!

Paulin Hountondji: To conclude, let me just add that from a methodological point of view, it is absolutely essential to distinguish between two levels of debate. One is the scientific and scholarly level. The other is the ideological level, necessary for historical reasons. Now the booklet on Oral Traditions by Louis-Jean Calvet, published in the *Que sais-je series*, from which the speaker quoted passages, operates on the ideological level. The speaker might also have cited another book by the same author, entitled *Linguistique et colonialisme*. It is very well known. In that book, Louis-Jean Calvet makes a vitriolic critique of what he calls 'glotophagy'. How does he define glotophagy? He defines it as the tendency to gobble up languages. French colonialism, in particular, had a tendency to suppress African languages, the languages of dominated countries.

Notes

1. The word 'chakatu' literally means 'firearm'. It refers to a practice whose underlying principles are known only to initiates. To the public it is something of a mystery. What is generally known is this: miscellaneous and unusual objects such as needles, razor blades, fishing hooks, nails and pieces of broken glass are inserted into a specially prepared piece of shinbone, along with sand, gunpowder and various other ingredients. The name of the intended victim is pronounced along with some incantations while the loaded shinbone is aimed at the sky. This, no doubt, is why the object is likened to a firearm. It is said that all these objects will penetrate the body of the victim no matter where he or she is.
2. See François Dossou, 'Critique du fétichisme de l'alphabet', Langage et devenir, Newsletter of the National Applied Linguistics centre (CENALA), Cotonou, Nos. 4 & 5, October 1988. pp.110-120. See also the daily newspaper EHUZU, Cotonou, 27 May, 3 June and 10 June 1987.

12

Graphic Representational Systems in Precolonial Africa

Albert Bienvenu Akoha

When we talk of graphic representational systems, we mean essentially writing. All definitions advanced by linguists, especially by grammarians, agree on this point. According to Marcel Cohen (1958:1), 'Writing consists of durable visual representations facilitating the transportation and preservation of language'.

James Février (1984:9) describes writing as 'a means currently used to give permanent form to articulate language, an essentially ephemeral phenomenon'. Writing, then, appears to be a 'major invention applied to' a product of the human mind, language, which itself may be considered an invention, an instrument helping to meet the need for communication and concerted action within the social group (Cohen 1958:1).

In precolonial Africa, as in the rest of the world, humans developed graphic representational systems as a means of imparting permanence to language. The basic quality of language is its double articulation. For, according to Martinet (1970:13), a statement or sentence, taken as an expression of human experience, can be broken down into a continuous chain of minimal linguistic units. Of this continuum, the smallest portion capable of expressing sense is the linguistic sign, to which Martinet gives the name of 'lexeme'. In the statement 'The woman works', for instance, woman is a lexeme. We can go a step farther and break this lexeme 'woman' down into appropriate phonetic units. In the process we see that our moneme comprises several distinct sounds: each such sound is a phoneme.

All natural languages function with a limited number of phonemes peculiar to them. It is the entire set of phonemes that constitutes the phonological system of a given language. Let us take the example of the French phonological system. It is made up of 16 vowels, 17 consonants and three semi-consonants. The Fon language, spoken in Benin, offers a different example: it has 16 vowels, 22 consonants and four 4 tones.

While every language has a limited number of phonemes, the number of lexemes or meaningful sounds is open-ended, because every language is capable of inventing new words to express new realities. One finding of analytical linguistics seems to be that graphic representational systems which emphasize the notation of sound units are invariably more economical and efficient than those dependent on notations of complete words or ideas. The history of writing is a difficult subject, and the attempt to trace its development is particularly problematic. As Cohen asserts: 'In those regions where writing originated in antiquity, we have no historical indications as to its beginnings' (1958:3). Charles Higounet (1976:17) reports that 'certain scholars have advanced the hypothesis that the writing systems of antiquity — Sumerian, Proto-Elamite, Egyptian, Proto-Indian, Chinese — had a common origin. In support, they put forward just one argument: the fact that all these were analytical languages, in the sense that they wrote down word units'. This, to put it mildly, is a shaky argument.

One thing is certain, though: writing appeared in different parts of the world at different times. The best way to determine the source of any writing system is to examine the dynamics of its internal development. Nevertheless, it is clear that interactions among peoples and cultures facilitated more or less intense borrowing and influence from more developed to less developed systems. If we examine the issue of the multiplicity of systems of graphic representation within the general context of the effort to give language permanent representational forms, it seems possible to rank various forms of writing along a scale leading from the depiction of ideas through the writing of words to the notation of sounds.

Stages of Writing

A world-wide survey of writing systems reveals four stages of development. The first or preliminary stage is that of symbolic writing. In his fourth book (Section 131 onwards), Herodotus gives a good example:

> The Scythian kings sent Darius a messenger carrying a bird, a mouse, a frog and five arrows. The Persians asked the messenger what these gifts meant. He replied that his only instructions were to deliver the gifts and to return as soon as possible. It was up to the Persians to figure out the meaning of the gifts. The Persians took counsel, and Darius concluded that the Scythians were signalling the surrender of themselves, their land and their waters. For, so he reasoned, the mouse was a land animal that ate the same food as man; the frog lived in water, while the bird much resembled a horse. As for the arrows, they signified that the Scythians were surrendering to him their weapons of war. Such was Darius's opinion. However, Gobryas, one of the seven killers of the Magi, was of an entirely different opinion.

To his mind the gifts meant:

> Unless you, Persians, become birds and fly through the air; or turn into mice and hide underground; or become frogs and leap into lakes; you shall be transfixed by these arrows, and never return home to your country (quoted by Gelb 1973:6-7).

The contradictory interpretations given this message are a good illustration of the limitations of communications systems based on the dispatch of symbolic objects. In any case, it is much handier to draw or make graphic representations of the objects in question. Humanity's store of 'primitive drawings' bearing messages is impressive. Some date from the depths of ages. They include rock paintings, stone carvings, cave paintings and line drawings, bas-reliefs and frescoes, etc. Taken together with tribal insignia, markings, emblems and assorted distinguishing images, they may be regarded as 'precursors of writing', writing degree zero, writing in the preliminary phase.

The second phase is what Cohen calls proto-writing. We prefer to call it the pictographic stage. At this stage, the tendency was to make writing coincide with articulate language, but still the correlation was only approximate. 'The intention was to use a written sign or group of signs to suggest — we cannot yet say to note — an entire sentence or phrase' (Février 1984:10).

Pictographs have been identified in various parts of the world at different times. We shall take two examples from the Fon language in the Republic of Benin:

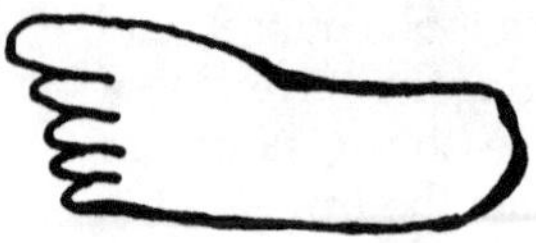

Pictograph 1

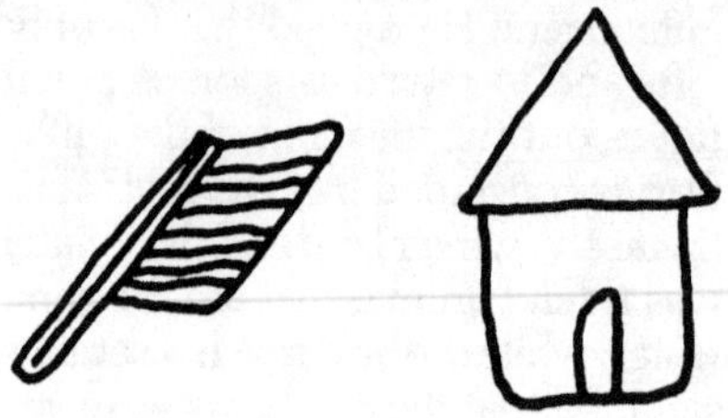

Pictograph 2

The first pictograph is a representation of a foot. It is given only one meaning by Fon convention: *Afo wèmyi mèmê*. This means: 'Visits are the greatest sign of friendship'. The axiom is used in times of sorrow, when someone shirks the duty of visiting a troubled friend with the excuse that he has no material help to bring.

The second pictograph is a representation of a broom and a house. The conventional message is equally unambiguous: *Akiza cé ma za hon towe to a o gbéfen na wu*. Translation: 'Unless my broom sweeps before your house, only weeds will grow there'. Long ago, among the Fon, only the mistress of a house or the favourite wife was expected to sweep the inside of a family compound and the space in front of it. By extension, when a woman was said to be the one to sweep a man's house, it meant she was his wife. The pictograph thus came to be used in the language of courting, with the meaning: 'I am the only woman who can make you happy. I love you to distraction'.

Février calls these prototypical writing systems synthetic. By that he means that 'their basic characteristic is that they aim at using a single image that the eye can encompass in one sweep, to suggest an entire statement, sentence or even a set of sentences' (1984:43).

At the third stage we come to the phenomenon that grammarians and linguists alike agree to call writing proper. 'The sign no longer stands for a phrase or sentence; it is a notation for a word'. This development is not the result of mere quantitative change. It is a significant 'leap' indicating really substantial progress from the previous level. Only mature reflection on the nature and function of language could pave the way to such progress. On this point, Antoine Meillet asserts that 'no drawing, pictograph or ideogram is adequate for the graphic rendition of a language'. Since the notation of words in a language requires breaking it down into component units, 'writing develops from synthetic forms to analytical or ideographic forms'. Charles Higounet gives us selected examples of analytical writing taken from Sumero-Akkadian writings from the third millennium BC (Higounet 1976:18).

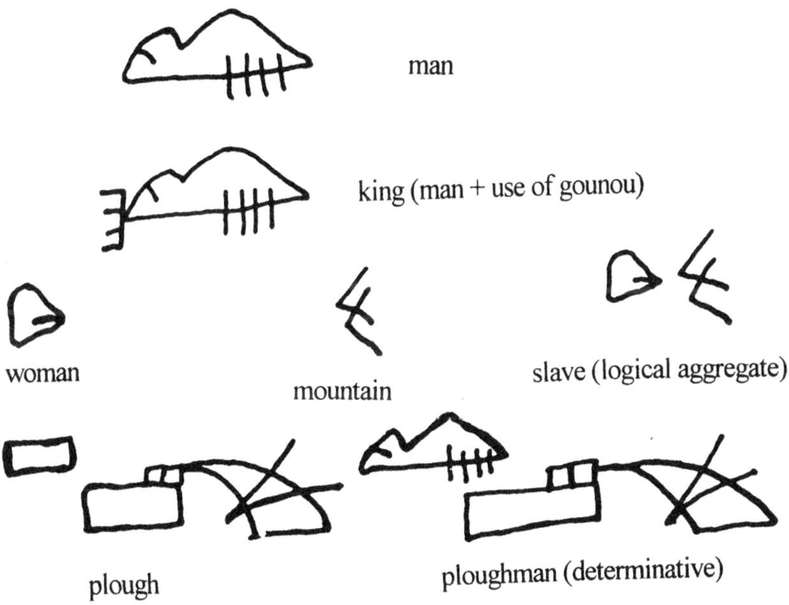

Sumero-Akkadian writing underwent a great deal of internal development. To avoid the infinite proliferation of signs designating words, use was made of *gounou,* a set of 'supplementary signs reinforcing the idea expressed by a given sign', as in the example of the word 'king'. Sumerian writing used other problem-solving techniques. These included logical aggregates, defined as 'the juxtaposition of two signs to express a new idea'; for example, the juxtaposition of the signs for 'woman' and 'mountain' to produce a new meaning: 'slave'. A further technique comprised determinatives. These were unpronounced signs inserted before words, indicating the category to which the specific usage belonged, and therefore complementing the normal meaning of the word. For example, the sign for 'plough', preceded by the determinative sign for 'man', meant 'ploughman'. On the other hand, preceded by the determinative sign for 'wood', it simply meant the plough. As we shall soon see, Egyptian writing was based on the same principle.

The fourth stage embraces all phonetic writing systems. Only profound reflection on the nature and function of writing over the centuries made the invention of writing possible. Such reflection inexorably led scholars to sound notation systems. The first people to abandon the use of signs representing sentences, phrases or words, and to take up the use of sound notations were indisputably the discoverers, in specific ways, of language as a doubly articulated phenomenon. In the process they found an efficient solution to the age-old problem of an economical system of graphic representational signs. Now as already pointed out, languages are generally made up of limited sets of consonants and vowels, supplemented occasionally by tones, accents, or both. To be able to isolate relevant linguistic elements and to create notational signs for them was a great liberating step forward. Because of the semiotic economy it makes possible, phonetic writing is the most efficient system of graphic representation known to humanity. Under the category of phonetic writing there are two sub-categories: syllabic writing and alphabetic writing.

Syllabic Writing

Here, as the name indicates, the basic unit of writing is the syllable. This form of writing occurs often among languages with a large proportion of monosyllabic words. We shall use selected examples from the Brahminic and Nagari writing systems of India to illustrate the workings of syllabic writing systems.

- Brahminic System (C. Higounet 1976:57).

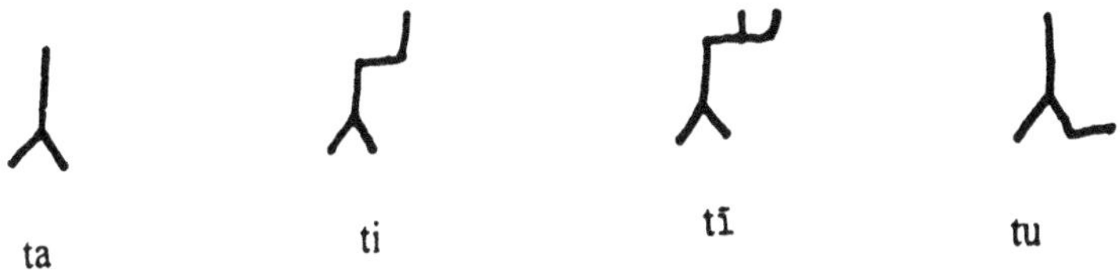

- Nagari System (C. Higounet 1976:58)

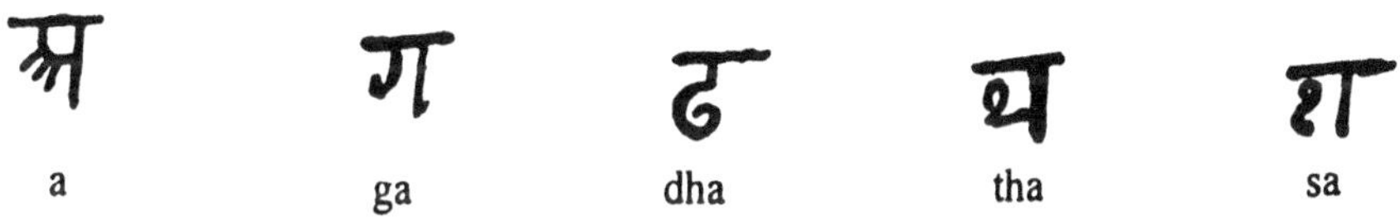

The Brahminic writing system comprises a total of four initial vowel signs (a, i, u, o) and 32 syllabic signs. The Nagari writing system was first used to write Sanskrit, a religious and scholarly language, before being used for Hindi, 'the lingua franca of Central India, whose use has steadily spread'. The name Nagari means 'urban writing'.

Historians of writing argue that Brahminic writing was based on the Semitic alphabet, but Février thinks instead that 'the inventors of the Brahminic system derived it from the Phoenician system'.

Syllabic writing systems are relatively efficient, but less so than alphabetic systems.

Alphabetic Writing

This is the type of writing system we use today. Prime examples are Greek and Latin. In French there are cases where words are pronounced differently from the way they are written. On the whole, however, French is written in a basically phonetic alphabet. All writing codes used for the transcription of African languages these days to facilitate their use in literacy programmes are derived from the international phonetic and Latin alphabets. They are all, in other words, phonetic, alphabetic systems.

There is no doubt that of all writing systems the handiest is the alphabetic system. The main reason is that it is the most economical. It is this quality that probably accounts for its wide dissemination, especially in the West.

We have just outlined the principal stages in what might be called humanity's long march towards phonetic writing. It should be pointed out that this development was not linear. The different systems we have described, along with variations on them, often existed side by side in different parts of the world. Sometimes they could be found in the same country. All historians of writing agree that civilizations often borrow, modify and develop writing systems. After this overview of the development of writing systems throughout the world and over the centuries we can now move on to identify and evaluate writing systems in precolonial Africa.

Graphic Representational Systems in Precolonial Africa

In many respects our knowledge of precolonial Africa is patchy. Still, historians of writing have identified numerous writing systems developed there. Together they cover the whole range of evolutionary stages as described above. An exhaustive inventory of African systems of graphic representation would make a long list indeed. Egypt alone presents such an array of special features in this domain that it would be tedious to list them all. We shall discuss each of the four stages outlined above, using for illustrative purposes only the most representative examples.

Prototypical Writing Systems in Africa

The type of phenomenon Herodotus described in his account of relations between Persians and Scythians had counterparts in Africa. In the old kingdoms of Dahomey and Oyo during the 17th century, objects with symbolic meanings were sent as messages. The Grammarian Gelb (1973:6) describes 'a very interesting custom, from a comparative viewpoint':

> During a siege of a Yoruba city mounted by a king of Dahomey, a Yoruba prisoner wishing to inform his wife of his plight sent her a stone, a piece of charcoal, some pepper, a maize twig and a rag. The intended message was as follows: the stone represented health, signifying that the prisoner's body had remained as tough and healthy as a stone. The pepper represented heat, signifying that the prisoner's spirit, anxious about its uncertain future, burned as painfully as pepper on the tongue. The maize twig represented thinness, signifying that the fire of captivity and suffering had dried up the prisoner's body as much as a drought-shrivelled maize shoot. The rag signified the tattered state of the prisoner's clothes.

Among the Fon, this method of sending messages is still used to this day, for instance, during *zindo* ritual ceremonies. As a rule, African symbolism is extremely rich. Among prototypical representational systems, we should mention sculpted staffs of office, carpets serving as maps, the Abomey bas-reliefs, and the popular system of Fa geomantic signs used among the Fon.

Sculpted staffs of office function as royal wands. They are sculpted with royal emblems, and those carrying them have the status of royal ambassadors plenipotentiary, and are expected to be treated as such (Adande 1962).

As the name carpet-maps implies, these were fabrics woven by spies sent by the Kingdom of Dahomey to reconnoitre countries earmarked for conquest. The stages of the campaign were as follows: Dahomean spies, known as *agbadjigeto,* were dispatched to targeted towns. For months or years they gathered intelligence on the customs and occult sciences of the target population, sending regular reports back to the Dahomean capital, Abomey. At the same time they sent back numbered pieces of woven fabric bearing drawings of various strategic locations in the target city or country. Back in Abomey, all the generals had to do was to put together the pieces of the puzzle making up the carpet-map, the centre-piece of their campaign plan.

After each campaign, outstanding deeds and courageous exploits, along with the honorific titles the king added to his roll, were given permanent form in bas-reliefs carved on palace buildings in Abomey. The motifs were normally war scenes such as the head of an enemy tied to a horse's neck, a soldier aiming at an enemy, an amazon hefting a hapless enemy soldier on her shoulder, etc. (Adande 1977 and Waterlote 1926).

Fa signs were another type of system used. According to Bernard Maupoil (1961:5), Fa is 'the god or spirit of divination, the intermediary between gods and men, ... a multi-purpose oracle'. The Fa priest, known as a Bokonon, meaning diviner, throws his sacred beads on a flat surface, where the lobes or beads take up various positions, open or closed. Each closed lobe is coded as two vertical lines, each open lobe as a single line. The resulting signs have the following configurations:

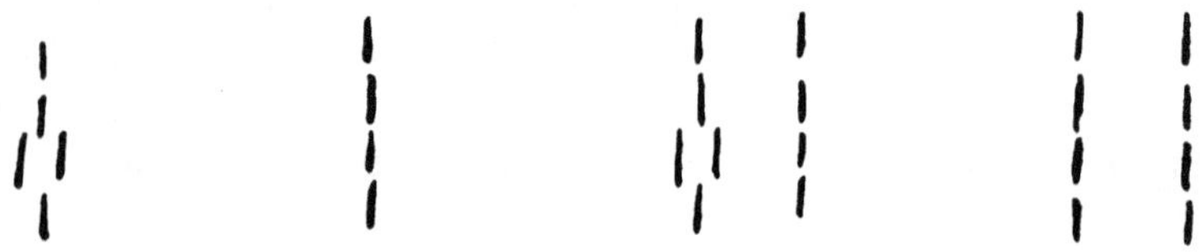

lèté gbé gbé-lèté gbé-mèji

At the end of the consultation session, the Bokonon traces out the signs occurring on a shard of calabash, then gives it to the seeker as a reminder. The seeker is free to obtain a second opinion from another diviner, to check the original interpretation. Very often, different diviners come up with exactly the same interpretation. This is evidence that Fa diviners or priests undergo an identical training course in which sign notation is an important component.

Non-alphabetical Writing in Africa

Apart from prototypical representational forms, Africa has had numerous non-alphabetical forms of writing. Under this category we shall list pictography, whose use is extremely widespread in Africa; Egyptian writing in its different forms, and the classical writing system of the Bamoun.

Pictography, the use of figurative drawings for communicating messages, appeared in several African cultures before and after colonial conquest. The pictographic systems of the Ashanti, Ewe and Fon people are among the most beautiful. We provided examples of these forms in the first part of this chapter. The following are further examples from the Ewe and Fon cultures:

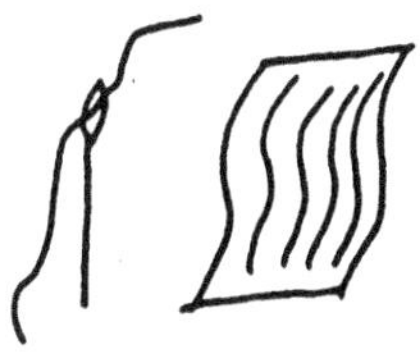

Pictograph 1

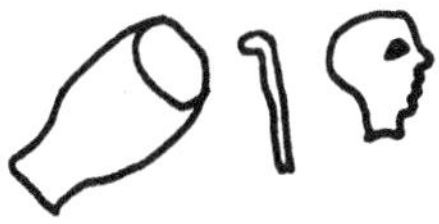

Pictograph 2

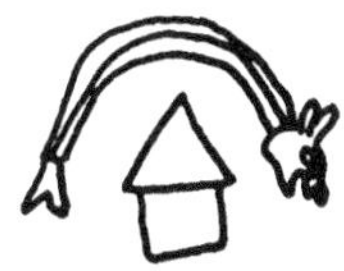

Pictograph 3

Pictograph 1 shows a threaded needle next to a piece of cloth. This is a graphic representation of an Ewe proverb: 'Whole cloth is made up of tiny threads'. This is similar to the proverb: 'Little drops of water make the mighty ocean'.

Pictograph 2 is from the Fon language. It shows a drum, a stick and a heart, signifying *Ta ce do gbè o ngida ce na do-nu do hun towé nu*. This translates as: 'If God gives me life, I shall make your heart resonate as a stick makes the drum resound'. This pictograph exploits the opening for a play on words offered by the fact that the Fon word *hun* means both 'drum' and 'heart' — conclusive proof that the Fon are familiar with punning in their linguistic notation.

Pictograph 3 shows a rainbow over a house. In Fon, the corresponding sentence is: *Xo émi do o gbé na gloo na huzu nyi bo na bla ta nu xwetowé.* This means: 'If you break your promise, I shall turn into a rainbow and surround your house'. It is used mostly to ratify blood pacts or secret accords between two or more parties. It constitutes a direct, dreaded threat of reprisals in case of any temptation to betray some trust or even simply to be negligent about its observance. There are many African countries in which pictographic art survived the colonial impact. In the Republic of Benin, Fon culture is an outstanding example. For detailed information, see Akoha (1987).

By every yardstick, Egyptian writing is the best known and most significant precolonial African writing system. It originated 3,000 years before the Christian era. Some consider it the oldest writing system in the world. About its veritable origins, however, nothing is known. As in the Sumero-Akkadian system, in Egyptian writing the basic unit is the word. The system is therefore known as a word-based writing system, with ideographic and analytic forms. In ancient Egyptian writing, graphic signs for words have some representational resemblance to the ideas expressed. Examples (cf. C. Higounet 1976:23).

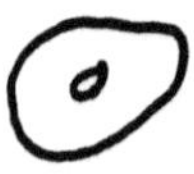

sun, weather

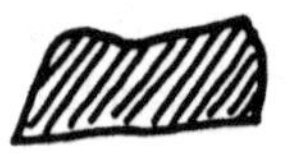

mountain

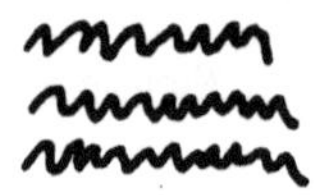

water, sea

This initial series belongs to the first grammatical category, that of nouns.

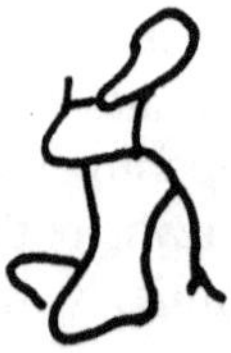

to eat

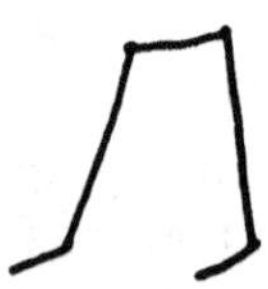

to go

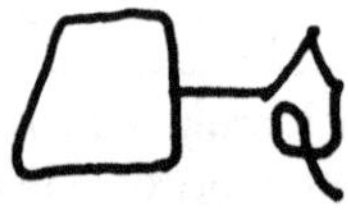

to fight

Egyptian writing was initially engraved on stone, but in time the transcription method changed. The characters used were simplified into so-called linear hieroglyphs, painted in ink on wooden sarcophagi or papyrus sheets. In the beginning the system was multidirectional. 'Characters could be written from top to bottom, left to right and right to left', with the objects drawn generally facing the beginning of the line.

We do not intend to get into a more detailed description of the formal characteristics of Egyptian writing. Suffice it to point out that Egyptian hieroglyphs or ideograms originally represented concrete realities such as the sun, the weather, mountains, seas, water, etc., as well as actions like eating, walking and fighting. Subsequently they evolved and were broken down into phonetic units, but the older forms also remained in use. Thus, at a certain period, signs used in Egyptian writing sometimes expressed words, sometimes sounds. Higounet, (1976:24-25) provides some examples:

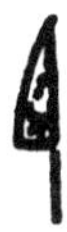 = i, j, = reed leaf

 = h = disk

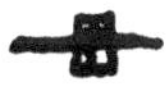 = s = bolt

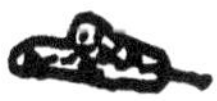 = d = hand

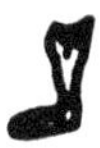 = b = leg

The revolutionary shift from word units to sound units was facilitated by the monosyllabic structure of Egyptian language. 'Thanks to the writing down of monosyllabic words, Egyptian writing progressed to the point of transcribing isolated syllables'. The social uses of writing determined the distinction between the two main forms of Egyptian writing, hieratic and demotic. In later times hieratic or sacred writing was the form of writing used by priests. It was a simplification of hieratic writing that led to the demotic (or popular) form at the beginning of the first millennium. In the Ptolemaic period (from 333 to 3 BC), demotic writing became the literary and administrative form. It remained in use until the end of the fifth century.

In its development, Egyptian writing straddled the word-based and the sound-based phases of writing systems. At the same time, it maintained certain pictographic features. For these reasons it provides an excellent overview of the development of different techniques for the transcription of articulate language. It had considerable influence, direct and indirect, on graphic representational systems in the sub-region.

The Bamoun writing this system was developed from scratch by African scholars commissioned by the Cameroonian King Njoya in 1900. It is a word-based writing system. Février (1984:536) provides some examples:

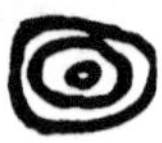 = Baka, Plate

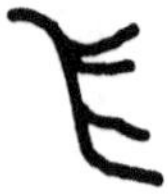 = Nyam, Horse

 = Yu, To eat

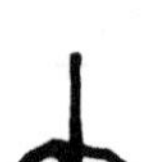 = Yúone, To see (2 eyes)

'Soon thereafter, the fact that most words were monosyllabic facilitated the use of rebus signs to represent them'. This in turn facilitated the use of a manageable number of signs in all. According to testimony recorded by Février (1984: 535), the number of graphic signs in the Bamoun system was estimated to be 348 in 1907. Under the impact of colonialism, Bamoun writing turned phonetic.

Phonetic Writing in Precolonial Africa

Technically, phonetic writing systems are superior. Africa has had a few phonetic systems, including the Vaï, Somali and Ethiopian systems.

The Mende and Vaï Systems

The Mende and Vaï languages belong to the same linguistic family, the great Mende group. Mende people live in Sierra Leone, while the Vaï are found on the Sierra Leonean and Liberian coasts.

Mende writing is purely syllabic. It comprises up to 190 characters, all monosyllables in which a consonant is linked to a vowel. This gives an indication of the richness of the Mende phonetic system. Some syllables are formed in regular fashion starting with the same sign. When the consonant is followed by the vowel a, this is indicated by a dot above the sign. Syllables ending in u are indicated by two superimposed dots. Syllables ending in i have no dots. The way vowels are transcribed here suggests some Arabic influence. However, Mende writing is derived more or less directly from Vaï writing.

The Vaï writing system became rather famous after publication of in-depth studies on it conducted by the linguistics scholars S.W. Koelle and M. Delafosse. Thanks to their research, we know that Vaï is a syllabic writing system, or at least that it has been syllabic since 1849. The system used 226 characters. Some, rarely used, dropped out of common usage. Occasionally, the same syllable might be represented by several different signs. The large number of signs was an indication of the richness of the Vaï phonetic system. It was also an index of the 'extreme precision' of this graphic system capable of recording the subtlest nuances of articulate speech. Vai writing goes from left to write. Even though the population is predominantly Muslim and familiar with Arabic script, the use of the Vaï system is widespread among them. Researchers trying to determine the origins of Vaï script have come up with numerous controversial hypotheses. It is clear, at any rate, that the shapes of characters in the Vaï script have undergone considerable change as a result of foreign contacts.

The Somali System

A Somali called Isman Yussuf is said 'to have designed an alphabet for the use of his compatriots, on which E. Ceruli offers some information' (Février 1984:528). Isman Yussuf spoke Arabic and could write it. In addition, he had a smattering of Italian and Latin. His writing system was directly based on these two sources. It consisted of 22 consonants ordered in the Arabic fashion, to which he added five characters representing vowel sounds. It was not a particularly original system, and never achieved much recognition.

Ethiopian Writing Systems

Several of Ethiopia's Semitic languages were transcribed with characters derived from the South Arabian alphabet. 'Classical Ethiopian, known as Ge'ez, a member of the Southern Semitic family, originated with a writing system that is still in use' (Higounet 1976:55). The system comprises 221 characters which together 'constitute a curious regression to syllabic forms after an excursion into the phonetic alphabet'.

Arabic Writing

Arabic writing is an offshoot of the Semitic tradition. It is a phonetic form, alphabetic to be precise. It might be even more accurate to call it a consonantal writing system. Little is known about this writing system. It would seem to be derived from Habatean writing, a system heavily influenced by Syriac. We do know, however, that the first records in Arabic, comprising the inscriptions of Ez-Zabad (+ 512-513), Harran (+ 568) and Oumm el Djima, were trilingual (Greek, Syriac and Arabic). We also know that they antedated Mohammed's arrival in Medina (+ 622, the Hegira). The subsequent expansion of Islam greatly facilitated the stabilization and spread of Arabic writing. Two main reasons have frequently been advanced to explain the international success of Arabic writing. The first is the Islamic injunction according to which 'The Koran, containing as it does the revealed truth of God, shall not be translated nor transcribed into any foreign tongue. Whoever aspires to knowledge of the Islamic religion must have an understanding, albeit of a rudimentary nature, of Arabic language and writing' (Février 1984:262).

Thus, the Arabic writing system, found in various regions of the world on account of its religious uses, has also served for the transcription of a wide range of languages including Persian, Turkish, Malagasy, Malay and Tamil. In Africa, Arabic script has been used to transcribe such languages as Berber and Kiswahili. It has been observed, however, that Arabic script is not altogether suitable for the transcription of non-Semitic languages. 'Diacritical marks therefore had to be used to help create many new signs, which did not have the same values in all languages. An example is the notation of g in Berber and Persian' (Février 1984:274). Similar problems were encountered in the transcription of such African languages as Kiswahili, the Bantu language used in East Africa.

Lastly, it must be remembered that it is not so much colloquial Arabic as classical (literal) Arabic that is 'understood and used from one corner of the Muslim world to the other'. That, at least in part, is the reason why certain countries intent on implementing cultural policies based on Arabization programmes now face so many problems.

African Societies and Writing Systems

Our brief overview of selected systems of graphic representation in Africa makes it clear that our continent has been through all stages of development in the art of writing, from synthetic forms through analytical and ideographic forms to phonetic writing. The question arises: why did Africa get isolated from the main current of ideas which propelled Europe into focusing on writing as the major means of communication? Why did the use of graphic representational systems get bogged down in Africa while in Europe and Asia it made rapid qualitative progress? We think Africa stagnated not so much because of any defect in the writing systems themselves, but because of the socio-historical conditions under which they evolved.

Origins and Development of Graphic Representational Systems

Scholars are yet uncertain about the exact origins of writing. They have therefore fallen back on more or less plausible hypotheses. Cohen, for instance, thinks that writing originated independently in various parts of the world. Others like Gelb are inclined to posit a common origin for all the writing systems of antiquity: Sumerian, Proto-Elamite, Egyptian, Proto-Indian, Chinese. Gelb, a renowned grammarian, goes so far as to argue that this original common writing system, which he calls

Proto-Sumerian, was a pictographic system dating back to the third millennium BC. The hypothesis sounds plausible enough. After all, we know that at the time, the Mediterranean area was unified, unlike our modern world. A writing system originating in the area might therefore have spread, wave-like, from region to region across countries and centuries. Different peoples have often borrowed writing systems developed by neighbours to transcribe their own language. Subsequent endeavours to find the best ways of adapting the borrowed methods have led to technical improvements that have enriched the universal pool of experience in the transcription of languages.

Let us note, right off, that Africa, through Egypt, was a founding participant in this great adventure. Better still, the Phoenician alphabet that influenced the Greek alphabet so greatly was itself, according to some scholars, 'a deformed variant of Egyptian hieroglyphic writing'. The argument is that this deformation happened slowly, through the agency of numerous intermediaries (Vendryes 1968:355).

Most historians have had to face, one way or the other, the issue of the origin of writing. Few, however, have paid any attention to the socio-historical conditions conducive to the social invention and development of graphic representational systems. In the absence of any thorough-going analysis of the issue, we might simply observe that as a rule, writing appears in a given society only when its organizational level and attendant practices make it necessary. The appearance of writing in Egypt, for instance, coincided with that country's unification around the year -2900. The expansion of Phoenician commerce necessitated the stabilization and spread of Phoenician writing. And the Arabic language and writing system did not really take off until the Hegira of +622, the date of Mohammed's arrival in Medina and the beginning of the Muslim era. Closer home, it was the determination to win expansionist wars that led to the use of carpet-maps by the Dahomean spies of Abomey, used to communicate strategic information to the kingdom's generals.

In short, writing invariably appears in a given society as a response to felt need. To meet that need, the society may develop its own system or borrow a foreign script. Within this historical and social dynamic, people initially use writing to meet imperative needs. This may mean the immortalization of what they consider most precious in their society, such as religious notions, philosophical ideas, literary texts, public accounts, legal decrees and political pronouncements. Once established in society, writing leads to profound changes in thought and habits, with correspondingly profound effects on social organization. The research of Goody (1979, 1986) provides definitive proof of this conclusion reached by several scholars, showing in specific ways (religious, economic, political, legal) the initial impact of writing on human social organization.

Writing, incidentally, has a tendency to get better with the passage of time, partly because it facilitates systematic thinking about language itself. The high proportion of monosyllabic words in the Egyptian language facilitated the advancement of the writing system from ideographic to phonetic forms. But there are other factors at play in the evolution of writing systems. The nature of materials used (such as clay tablets, stone slabs, wooden sarcophagi, leather parchment or papyrus) is important, as is the sacred or secular status of the script.

The spread and influence of writing systems, however, has little to do with their intrinsic perfection. The key factor here seems to be the economic and political power of the society using a particular writing system as its means of communication. The Greeks and Romans exported their writing systems thanks to imperial states established by military force. The Latin script and language owed their spread and prestige in Europe to the triumph of Christianity in that region of the world. Arabic owed a similar boost to Muslim expansion. Likewise, colonialism lifted such languages as English, French and Spanish to the status of international languages. In the process, it also conferred world-wide fame and prestige on the Latin alphabet. In sum, Goody is quite right when he argues that 'the social structure undergirding acts of communication is often of prime importance.... Nevertheless, it is no accident that the decisive developmental stages of what we now term 'science' have invariably followed pivotal changes in communications techniques: writing in Babylon, the alphabet in ancient Greece, the printing press in Western Europe' (Goody 1979:107).

The Decline of African Writing Systems

Strictly speaking, the issue of the stagnation or disappearance of African writing systems falls more under the disciplines of history and archaeology than under linguistics. Africa in antiquity was among the pioneers in the invention of writing. The continent has gone through the entire range of possible stages in the development of writing. Yet somewhere along the way Africa seems to have lost the knack of writing, falling so far back that certain scholars unblinkingly present it as the continent of 'civilizations without writing'. Available evidence exposes the crudeness of such conclusions. It is a fact that several African cultures were literate, and that some actually kept up their writing skills in various forms. Still, it is important, in any historical approach to causal factors, to take care not to lose sight of fundamental differences between societies which stressed the use of writing as a means of communication, and those in which oral forms of communication remained dominant.

There is every reason to believe that the current gap between Africa and the so-called 'literate civilizations' has not always existed. One example, as we have seen, was that of ancient Egypt. Further, in the period when Europe was going through its Middle Ages, the African cities of Djenne and Timbuktu were brilliant centres of learning, according to historians. Suret-Canale (1973:187) points out that in the sixteenth century, during the reign of Askia Mohamed, 'renowned doctors and writers from the Maghreb did not look down on opportunities to come for courses given by their black colleagues in Timbuktu'. The same scholar, author of *L'Afrique Noire, géographie, civilisation et histoire,* adds that in Timbuktu, 'there were 150 to 180 Koranic schools, with the best known counting over 100 pupils, sometimes even more than 150' (1987:181).

Against this background, we link the marginalization of Africa to the invention of the printing press and the intensification of the slave trade by the West from the fifteenth to the nineteenth century. For while, with the invention and spread of the printing press, the West took some great qualitative strides forward in science and technology, Africa, pushed into defensive postures and withdrawal, had to absorb the devastating impact of the slave trade for four centuries. In his work the historian Inikori (1979) does not focus directly on the loss of writing by African civilizations; nevertheless, his findings provide convincing proof of the causal relationship between the installation of the Slave Trade and the cultural and scientific marginalization of Africa. 'The demands of the Slave Trade', he observes, 'were such that they could in no way be conducive to the improvement of infrastructural systems in the affected states' (1979:78). He adds later, citing work done by Peter Morton: 'The wars and raids necessitated by the Slave Trade pushed populations to settle in easily defensible locations. Sites thus chosen because of the presence of natural obstacles were inaccessible. This meant that ease of communication was sacrificed. Indeed, areas that under peaceful conditions would have been excellent for construction (and farming) were abandoned. The resulting settlement patterns encouraged subsistence farming and discouraged peaceful trade. *Worse still, in hiding from slave raiders, the populations also missed the swirl of new ideas in the world'* (italics ours). Inikori concludes that in this way the slave trade slowed down economic development in Africa by preventing the 'expansion of normal exchanges between Africa and the rest of the world at a time (1451 — 1870) when these exchanges were a powerful motor for economic development in a number of countries' (1979:79).

In conclusion, let us observe that writing is not simply the recording of speech. It is also a technique for breaking down language into serial component units. Simultaneously, writing is also the outcome of this analytical breakdown. Incidentally, the presence of writing in a given society is not sufficient to ensure that the society in question can take full advantage of scientific advances made possible by the communications medium of writing. The medium has to spread. And it is only under those conditions that writing becomes a powerful motor ensuring scientific progress. In his analysis of the social impact of alphabetical writing, Goody notes, quite rightly, that its use 'necessarily affects relationships between individuals as well as the development of storage capacities, analytical capabilities and creative potential in the field of knowledge'.

Because it gave hitherto oral statements a semi-permanent form, writing, to quote Goody (1979:86-87) once again, provided a new way to examine rhetoric. This new resource, by helping to expand the range of critical activity, encouraged rational and skeptical attitudes and logical thought (to return to these arguable dichotomies). Opportunities for critical thinking increased because people could now actually look at the content of all discourse. Concurrently, there was a tremendous increase in the capacity to accumulate knowledge, especially abstract knowledge'.

It is understandable, then, that Africa, by missing the opportunity to develop writing at a decisive turning point in history, no doubt on account of the slave trade, got stranded beside the mainstream of ideas changing the world so profoundly ever since the Middle Ages. It is to be hoped that coming advances in archaeological and historical research in Africa will sooner or later provide us with definitive answers to questions confronting the scientific and scholarly community as to the reasons for and antidotes to the stagnation and sclerosis of writing systems in Africa.

Discussion

The following is a transcript of the discussion which took place after the presentation of this chapter at the National University of Benin seminar.

Abel Yakpa: Modern writing systems make it possible for speakers of different languages in any country or region to communicate with each other. I'd like to know if, with the writing systems of the past, such regional intercommunication was possible.

Bienvenu Akoha: First of all, it is not entirely accurate to say that people speaking different languages can understand each other. Let us take specific examples. Nowadays we can say there is a partial sort of mutual comprehension between Gun and Fon speakers. I doubt very much, however, if the same can be said of Fon speakers and speakers of Batonu or Ditamari. That said, we have to qualify the degree of incomprehension. Mutual comprehension occurs, to varying degrees, between languages of a single family. But let me address the question: did past writing systems enable people to understand each other then?

Absolutely. I talked of developments dating back to the third, second and first millennia BC. Those were ancient times. In the second millennium BC, for instance, Sumero-Akkadian was the international language used in Western Asia and the regions of Babylon, Mesopotamia, etc. Later, at the time of the Persian Empire, the Persian language and script became the standard, indeed the compulsory lingua franca. Even non-Persians used it for purposes of communication. The situation was similar under the Roman Empire. Whoever wanted to communicate then used Latin, which was the international language of the time. In its day, Egyptian too had served as an international language. There was a period when Phoenician was heard as an international language, especially in commercial circles, where the Phoenicians excelled.

We need to guard against hasty assumptions of mutual comprehension, however. The situation then was no different from our present situation. Today, everywhere you turn, you bump into Americans. This confers tremendous prestige on the English language. Some of you here are Ditamari speakers. You use English to communicate with others, and yet it cannot be said that Ditamari and English are mutually comprehensible.

Ignace Djenontin: You spoke of different types of writing such as the Bamoun and Egyptian scripts, etc. Then you began to list prototypical writing systems. I would like to know if you listed African systems in the order of their appearance. You promised to tell us the order in which those writing systems occurred.

Bienvenu Akoha: I did not undertake to describe African writing systems in any particular order. If you assumed that the order in which I mentioned them was chronological, that was a mistake. They did not appear in a linear array. What I did was to classify various systems on a qualitative scale determined by the purpose of writing, which is the representation of language. I said that the closer a writing system got to the phonetic standard, the higher its quality. The reason is that any language has only a very limited number of sounds. Any language which can be written using sound notation only, therefore, achieves a very substantial economy. For example, you will have noticed what a vast range of sentences and words in the Fon language can be represented with only 22 consonants, 16 vowels and four tones. If, by contrast, you were to use a writing system capable only of representing whole sentences, you would very quickly reach a limit. Systems using only whole words may be slightly less cumbersome, but they still are limited. The number of words in any language is open-ended.

If your system uses syllables, you are luckier because it is more manageable. But you are still in trouble. You get out of the woods only when you succeed in using a system based on sound notation. That, to my recollection, is what I said. I also tried to demonstrate that it is wrong to suppose that Africa had only prototypical forms of writing, leaving the development of the most sophisticated system — phonetic writing — to Europe. I showed that all the different stages of writing occurred in the West as well as in Africa. But in the end something happened. Africa did not surge forward on the strength of its writing systems, using science and technology, the way the West did.

Epiphane Hougnon: Listening to you, one gets the impression that Africa had quite a few writing systems. One wonders, then, how come these writing systems disappeared while the French, English and Chinese systems, for instance, were able to dominate history.

Moukadam Bourama: First, how and in what way can the reconstruction of the past help in the development of Africa today? Second, there has been some talk of a project to adopt a single official language for Africa, possibly Kiswahili. How far has that project gone? And what do you think of the idea?

Geoffroy Botoyiye: How would the speaker rate the quality of Swahili script? I ask because of reports of a desire to make that language the official language for all Africa.

Bienvenu Akoha: The Arabic writing system has stood the test of time. Egyptian writing goes too far back in time. There were successive invasions: Greek, Roman. You know, at that time every invasion meant total destruction. Everything was smashed. Remember the notorious dictum about Cartage having to be destroyed? The practice was for the victor to leave not a single stone on top of the other. Such practices were mainly responsible for the disappearance of ancient civilizations. Closer to our own time, there was colonialism. There are other possible reasons: the climate, migratory movements, perhaps. There were major movements of African populations from the Nile Valley. A great deal got lost in the process.

The Chinese, far off in their own world, did not suffer the same invasions as Africans did. Talking about development in Africa, the axiom 'Know thyself' is even more pertinent today. The fact is that imported development models guarantee no development whatsoever. I think it is important for us to regain confidence in ourselves, trust in our own values. The rediscovery of our own writing systems is part of the development process.

The project of a single language for all Africa is a matter of enormous controversy. For my part, I do not think any language is intrinsically endowed with particularly desirable qualities. The only way any continent acquires a single language is through political happenstance. If today a great Swahili emperor conquered Africa from Zaire to Senegal and imposed his language, Kiswahili, as the official language, everyone would protest, saying 'We have to defend our autonomy. I'm a Fon... I'm an Ibo'. But a century later, everyone would be speaking Kiswahili. Two, three, four centuries, a millennium later, and the process would be complete. Kiswahili would have become the African language, because over the generations, resistance would have died down. Invariably, it is political contingencies and the development process which determine which language a continent speaks. As for the Kiswahili project, it is in neutral. It will stay there a long time. Like the Pan-African movement, the project of a Pan-African language has had its ups and downs. If Pan-Africanism succeeds, I am certain the movement to give Africa a single language will also succeed. If, on the other hand, the Pan-African movement fails, I am sure we shall remain bogged down for a long time in our separate linguistic peculiarities. I am not unduly pessimistic. I think that in future, our children will meet our challenges, I just don't think we ourselves can do that now.

A great scholar, Cheikh Anta Diop, once said: 'Ancient Egyptian is for us Africans the equivalent of Indo-European'. It is a working hypothesis, and it requires backing up. Cheikh Anta Diop himself tried to provide supporting evidence, but in scholarly terms his arguments were weak. Obenga took up the challenge, only to run into problems because his basic methodology depends exclusively on written texts. The trouble is that to prove the thesis that the Egyptian language is the common heritage of all Africans, various languages have to be studied comparatively, and they are mainly oral. That is the crucial problem blocking Theophile Obenga's researches. If we look at the issue in perspective, however, the problem is perfectly normal. After all, it was not until the 19th century that European grammarians and other scholars were able to prove that European and Indian languages had a single source, now termed Indo-European.

Ms Wiesermann: I found the answers to questions interesting, especially those concerning the reasons why African writing systems disappeared while those of Europe thrived. I do not want to talk of Chinese, since the situation there is different. But the development of writing systems or written languages has been enormous. The reason was that at a certain time in Europe all educated persons spoke, read and wrote Latin. People were motivated to learn Latin because it was integrated into the school system.

But the second problem that has to be solved is to remove obstacles to literacy by motivating people. This is where religion comes in. It helps to motivate people strongly enough to take the trouble to learn to read and write.

Paulin Hountondji: Popular interest in the use of writing for religious purposes is a pretty new phenomenon. Before Jesus Christ the phenomenon was unknown, except in Israel where the Old Testament was commonly read in Hebrew. That was not the case with regard to Greek or Greco-Roman civilization before Jesus Christ. The situation was quite different before Caesar. I remember a comment made by Claude Levi-Strauss in *Tristes Tropiques* in a chapter entitled 'Lessons of Writing'. According to him, the development of writing went hand in hand with the reinforcement of the system of domination. Yet, in practice, it has been observed that writing eventually operated as a checking mechanism. I am also reminded of a small book by a French geographer. Its title said: *The Primary Purpose of Geography is War*.

What Mr Akoha just said was in a sense proof of that statement. The use of carpet-maps in the ancient Fon civilization to make secret maps of enemy territories demonstrates clearly how the practice of writing can sometimes become a vital necessity. In wartime, belligerents who do not know how to read or write were stimulated to learn, if only to make detailed maps of the field of operations. Such items of information are interesting in themselves, but ultimately they are inadequate explanations, and the question remains unanswered.

It is extremely important to establish the fact that the reasons why writing developed so differently in Europe and Africa are not traceable to the nature of the writing systems themselves but to external causes. That said, we still have to determine precisely what those external causes were. Might religious reasons have been among them? Certainly. Military factors? Political and administrative factors too, no doubt. Still, what are the ultimate reasons for Europe's grand take-off and the stagnation of African civilizations? Whatever we might say, it is an enigma.

I think we still need to conduct in-depth , complementary research on the social and political conditions for scientific development or take-off, to use the term just employed by Akoha. Incidentally, we know that for a long time, Chinese science was apparently far in advance of Western science. That advance lasted at least until the fifteenth century. Some extremely important work has been done on the topic. An interesting example is the small book by the English scholar, Joseph Needham.

According to Needham, until the seventeenth century at least, Chinese science was considerably more advanced than Western science and technology. That is why nowadays we hear it said so often that it was the Chinese who invented the compass, gunpowder, etc. But Needham shows that what was involved was not a simple series of individual borrowings. In the actual historical situation, these inventions were an integral part of a powerful scientific and technological movement. That fact is of extreme significance.

What happened, then, in the sixteenth and seventeenth centuries? The new development was Galileo's science. It was a scientific revolution, the inspiration for modern science. The key components were physics and mathematics; the underlying hypothesis was that reality could be hypothetically structured as a mathematical model. From that point on, everything changed. All this still merely postpones the answer to our question: why did the scientific hypothesis originate only in Western culture?

Now let me turn to writing. A while back, Akoha mentioned an extremely interesting text by Herodotus about gifts supposedly sent to the Persians by the Shiite king. As he pointed out, the objects could be interpreted variously. In that particular instance, there were conflicting interpretations, as he showed. Then he described a set of Fon pictographs, but in this case proceeded to give us just one meaning. He said the drawing of a broom in front of a house meant: 'Unless my broom sweeps before your house, only wild plants will grow there'. That was interpreted to mean: 'Only I can make you happy'. My question, is this: how can you be sure, after what you told us concerning the Shiites and the Persians, that this was the only possible interpretation?

Bienvenu Akoha: The two cases were not identical. In the case of the Shiites and Persians, actual objects were sent. In the Fon case, there were images of objects. The transition from object to image involves a qualitative break, because in the first place it is no longer necessary to carry the broom and the house along just to communicate a message. The image is adequate to the purpose. The shift is in itself a step towards writing.

As to the question why there is only one possible meaning for the images described, the reason is that they represented a proverbial saying, and in all civilizations proverbs comprise fixed conventional formulae. A proverb is a localized statement given rhythmic cadences for mnemonic purposes. This makes proverbs supremely special statements, the height, in short, of rhetoric. In the culture in question, only proverbs, given their sublime status, were considered important enough to be set down in writing. As you know, proverbs are limited in number.

Paulin Hountondji: I find the answer satisfactory. It reinforces the point I wanted to raise. Pictographic writing, understood in the way you have thus explained, can only give us information we already possess. It is merely the illustration of a proverb, an institutionalized statement. The meaning is not, a priori, the only one possible. But of all possible interpretations, that is the one agreed on by communal habit, convention and custom. In the choice of meaning, there is something altogether empirical, accidental, artificial. The pictograph, in other words, has no heuristic value, strictly speaking. Its value is simply illustrative. I repeat: pictographs do not convey new information. They tell us what we already know. I cannot understand a particular pictographic message unless I already know the proverb it illustrates. In this particular case, the proverb says: 'If I don't sweep before your house, only wild plants will grow there'.

Here we come to the major problem of the value, the comparative productivity of different writing systems. Now when you say that we in Africa have known all stages of the writing process, including alphabetic writing, I agree. Still, I feel we came to the alphabetic phase rather late. In discussing ancient Egyptian, you said it progressed towards syllabic writing, and even took some initial steps towards phonetic writing. The problem is that these were only initial steps. Is it not possible to identify, quite apart from causes external and extrinsic to the writing systems, any causes internal to these writing systems themselves to explain the difference in evolution between Western culture and ours with regard to writing?

Bienvenu Akoha: Let us agree, first of all, that writing is a most complex phenomenon. Different writing systems interlace, and patterns of progression are not linear. I am practically certain that it was their contacts with Egypt that helped the Greeks develop a phonetic writing system. Why not? And then after the Greeks had developed their alphabetical system, there was nothing wrong with the idea of Egyptians going in their turn to borrow it and bring it back to Africa.

That is why I have consistently refused to blame the writing systems themselves for the stagnation of one society or the advancement of another. What goes on is a reciprocal process in which each party borrows from others. That was the gist of my argument. As you pointed out, the Greek language had a phonetic writing system well before Socrates, some five or six centuries before Jesus Christ. China does not have a phonetic writing system, yet it was more advanced than Europe until the sixteenth century. And what you term the take-off of the West did not begin until the Copernican and Galilean revolution in science, a recent development. Don't forget, in the seventeenth century they burned Galileo for his ideas. My point is that the Chinese were able to achieve so much with their system. How?

Ms Wiesermann: As far as the Chinese are concerned, we have to admit that the efficiency of a writing system is important. That is clearly an internal factor. I believe it is important, and I believe China itself provides support for this hypothesis. It is true that China was ahead of Europe at a certain period. But we always have to remember that in China, as in all ancient cultures, only a tiny circle of scholars was literate. That gave them an instrument of scientific scholarship, a working tool. But the key point is that the literate population was tiny.

Second, a tremendous proportion of their intellectual capacities was wasted in learning this writing system. There is a marked difference there from basically easy writing systems with a manageable number of rules. It makes reading less of an ordeal. Such an easy writing system obviously enables many more potential scholars and scientists to contribute to the development of science. On the other hand, a difficult writing system ties up a considerable part of the intellectual potential of the literate population in the reading and writing process itself. What is left over is so little that eventually people forget that reading and writing are means, not ends in themselves.

We know now, for instance, that in order to read Chinese documents one had to assimilate 3,000 symbols. That is only at the basic level, equivalent to our primary school level. To become an expert scholar one had to assimilate no less than 30,000 symbols. Think of the sheer amount of intellectual energy consumed simply by the writing system.

The Chinese have abandoned this complex system. Why? Precisely because the information explosion shaking the world today leaves little room for an intellectual communications system so cumbersome that it crams our minds with useless details. That is why the Chinese, determined now to modernize their society, have taken the first step of simplifying their writing system. They have not completely dropped the old system. They still have scholars familiar with the old symbolic system. But for the conduct of practical business they use a new system. Incidentally, like everyone else in the world today, the Chinese are learning English. That is because if you want to study science today there are no two ways about it: you have to learn English. That is the dominant language today. German used to be important, but it lost out long ago.

My point, then, is that it seems quite inaccurate to say simply that the writing system itself has no influence whatsoever. It does have an impact. Easy writing systems can be learned by a larger number of people, and that can affect development. Why do we have so many scientists and scholars in Europe and the United States? Because everyone there is literate. Literacy is the bedrock. Reading and writing do not constitute the essence of what they know. Literacy is simply the instrumental basis that enables them to acquire other knowledge. It is the foundation on which they can build all sorts of intellectual structures.

Paulin Hountondji: No. As far as language is concerned, yes. I'm simply talking about writing systems as related to spoken languages. Let me make myself clear. I'm not talking of the complexity of the spoken language itself. All I'm talking about is the writing system linked with the spoken language. On this point I find that of all languages known to me, French is extremely complex. But what I want to say is that one reason for the information explosion today is that none of us, on our own, can assimilate all data even in our own fields. The process requires inputs from a lot of people.

Bienvenu Akoha: I agree perfectly with what Wiesermann just said. I would simply like to add this point. Let us look at the example of the French revolution of 1789, which led to the establishment of universal education in France. That was a key factor. After all, before the revolution, the French writing system was phonetic. But due to the social system, only a particular class, in fact only a tiny caste within that society, had access to it. So there certainly was an external factor quite apart from the language.

Paulin Hountondji: This question is for Wiesermann. What is the instructional language used for higher education in China today?

Ms Wiesermann: They are shifting increasingly towards English. They still think in Chinese, but they are moving closer to English. Faculty members are moving closer to English.

Paulin Hountondji: Beyond all the different issues raised at this seminar, one question provides a constant refrain: What are we to do, here and now, with these endogenous writing systems? What are we to do to meet our needs and requirements today?

Bienvenu Akoha: I have no qualms whatsoever about dropping these old systems and using phonetic writing. The Latin alphabet is suited to our world. Universal science has revealed that it is the best system for linguistic transcription. On this point most linguists agree.

Paulin Hountondji: It is with the greatest pleasure that I express my appreciation, and that of the audience, I am sure, for Mr. Akoha's contribution. The road to interdisciplinary research is more arduous than the other road, that of compartmentalized isolation. But it is worthwhile to follow it, and we must have the courage to try it.

Bibliography

Abe, Ndoumy Noël, 1991-1992, *La médecine africaine et la médecine officielle en Côte d'Ivoire: une approche stratégique de collaboration*, thèse de doctorat de 3e cycle sociologie et anthropologie médicales, Abidjan, Université nationale, 699pp.

Abimbola, Wande, 1968, 'Ifa as a Body of Knowledge and as an Academic Discipline', *Lagos Notes and Records*, 2,1.

Abimbola, Wande, 1975, *Sixteen Great Poems of Ifa*, Niamey, Celhto, 468pp.

Abimbola, Wande, 1976, *Ifa: An Exposition of Ifa Literary Corpus*, Ibadan, Oxford University Press, Xii + 256pp.

Abimbola, Wande, 1977, *Ifa Divination* Poetry, New York, Nok Publishers.

Abraham, William, E., 1962, *The Mind of Africa*, London.

Abraamsson, H, 1955, *The Origin of Death, Studies in African Mythology* (Studia Ethnographica Upsaliensia, 3, New York, Arnos Press, 1977).

Adam, Jerôme, 1987, «Sagesse Olamba (Haut-Ogooué)», *Muntu*, revue scientifique et culturelle du CICIBA, 7:109-119.

Adam, Kolawolé, Sidirou, and Boko, Michel, 1983, *Le Bénin*, Sodima/Edicef, Paris.

Adande, A., 1962, *Les récades des rois du Dahomey*, Dakar, IFAN.

Adande, Sénou Alexandre, 1984, *Le maïs et ses usages au Bénin méridional*, Dakar-Abidjan-Lomé, Agence de coopération culturelle et technique, Les Nouvelles éditions africaines.

Adande, A., 1981, «Un exemple de recherche archéologique: enquête réalisée par les élèves de l'école publique de Bensékou», in: *Recherches pédagogie, culture*, Vol. IX, No. 55, sept-décembre, pp. 81-82.

Adande, A. et Metinhoue, G., n.d., *Potières et peterie de Sè*, Cotonou, Université nationale du Bénin, 59 pages ronéotypées.

Adande, A., 1983, «Notes AND questions à propos de la métallurgie du fer dans la région du Golfe du Bénin pendant la période pré-coloniale», Communication au Colloque sur *La métallurgie du fer avant la méthode indirecte, à Madagascar, en Afrique et en Europe*, Centre de Recherches Africaines, Université de Paris I.

Adande, A., 1988, *Les origines lointaines des peuples de la République du Bénin: Problèmatique et perspectives de recherche*, Communication au séminaire sur l'histoire du Bénin, Université Nationale du Bénin, Cotonou, 34 pages dactylographiées + 2 cartes.

Addea Mensah, I.; F. G. Torto; C. D. Dimoneyeka; I. Baxter and J. K. M., Sanders, 1977, 'Novel amide-alkaloids from the roots of Piper guineense', *Phytochemistry*, 16:757-9.

Adesina, S. K.; B. J. Oguntimein and D. D. Akinwusi, 1980b, 'Phytochemical and Biological Examination of the Leaves of *Acalypha wikesiana* (red acalypha)', *Quarterly Journal of Crude Drug Research*, 18:45-8.

Adjanahoun, E.J.; Ahyi, A.M.R.; Aké Assi L., 1980, «Médecine traditionnelle et pharmacopée: contribution aux études ethnobotaniques et floristiques du Niger», Rapport présenté à l'ACCT, Paris, ACCT, 243p.

Adjanohoun, E. J., 1980, *Médecine traditionnelle et pharmacopé, contribution aux études ethnobotaniques et floristiques au Niger*, ed. Agence de Coopération culturelle et technique, Paris, I vol, 250p.

Adjido, C.T., 1972, *Le mythe et l'homme*, Edit. Gallimard, Paris.

Adjido, C.T., 1984, «Psychologie médicale et pratiques traditionnelles», in *Revue de psychologie médicale*, Mai, VI. 16, No. 7.

Adler, A., and A. Zempléni, 1972, *Le bâton de l'aveugle: Divination, maladie et pouvoir chez les Moundang du Tchad*, Paris, Herman, 224p.

Adler, A., 1977, *Faiseurs de pluie, faiseurs d'ordre. Reflexion sur les rapports de la magie et du pouvoir en Afrique Noire*, Paris, pp. 46-49.

Adokonou, B., 1987, «Religions et médecines africaines traditionelles», Communication aux *V*[èmes] *Entretiens de médecine aéronautique et tropicale*, Cotonou, 20-28.

Agboka, Lucien (Evêque Béninois), 1987, Allocution d'accueil à l'assemblée générale des médecins, dentistes et pharmaciens catholiques du Bénin, Séminaire St-Paul de Djimè, Abomey, le 8 août.

Aguessy, Honorat, 1985, «Religion africaine et rapports de forces», in: *Cultures africaines*, (Documents de la réunion d'experts sur *Les survivances des traditions religieuses africaines dans les Caraïbes et en Amérique Latine*), Paris, UNESCO, CC-86/WS/24, pp. 230-244.

Aguessy, H., 1989, «Technologies endogènes et développement de l'Afrique noire. Bilan de recherches déjà effectuées et perspectives d'avenir», in: *Actes de la 14*[e] *Conférence Biennale de l'Association Scientifique Ouest Africaine*, Cotonou, MEPS, 17-15 septembre, pp. 15-29.

Ahyi, R. G., 1987, «La psychiatrie en Afrique noire», in *51è Entretiens de Médecine Aéronautique et Tropicale*, 20-27 February, Cotonou (Bénin).

Ainslie, J. R., 1937, *A list of Plants used in Native Medicine in Nigeria*, Imperial Forestry Institute, Oxford, No. 7, 109p.

Ajisafe, A.K., 1945, *Laws and Customs of the Bénin People*, Lagos, Kashand Klane bookshops, 101p.

Aké, Assi L., «Les surprenantes vertus de la Kola», in *Balafon*.

Akindélé, A. et Aguessy, C., 1953, *Contribution à l'histoire de l'ancien royaume de Porto-Novo*, Dakar, IFAN, 168 p.

Akoha, A.B., 1987, «Les pictogrammes en pays fon», *Langage et Pédagogie* No. 8, Cotonou, UNB-CE.BE.LA.E, 110p.

Alain, M. E.; Massal, R.; Touzin and L. Porte, 1949, «Le traitement de l'amibiase par la conessine. Résultats d'une expérimentation faite à l'hôpital Michel Lévy, Hôpital d'instruction de l'Ecole d'Application du Service de Santé des troupes coloniales», in: *Médecine Tropicale*, 9, 5-38.

Alapini, Julien, 1950, *Les noix sacrées* (Etude complète de Fa-Ahidegoun génie de la sagesse et de la divination au Dahomey), Monte Carlo, Regain, 127p.

Alexander, J. and D. G., Coursey, 1969, 'The Origins of Yam Cultivation', in: P J, Ucko and G W, Dimbleby, eds *The Domestication and Exploitation of Plants and Animals*, Chicago, Aldine, 405-25.

Alexandre, Pierre, 1961, «Problèmes linguistiques des Etats Négro-africains à l'heure de l'indépendance», in: *Cahiers d'études africaines*, No. 36, pp. 177-195, Paris, Mouton.

Amon d'Aby, F. J., 1960, *Croyances religieuses et coutumes juridiques des Agni de la Côte d'Ivoire*, Paris, Larose.

Anderson, E., 1960, 'The Evolution of Domestication', in Sol Tax, ed., *Evolution Darwin*, Vol. 2, 67-84, Chicago, University of Chicago Press.

Anderson, E., 1967, 'The Bearings of Botanical Evidence on African Culture History', in C. Gabel and N.R. Bennett, eds. *Reconstructing African Culture History*, Boston, Houston University Press, 169-180.

Angelot, P., 1977, *Africanalinguistica VII Tervuren*, Musée royal de l'Afrique central.

Anonyme, 1954, *L'invention humaine: Technique morale, science, leurs rapports au cours de l'évolution* (exposés et discussions), Paris, Albin Michel, 255p.

Anonyme, 1960, *Mythe, Dreams and Mysteries, The Encounter Between Contemporary Faiths and Archaic Realities*, New York, Harpen and Brothers, 256p.

Anonyme, 1960, «Le fer de Fort Gouraud», in: *Industries et travaux d'outre-mer*, No. 75, février, pp. 96-98.

Anonyme, 1969, «Le fer en Afrique», in: *Moniteur Africain*, No. 422, 30 octobre, p. 12.

Anonyme, 1969, *Witchcraft and Healing*, (Centre of African Studies, University of Edimburg, 14th and 15th February), Edimburg, Center of African Studies, 87p.

nonyme, 1971, «Le minerai de fer en Afrique», in: *Industries et travaux d'outre-mer*, No. 206, janvier, pp. 32-37.

Anonyme, 1973, «Les mines de fer du Libéria», in: *Industries et travaux d'outre-mer*, No. 238, septembre, pp. 787-790.

Anonyme, 1976, «Théories et méthodes en linguistique africaine», (communication du 11ème congrès de la société de linguistique d'Afrique occidentale), Yaoundé, ed. Luc Bouquiaux, 172p.

Anonyme, 1977, «Médecine traditionnelle et médecine moderne» (Dossier), in: *AGECOP liaison*, No. 36, juillet, pp. 3-17.

Anonyme, 1979, «Technologie traditionnelle - Technologies combinées», in: *Environnement Africain*, Dakar, ENDA, Vol. III, No. 3-4, 475p.

Anonyme, 1979, «L'enfant en milieu tropical», in: *Médecine traditionnelle*, No. 122, pp. 4-31.

Anonyme, 1980, «Colloque international sur les traditions orales du Gabu», 19-24 Mai, Dakar, *Fondation Léopold Sédar Senghor*, 32p.

Anonyme, 1983, «Médecins et santé», Paris, ORSTOM, in: *Cahiers ORSTOM*, Série sciences humaines, Vol. XVIII, 4, 1981-1982, 592p.

Anozie, F., 1979, 'Early Iron Technology in Igboland (Lejja and Umundu)', in: *Perspectives on West Africa's Past, West African Journal of Archaelogy*, Vol. 9, 119-143.

Anquandah, J. R., 1965, 'Ghana's Terracotta Cigars', in *Ghana Notes and Queries, 7, 26.*

Anton, R. and P. L., 1968, «Duquenois, L'emploi des cassias dans les pays tropicaux et subtropicaux examinés d'après quelques uns des constituants chimiques de ces plantes médicinales», *Plantes médicinales et l'hytothérapie, 2,* 255-68.

Anyinam, Charles, 1989, 'Traditional Medical Practice in Contemporary Ghana: A Dying or Growing «Profession»?: A Response to Ahiakpor', in: *Canadian Journal of African Studies*, Vol. 23, No. 1, pp. 297-299.

Ardant du Req (Colonel), 1930, *Etude comparative sur la divination en Afrique et à Madascar*, in: Bulletin Com. Hist. et Scientif. AOF, T. 13, pp. 9-25.

Ardrey, R., 1976, *The Hunting Hypothesis: A Personal Conclusion Concerning the Evolutionary Nature of Man*, New York, Athenaeum.

Armartte, Bailly, Baruk, Blanchard, 1984, *Le sujet et l'objet: confrontations*, (Séminaire d'interrogations sur les savoirs et les sciences), Paris, CNRS, 266p.

Arora, R. B., C. N., Mathor and S D S, Seth, 1962, 'Anticoagulant and Cardiovascular Actions of Calophyllolide, and Indigenous Complex Coumarin', *Archives Internationales de Pharmacodynamie*, p 139-75.

Aschmann, H., 1968, Comment on 'The Origins of Agriculture', *Current Anthropology* 9, 494-495.

Asuni, T., 1961, *Suicide in Western Nigeria*, in *First Pan-African Psychiatric Conference* (Abeokuta, Nigeria, 12-18 October, 1961), *Conference Report*, ed. T. A. Lambo, Ibadan, Nigeria: Government Printer, pp. 164-75.

Atiwiya, G., 1971, Le «Zebola» (thérapie traditionnelle des maladies mentales dans un cadre urbain), *Psychopathologie Africaine*, 7(3) 389-416.

Attisso, Michèle, A., 1968, *Rapport général et analyse du premier symposium inter-africain sur les pharmacopées traditionnelles et les plantes médicales africaines*, (Dakar 25-29 mars 1959), Dakar Faculté Mixte de Médecine et de Pharmacie, 94 p.

Audebeau, M. C., 1919, «L'agriculture égyptienne à la fin du XVIIIe siècle», *L'Egypte contemporaine* 10, 132-169.

Aujas, I., 1927, *Les rites du sacrifice à Madagascar*, Tananarive, mémoires de l'académie malgache, fascicule 2, 88p.

Awouters, F., C. J. E., Niemeegers, F. M., Lenaerts and P. A. J., Jansen, 1978, 'Delay of Castor Oil Diarrhaea in Rats: A New Way to Evaluate Inhibitors of Prostaglandin Biosynthesis', *Journal of Pharmacy and Pharmocology*, 30, 41-5.

Ayats, H., 1968, «Essai de différenciation statistique, selon des citères socio-culturels, d'une population de schizophrènes hospitalisés, délirants et non délirants», in: *Deuxième Colloque Africain de Psychiatrie* (Dakar, Sénégal, 5-9 mars, 1968), Compte rendu, Paris, Audecam.

Ayensu, E. S., 1978, *Medicinal Plants of West Africa*, Reference Publications Inc. Alsona, MI, I Vol, 330pp.

Ayim, J. S. R., D. Dwuma Badu, N. Y., Fiagbe, A. M. Aleya, D. J., Statkin, J. E., Knapp and P. L., Schiff, Jr, 1977, 'Constituents of West African Plants XXI, Tiliafunimine', a new imino bisbenzylisoquinoline alkaloid from *Tiliacora funifera*. *Lloydia*, 40, 561-5.

Ayodélé, Tella, 1976, «Les pratiques médicales traditionnelles en Afrique», in: *Ethiopiques*, (numéro spécial) novembre, pp. 168-175.

Ba, A. H., 1965, *Textes sacrés d'Afrique noire* (Collection UNESCO d'oeuvres représentatives; Série africaine), ed. G. Dieterlen, Paris, Gallimard, pp. 7-13 (Préface).

Baasher, T. A., 1961, 'Some Aspects of the History of the Treatment of Mental Discorders in the Sudan', Paper distributed at the First Pan-African Psychiatric Conference, Abeokuta, Nigeria, 12-18 Nov.

Baker, H. G., and N. W., Simmonds, 1953a, 'The Genus Ensete in Africa', *Kew Bulletin*, 3, 405-416.

Baker, H. G., 1962, 'Comments on the Thesis that there was a Major Centre of Plant Domestication Near the Headwaters of the River Niger', *Journal of African History* 3, 229-233.

Balandier, G., 1955, *The Sociology of Black Africa: Social Dynamics in Central Africa*, trans. D. Garman, New York, Praeger.

Baranger, P., 1952, «Notes sur les colliers thérapeutiques», in: *Notes Africaines*, No. 55, juillet, pp. 93-94.

Bareteau, Daniel, 1978, *Inventaire des études linguistiques sur les pays d'Afrique noire, d'expression française et de Madagascar*, Paris, SELAF, 624p.

Barros (de), Ph, 1985, *The Bassar: Large Scale Iron Producers of the West African Savanna*, Ph. D. Dissertation, University of California at Los Angeles.

Barros (de), Ph., 1986, 'Bassar: A Quantified, Chronologically Controlled, Regional Approach to a Traditional Iron Production Centre in West Africa', in: *Africa*, 56 (2), 184-174.

Barros (de), Ph., 1988, 'Societal Repercussion of the Rise of Large Scale Traditional Iron Production: A West African Example', *The African Archaelogical Review*, 6, 91-113.

Bascom, William, R., 1942, 'The Sanctions of Ifa Divination', London, *The Royal Anthropological Institute of Great-Britain*, pp. 43-54.

Bascom, William R., 1969, *Ifa Divination: Communication between Gods and Men in West Africa*, Bloomington, Indiana University Press.

Bastide, R., 1956, «La causalité externe et la causalité interne dans l'explication sociologique», *Cahiers Internationaux de Sociology*, 21, 27-99.

Bateson, Gregory, 1974, *Steps on Ecology of Mind*, New York, Ballantine.

Battestini, Simon, P., 1991, 'Reading Signs of Identity and Alterity: History, Semiotics and a Nigerian Case', in: *African studies*, review, Vol. 34, No. 1, April, pp. 99-116.

Bauer, Dan, F., and John Hinnant, 1980, 'Normal and Revolutionary Divination: A Kuhnian Approach to African Traditional Thought', in: *Explorations in African Systems of Thought*, ed. Ivan Karp and Charles S. Bird. Bloomington: Indiana University Press, 213-36.

Beattie, John, and John Middleton, 1969, eds, *Spirit Mediumship and Society in Africa*. London, Routledge, Kegan and Paul.

Beaumont, P. B., *et al.*, 1978, 'Modern Man in Sub-saharan Africa Prior to 49,000 Years B.P.", *South African Journal of Science*, 74, pp.409-19.

Beauquesne, L., 1947, «Le Samagoura» (*Swartzia madagascariensis*), Légumineuse africaine. *Annales pharmaceutiques françaises*, 5, pp.470-83.

Bedaya, Ngaro, S., 1984, «L'aide apportée à la pénétration de la pratique médicale moderne par la prise en considération des pratiques superstitieuses en brousse», Bull Ac Nat Médecin, No. 9, 168p., 10-19.

Bedaya, Ngaro, S., 1984, «L'aide apportée à la pénétration de la pratique moderne par la prise en considération des pratiques superstitieuses en brousse», Bull AC Nat Médecin, No. 9, pp.10-19.

Beliquini, H. M., 1946, *Cultivation of Egyptian Crops* (In Arabic), pt I. Cairo: Matba't el'Oloum.

Bell, R. H. V., 1971, A Grazing Ecosystem in the Serengeti. *Scientific American*, 225, pp.86-93.

Benoist, J., 1975, «Médecin, maladies et guérisseurs dans une société polyethnique», in: *Environnement Africain*, Vol. 1, No. 4, pp.43-69.
BEP, Oliver-Bever, 1986, *Medicinal Plants in Intertropical Africa*, Cambridge University Press.
Berentjes, B., 1968, Comments on 'The Origins of Agriculture', *Current Anthropology* 9, p.495.
Berge, D. A., Van den, M., Ieven, F., Mertens, A. J. Vlietinek and E., Lammens, 1978, Screening of Higher Plants for Biological Activities II, Antiviral Activity, *Lloydia* 41, 463-71.
Bernard, A. M., 1962, «Le mystère du nom», *Lectio Divina*, No. 35.
Bernis, J., 1975, *L'immagination*, PUF, Paris.
Bertho, J., 1936, «La science du destin au Dahomey», in: *Africa*, juillet, vol. 9, No 3, pp. 339-378.
Bertho, J., 1945, «Vestiges de la fabrication du fer au Bas-Dahomey», *Notes Africaines*, No. 28, octobre, 9-10.
Bertho, J., 1949, «Langues rituelles du bas-Dahomey», in: *Notes Africaines*, No. 43, juillet, pp. 99-100.
Bertho, J., 1949, «Notice sur le Pila-Pila du Dahomey», in: *Notes Africaines*, No. 43, juillet, pp. 74-77.
Bertho, J., 1950, «Coiffures, masques à franges de perles chez les rois Yoruba du Nigéria et du Dahomey», in: *Notes Africaines*, No. 47, juillet, pp. 71-74.
Bertho, J., 1950, «Habitations à impluviums dans les régions de Porto-Novo AND Kétou (Dahomey)», in: *Notes Africaines*, No. 47, juillet, pp. 74-75.
Bertho, J., 1951, «Instruments de musique des rois de Nikki au Dahomey», in: *Notes Africaines* No. 52, pp. 99-101.
Bertho, J., «Le Gbadou chez les Adja du Togo et du Dahomey», in: *Première conférence internationale des Africanistes de l'Ouest*, Comptes-rendus T. II, pp. 331-350.
Bertho, J, Quatre dialectes mandé du nord Dahomey et de la Hiveria anglaise, in: Bulletin de l'IFAN, Tome XIII, No. 4, octobre 1951, pp. 1265-1271.
Bertho, J., 1951, «Trois états linguistiques du moyen Dahomey. The shummbuli, la Bzantche et le Basila», in: *Bulletin de l'IFAN*, Tome XIII, No. 3, juillet, pp. 872-892.
Bertrand, M., 1984, «Automédication et guérison: approche psychopathologique à travers les aspects traditionnels et actuels de la médecine en Limousin», *Mémoire de CES de Psychiatrie*, Limoges.
Beverige, W. I. B., 1977, *Influenza: The Last Great Plague*, Heinmen, London.
Bézanger-Beauquesne, L., M., Pinkas, M., Torck and F., Trottin, 1980, *Les Plantes Médicinales des Régions Tempérés*, Maloine, Paris.
Bindzingre, Nicole, 1983, «Analyse AND comptes-rendus», in: *Cahiers d'Etudes Africaines*, T. XXIII-3, No. 91, pp. 357-359. (cr. de: Sargent (Carolyn

Fishe, The Cultural context of therapeutic choice obstétrical care decisions among the Bariba of Benin, Dordrecht - Boston - London, D. Reidel, 1982, 192p.).

Binford, I. R., 1980, 'Willow Smoke and Dogs' Tails: Hunter-hatherer Settlement Systems and Archeological Site Formation', *American Antiquity*, 45, 4-20.

Binsbergen, Wim van, and Matthew Schoffereers, 1985, 'Introduction: Theoretical Explorations in African Religion', In: *Theoretical Explorations in African Religion*, ed. W. van Binbergen and M. Schoffeleers, 1-49, London, Routeledge, Kegan and Paul.

Bismuth, H. et Ménage, C., 1860, Les boissons alcooliques en AOF, in: *Bulletin IFAN*, T. XXIII, série B, No. 1-2, pp. 60-111.

Bisson, M. S., 1975, 'Copper Currency in Central Africa: The Archaeological Evidence', *World Archaeology*, 6, 272-92.

Blaise, H., 1932, *Les Crossopteryx africains*. Thèse de Doctorat en Pharmacie, Université de Paris.

Bleger, J., 1981, *Symbosis and Ambiguity*, PUF, Paris.

Blier, Suzanne Preston, 1983, 'African Geomancy: Art and the Idiom of Knowledge Revelation', Paper presented at the *African Studies Association* meeting, Boston.

Boeuf, C.F., 1957, «L'industrie autochtone du fer en Afrique occidentale française», in: *Bulletin Com. et His. et Scient*. AOF, Tome 20, pp. 402-464.

Bohanna, Paul, 1975, 'Tiv Divination', in: *Studies in Social Anthropology*, ed: J H M, Beattie and R G, Lienhardt, Oxford: Clarendon Press, 149-66.

Bohumil, Holas, 1941, «Pour faire tomber la pluie (nord du Togo)», No. Notes, in: *Notes Africaines*, No. 41, pp. 13-124.

Boll, M., 1971, *L'exploitation du hasard*, «Que Sais-je», No. 57, PUF, Paris.

Bosrup., E., 1965, *The Conditions of Agricultural Growth: The Economies of Agrarian Change under Population Pressure*. Chicago: Aldine.

Bouchud, J., 1975, «La faune de Medjez II. In H. Camps-Fabrer, Un gisement capsien de facies sétifien: Medje: II, El Eulma (Algérie), Paris, CNRS, 337-391.»@REFERENCE = Bouquet, A., 1949, «Sur un traitement africain des différentes affections occulaires», in: *C.N. Seances Acad. Sc.*, T. 226, No. 4, janvier, pp. 353-361.

Bouquet, A., 1969, *Féticheurs et Médecines Traditionnelles du Congo-Brazzaville*, ed. ORSTOM, Paris, I vol., 282pp.

Bouquet, A., 1972, *Plantes médicinales du Congo-Brazzaville*, Doctorat. Publ. No. 13 ORSTOM, 112pp. and in Travaux Labo. Matière Médicale.

Bouquet, A. and M. Debray, 1974, *Plantes Médicinales de la Côte d'Ivoire*. Document ORSTOM No. 32, 232pp.

Bouquiaux, J., 1976, *Théorie et méthodes en linguistique africaine* (communication au 11ème congrès de la société de linguistique d'Afrique occidentale, SIA Yaoundé, Avril 1974), Paris, SELAF-ORSTOM, 172p.

Bourguignon, E., 1966, «Divination, transe et possession en Afrique transharienne», in: *La divination* (vol. 2), ed. A. Caquot & Beibovici, Paris, Presses Universitaires de France, pp. 331-58.

Bourlière, F., 1963, *Observations on the ecology of some large mammals,* in: F C, Howell and F, Bourlière, eds. *African Ecology and Human Evolution.* Chicago, Aldine, 43-54.

Bower, J. R. F., 1977, 'Preliminary Report of a Study of Prehistoric Cultures of the Serengeti National Park', *Nyame Akuma* 11, 20-27.

Brand, Robert, 1976, *Les hommes et les plantes: l'usage des plantes chez les Wéménou du Sud Dahomey,* in: Génève Afrique, vol XV, No. 1, pp. 15-44.

Brand, R.B., 1985, *Les hommes et les plantes, L'usage des plantes chez les Wéménous du sud-Bénin,* Curare, 3, 257-275.

Brentjes, B., 1968, Comments on 'The Origins of Agriculture', *Current Anthropology* 9, 495p.

Bronson, B., 1972, 'Farm Labour and the Evolution of Food Production', in: B. Spooner, ed. *Population Growth: Anthropological Implications.* Cambridge, Mass, MIT Press, 190-218p.

Bronson, B., 1975, 'The Earliest Farming: Demography as Cause and Consequence', in: S. Polgar, ed. *Population, Ecology, and Social Evolution.* The Hague, Mouton, 33-78.

Brothwell, D. R., 1974, 'The Upper Pleistocene Singa Skull, A Problem in Paleontological Interpretation', in: W. Bernhard and A Kandler, eds., *Bevölkerungsbiologie*: 534-45, Stuttgart: G. Fischer-Verlag.

Brunken, J., J. M. J. de Wet, and J.R. Harlan, 1977, 'The Morphology and Domestication of Pearl Millet', *Economic Botany* 31 (2), 163-174.

Buakasa, G., 1971, *La Kindoki et les Nkisi*. Thèse de 3e cycle, Université de Paris (EPHE).

Buckland, A. W., 1878, 'Primitive Agriculture', *Journal of the Anthropological Institut* 7, 2-18.

Busson, F., 1965, *Plantes alimentaires de l'Ouest Africain*. Lecomte, Marseille, I vol. 568pp.

Buxton, Jean, 1973, *Religion and Healing in Mandari*. Oxford, Clarendon Press.

Caiment-Leblond, J., 1957, *Contribution à l'étude des plantes médicinales de l'AOF,* Thèse de Doctorat en Pharmacie, Université de Paris.

Calame-Griaule, G., 1965, *Ethnologie et langage: La parole chez les Dogon*, Paris, Gallimard.

Calme-Griaule, Geneviève, 1974, *La tradition orale,* in: 10-12, mai-août, pp. 4-12.

Calvet, L.F., 1980, «Linguistique et ethnocentrisme», in: *Recherche pédagogiques et culture*, No. 46, mars-avril, pp. 22-24.
Calvet, L.J., 1974, *Linguistique et colonialisme*, Payot, Paris.
Calvet, L.J., 1984, *La tradition orale*, «Que sais-je?» PUF, Paris.
Calvet, Maurice, 1968, *De l'oralité à l'écriture*, Dakar, CLAD, 25p.
Camps, G., 1969, *Amekni: Néolithique ancien du Hoggar*. Centre de Recherches Anthropologiques, Préhistoriques et Ethnographiques, Mémoire 10, Paris, Arts et Métiers Graphiques.
Camps, G., 1974, *Les civilisations préhistoriques de l'Afrique du Nord et du Sahara*. Paris, Doin.
Caquot, A. & Leibovici, M., 1968, eds., *La divination*. Paris, Presses Universitaires de France.
Carolier, P., 1916, La linguistique et l'origine des mythes, Paris, Sansot, 67p.
Carothers, J. C., 1947, 'A Study of Mental Derangement in Africans, and an Attempt to Explain its Peculiarities, More Especially in Relation to the African Attitude to Life', *J. Ment. Sci.*, 93, 548-07.
Carothers, M. C., 1970, *The African Mind in Health and Disease: A Study in Ethnopsychiatry* (World Health Organization Monograph Series, No. 17, 1953), New York, Negro Universities Press.
Carter, P. L. and C. Flight, 1972, 'A Report on the Fauna from the Sites of Nteresco and Kintampo Rock Shelter Six in Ghana with Evidence for the Practice of Animal Husbandry During the Second Millennium B.C.' *Man* 7, 277-282.
Carter, P. L., and Vogel, J. C., 1974, 'The Dating of Industrial Assemblage from Stratified Sites in Eastern Lesotho', *Man* (N.S.), 9, 557-623.
Carveth, Dead, 1925, *Man and his Superstitions*, Cambridge, University Press, 278p.
Cassiber, Ernst, *La philosophie des formes symboliques*, Paris, ed. de Minuit, 1977-1982 (3 vol.) Vol 1. *Le langage*, 1977, 356p., Vol. 2. *La pensée mythique*, 1979, 342p., Vol. 3, *la phénoménologie de la connaissance*, 1981, 609p.
Cauvin, Jean, 1980, *L'image, la langue et la pensée*, Saint-Augustin, Anthropos institut, (2 vol.) (Vol. 1, 704p.), (Vol. 2, 750p.).
Cazeneuve, J., 1971, *Sociologie du rite*. Paris, Presses Universitaires de France.
Chaavane,Bruno, A., 1952, «Bibliographie de l'âge des métaux en Afrique occidentale», in: *Bulletin de l'IFAN*, T. XIV, No. 2, avril, pp 545-595.
Charmar, P. C., 1973, «Monographie d'une sebkha continentale du Sud-Ouest Saharien: la sebkha de Chemchane» (Adrar de Mauritanie). *Bulletin de l'Institut Fondamental d'Afrique Noire* 35A, 207-43.
Chauveau, Jean-Pierre, 1984, «Une entreprise interdisciplinaire dans le domaine de la métallurgie africaine», in: *Cahiers d'Etudes Africaines*, T XXIV, No. 95, pp. 371-376.

Chavane, Bruno, A., 1952, «Bibliographie de l'âge des métyaux en Afrique occcidentale», in: *Bulletin de l'IFAN*, T. XIV, Avril, pp. 545-595.

Chevalier, A., 1938, «Le Sahara, centre d'origine des plantes cultivées», *Société de biogéographie*, Mémoires 6, 307-22.

Chevalier, A., 1947, «Les Mostuea africains et leurs propriétés stimulantes», *Revue de Botanique Appliquée et d'Agriculture Tropicale*, 27, 104-109.

Chevalier, A., 1928, «Notes sur l'exploration botanique de l'Afrique occidentale française (gorli)», *Revue de Botanique Appliquée*, 643-58.

Cjalendar, P., Chalendar, G., 1977, «Pharmacopée traditionnelle et médecine moderne», in: *L'Afrique Littéraires et Artistique*, No 45, 9ème Trim, pp. 63-73.

Clark, J. D., and A. Stemler, 1975, 'Early Domesticated Sorghum from Central Sudan', *Nature* 254, 588-91.

Clark, J. D., and A. Stemler, 1976, 'African Origins of Man the Toolmaker', in: *Isaac and McCoiwn*, 1-53.

Clark, J. D. and A. Stemler, 1980, 'Human Populations and Cultural Adaptations in the Sahara and Nile During Prehistoiric Times', in: *Williams and Faure*, 527-82.

Cohen, M., 1958, *La grande invention de l'écriture et son évolution*, Paris, Imprimerie Nationale, Librairie C. Klincksieck, 3 vol. 471p. + 228p. + 95 planches.

Cohen, Marcel, 1963, *L'écriture et la psychologie des peuples*, Paris, Arnaud Colin, 318p.

Collectif, 1975, *Mia hièn enu do àjágbèmè* (comptons en aja) document relatif à la numératon décimale, Porto-Novo.

Collomb, H. & Zwingelstein, J., 1962, «Les états dépressifs en milieu africain» (Dakar), *Information Psychiatrique*, 6, juin, 515-27.

Collomb, H., 1965a, «Assistance psychiatrique en Afrique» (expérience sénégalaise), *Psychopathologie Africaine*, I(1), 11-84.

Collomb, H., 1965b, «Bouffée délirantes en psychiatrie africaine», *Psychopathologie Africaine*, 1(2), 167-239.

Collomb, H., 1966, «Aspects particuliers de la psychiatrie africaine», in: *Cliniques africaines*, ed. M. Payet, P. Pène, M. Sankalé *et al.* Paris, Gauthier-Villatrs, pp. 419-31.

Colomb, H., 1973, «Psychothérapies en Afrique», *Neuvième Congrès International de Psycothérapie*, Oslo, 25 juin.

Colomb, H., 1975 «Psychiatrie moderne et thérapeutique traditionnelle», *Ethiopiques*, 2, 40-54.

Colomb, H., 1975, «Agressivité AND mort socio-somatique», *Third Congress of the International College of Psychosomatic Medecine*, Roma, September, 15-19.

Colomb, H., 1977, «Les modèles de la psychiatrie africaines», *Transcultural psychiatry symposium*, La Havane, 20-26 février.

Colomb, H., 1977, «Sorcellerie: Anthropophagie et relation duelle», Congress of Psychanalysis on *Madness*, Milan, 1-4 December, 1976, Inda Follia, Feltrinelli edt. Milano, vol. 1, 82-90.

Colomb, H., 1977, «Violence, sacrifice et thérapeutique», *Collège International de Psychanalyse*, Malam, 24-26 novembre.

Colomb, H., 1978, «La sorcellerie: antropohagie, Genèse et fonction», in: *Transculture Psychatry*, Montréal.

Colson, E., 1948, 'Rain Shrimes of the Plateau Tongo of the Northern Rhodesia', in: *Africa*, octobre, Vol. 18, pp. 272-283.

Connah, G., n.d., *Polished Stone Axes in Benin*, Lagos.

Connah, G., 1975, *The Archeology of Benin*, Oxford.

Cornevin-Calme Oriane Lacroix, 1973, Colloques sur la collecte des traditions orales, in: *C.R. Trim de l'Acad. des Sciences d'Outre-Mer*, Tome XXXII, No. 3, pp. 323-360.

Coulmas, Florian, 1984, Linguistic Minorities and Literacy: Language Issues in Developpint Countries, Houston, 153p.

Cousteix, P.J., 1962, «L'art et la pharmacopée des guérisseurs du Cameroun», Paris, DP. TAIB, 145p.

Crawford, J.R., 1967, *Witchcraft and Sorcery in Rhodesia*. London: Oxford University Press.

Dacruz, C., 1954, Les instruments de musique dans le bas-Dahomey, in: Etudes Dahoméennes, No. 12, pp. 1-79.

Dalziel, J. M., 1937, *The Useful Plants of West Tropical Africa*. Crown Agents, London.

Daninos, Guy, 1978, «De l'importance de la littérature orale en Afrique noire et en particulier au Congo», in: *L'Afrique Littéraires et Artistique*, No. 48, 2ème trimestre, pp. 2-19.

Danzel (Th. W), 1947, *Magie et science secrète - Art divinatoire*, Paris, Payot, 193p.

Dark, P. F. C., 1973, *An Introduction to Benin Art and Technology*, Oxford.

Darwish Sayed, M., 1980, 'Traditional Medicine in Health Carte, *Journal of Ethnopharmacology*, 2, 19-22.

Davies, O., 1961, 'The Invaders of Northern Ghana', *Universitas* 4, 134-36.

Davies, O., 1962, 'Neolithic Cultures of Ghana', in: *G. Mortelmans and J. Nenquin*, eds., *Actes du quatrième Congrès de préhistoire et de l'étude du Quartenaire*. Tervuren, Musée Royale de l'Afrique Centrale, 291-302.

Davies, O., 1966, 'The invasion of Ghana from the Sahara in the Early Iron Age', in L.D. Cuscoy, ed, *Actas del Quinto Congreso Panafricano de Prehiustoria y de Estudio del Cuaternaria* 2 Tenerife, 27-42.

Davies, O., 1967, *West Africa before the Europeans,* London, Methuen.

Davies, O., 1968, 'The Origins of Agriculture in West Africa', *Current Anthropology* 9, 479-482.

Davies, O., 1960, The Neolithic Revolution in Tropical Africa, *Transactions of the Historical Society of Ghana* 4(2), 14-20.

Davis, S., 1955, 'Divining Bowis, Their Uses and Origin: Some African Examples and Parallels from the Ancient World', *Man* 55 (143), 132-35.

De Wet, J. M. J., and J. R. Harlan, 1971, 'The Origin and Domestication of Sorghum Bicolor', *Economic Botany* 25, 128-35.

Debaille, G. and P., 1953, «Petard, Notes préliminaires sur les plantes antisydentériques du Soudan et de la Haute Volta», *Bulletin Médical de l'AOF*, 10, 11-14.

Degert, Françoise, 1974, *Le fer dans l'Afrique de l'Ouest des origines à 1850,* (Mémoires de Maîtrise), SLND, Paris, Université, 91p.

Delaveau, P. A. Desvignes, E. Adoux and A.M. Tessier, 1979, «Baguettes frotte dents d'Afrique occidentale, Examen chimique et microbiologique», *Annales pharmaceutiques françaises*, 37, 185-90.

Deluz, A., Lecour-Grandmaison, C., Rete, A., Laurentin, 1978, *La natte et le manguier*, Paris, Mercure de France, 1978, 248p.

Dembele, Magognime, Urbain, 1974, «De la tradition orale à la littérature», in: *Etudes Maliennes*, No. 11, septembre.

Denoël, A., 1958, *Matière Médicale Végétale*, 2 vols., Presses Universitaires, Liège.

Derrida, J., 1967, *De la grammatologie*, Ed. de Minuit, Paris.

Derrida, J., De la grammatologie, Ed. de Minuit, Paris, 1967.

Desjeux, Dominique, 1984, «Les religions agraires en Afrique Noire: la lutte de l'ordre et du désordre», in: *Le mois en Afrique*, No. 225-220, octobre-novembre, pp. 120-131.

Desanti, H., 1945, *Du Danhome au Bénin-Niger*, Paris, Larose, 260p.

Dessens, Henri, 1963, *Physiciens et sorciers faiseurs de pluie*, (conférence donnée au Palais de la découverte le 25 mai 1983), Paris, Université, 20p.

Devisch, René, 1985, 'Perspectives on Divination in Contemporary sub-Saharan Africa', in: *Theoretical Explorations in African Religions*, ed., W. Van Binsbergen and M. Schoffeleers, 50-83, London, KPI/Routledge, Kegan and Paul.

Devish, Renaat, 1985, «Compte rendu», in: *Canadian Journal of African Studies*, Vol. 19, No. 1, pp. 250-251.

Devisse, J., 1984, «L'histoire chez les autres», in: *Actes du Colloque national sur l'histoire et son enseignement*, 19-20-21 janvier, Montpellier, France, p. 57.

Devisse, Jean, 1984, «L'histoire chez les autres», paper presented at the *National Colloquium on the Study and Teaching of History*, Montpellier, 19-21 January, p. 57.

Devisse, Jean, 1985, *Sur l'oralité: perplexité d'un historien*, CNRS Monograph Series No.3.

Diabaté, Henriette, 1980, «La Sannvinv, sources orales et histoire, essai méthodologique», *Nouvelles éditions africaines*, Abidjan.

Diagne, P., 1976, *Langues africaines et impérialisme*, Dakar, P. Diagne, 218p.

Diasdado Decaso, Gordano, Plehman, 1968, «Mauvais guérisseur et génie protecteur». Evolution d'un Etat dangereux d'angoisse aigu, résolu en un retour aux cultes traditionnels N'zima, in: *Psychopathologie africaine*, Vol. IV, No.3, pp. 383-417.

Diemé, Sébastien, 1992, *Contribution à l'étude de la pharmacopée traditionnelle diola*, (Thèse), Dakar, Pharmacie, 66 p.

Dieng, Amady, Aly, 1989, «Hommage à Cheikh Anta Diop, 1923-1926, un bilan critique de l'oeuvre», in: *Canadian Journal of Africain Studies*, Vol. 23, No. 1, pp. 151-1456.

Dieterlen, G., 1951, *Essai sur la religion bambara*. Paris, Presses Universitaires de France.

Dieu, M., Renaud, P., Tadajen, M. Breton, R., 1983, *Atlas linguistique de l'Afrique centrale, structures et méthodes*, Paris-Yaoundé, ACCT-CEDETOLA, 190p.

Dika Akwa, 1971, *La sphère du sacré en Afrique*. Thèse de 3e cycle, Université de Paris (VII).

Diki Kidiri, Marcel, «Réflexions sur la graphématique», in: *Cahiers d'Etudes Africaines*, Vol. XXIII - I - 2, No. 89-90, pp. 169-174.

Dim Debbson, A.A., 1934, *Le secret des sorciers noirs*, Paris, Librairie Emile Boury, 298p.

Diop, C.A., 1973, «La métallurgie du fer sous l'Ancien Empire égyptien», *Bulletin de l'IFAN*, série B, T. XXXV, No. 3, Juillet, 532-547.

Diop, C.A., 1974, *Les fondements culturels, techniques et industriels d'un Futur Etat Fédéral d'Afrique Noire*, Présence africaine, 126p.

Diop, C.A., 1975, «L'antiquité africaine par l'image», in: *Notes Africaines*, janvier-avril, No. 145-146, Dakar, Université de Dakar, IFAN, NEA, 66p.

Diop, C.A., 1976, «L'usage du fer en Afrique», in: *Notes Africaines*, No. 152, octobre, 93-95.

Diop, C.A., 1979, *Nations nègres et culture*, Paris, Présence africaine, 572p.

Diop, L.M., 1968, «Metallurgie traditionnelle et âge du fer en Afrique», *Bulletin de l'IFAN*, série B, T. XXX: 10-38 + 6 fug.

Diop, M. et Collomb, H., 1965, «Pratiques mystiques et psychopathologie», in: *Psychopathologie Africaine*, No. 2, p. 304-382.

Diop, M., 1967, «La dépression chez le Noir africain», *Psychopathologie Africaine*, 3(2), 183-94.

Diop, M., Zempleni, A., Martino, P. & Collomb, H., 1964, «Signification et valeur de la persécution dans les cultures africaines», in: *Congrès de Psychiatrie et de Neurologie de Langue Française* (Marseilles, 7-12 sept., 1964), Comptes rendus, ed. P. Warot, Paris, Masson, pp. 333-43.

Diop, Marie-Louise, 1968, «Métallurgie traditionnelle et âge du fer en Afrique», in: *Bulletin IFAN*, Tome XXX, série B, No. 1, pp. 1038.

Dolto, F., 1984, *L'image inconsciente du corps*, Paris.

Dossevi, Othniel, 1979, *Problèmes posés par les textes transcrits de l'oralité*, Dakar, Ann. Fac Lettres et Sciences Humaines, pp. 131-169.

Douglas, Mary, 1970, *Witchcraft Confessions and Accusations*. Association of Social Anthropologists, 9, London, Tavistock Publications, Monographs.

Douglas, Mary, 1984, 'Animals in Lele Religious Symbbolism', *Implicit Meanings: Essays in Anthropology*, 27-46, London, Routledge, Kegan and Paul, 27-46.

Dubois Jean *et al.*, 1973, *Dictionnaire de Linguistique*, Paris, Larousse.

Ducros, Oswald, 1984, *Le dire et le dit*, Paris, ed. de Minuit, 233p.

Dugast, S., 1988, «La pince et le soufflet: deux techniques de forge traditionnelles au nord Togo», *Journal des Africanistes*, T. 56, fasc. 2, 29-53.

Dunglass, E., 1957, *Contribution à l'histoire du moyen Dahomey* (Royaume d'Abomey, de Kétou, et de Ouidah) Tomes I, II, III, Porto-Novo, Centre IFAP, 185p., 152, p. 118.

Duteil, Armel, 1981, *La sorcellerie pourquoi?*, Paris, CIM, 166p.

Ekong, D. E. U. and O. G. Idemudia, 1967, 'Constituents of Some West African Members of the Genus Terminalia', *Journal of the Chemical Society*, 863-4.

El Kheir, Y. M. and A. M. Salih, 1979, Investigation of the Nature of the Molluscicidal Factor of *Croton Macrostachys*. 2nd OUA/STRC *Inter-African Symposium on Traditional Pharmacopoeia and African Medicinal Plants*, Publication No. 115, OUA/STRC Lagos.

El Said, P.; Sofowara, E.A. and T. Olaniyi, 1968, Study of Certain Nigerian Plants used in Fever. Communication at the *Inter-African Symposium on Traditional Pharmacopoeia and Medicinal Plants*, Dakar.

Eliade Mircea, n.d., *Essai sur le symbolisme magico-religieux*, Paris, Gallimard, 239p.

Eliade, Mircea, 1951, *Le Chamanisme et les techniques archaïques de l'extase*, Paris, Payot.

Eliade, Mircea, 1957, *Mythes, rêves et mystères*, Paris, Gallimard.

Eliade, Mircea, 1983, *Le sacré et le profane*, Paris, Gallimard, 186p.

Ellenberger, Victor, 1958, *Afrique avec cette peur venue du fond des ages - Sorcellerie: initiation - exorcisme*, Paris, Amiot Dumont, 261p.

Engekhard, P., Robineau, L., 1981, *La pharmacopée composante de l'économie de santé au Sénégal*, Dakar, ENDA-UNICEF, 95p.

Epstein, H., 1971, *The Origin of the Domestic Animals of Africa*. New York, Africana Publishing Co.

Erivwo, Sam, 1979, 'Epha Divination System among the Urhobo of the Niger Delta', *African Notes* (Ibadan) 8(1), 21-25.

Erny, P., 1972, *L'enfant et son milieu en Afrique noire*. Paris, Payot.

Evans-Pritchard, E. E., 1937, *Witchcraft, Oracles and Magic among the Azande*. Oxford, Clarendon Press (trad; française: *Sorcellerie, oracles et magie chez les Azande*, Paris, Gallimard, 1972, 642p).

Fabvre, Lucien, 1948, «Sorcellerie, sottise ou révolution mentale?», in: *Annales économies, sociétés, civilisations*, No. 1, janvier-mars, pp. 9-15.

Faegri, K. and J. Iversen, 1964, *Textbook of Pollen Analysis*. New York, Hafner.

Fagan, B. M., 1968, Comment on 'The Origins of Agriculture', *Current Anthropology* 9, 946p.

Fage, J. D., 1961, 'Anthropology, Botany and the History of Africa', *Journal of African Hisqtory* 2, pp.299-309.

Fall, Makhoumy, 1978, *Le rôle du devin en Grèce classique dans la conduite de la guerre et dans les sociétés traditionnelles de l'Afrique de l'ouest: Etude comparée*. Dakar, Université, 124 p. (Mémoire maîtrise histoire).

Février, J., 1984, *Histoire de l'écriture*, Paris, Payot, 615p.

Finnegan, Ruth, 1970, *Oral Literature in Africa*, Oxford, Clarendon Press, 558p.

Fischer, Eberhard, and Lorenz Homberger, 1986, *Masks in Guro Culture, Ivory Coast*. Zurich, Museum Rietberg and New York, Center for African Art.

Fleuret, A., 1979, 'The Role of Weld Foliage Plants in the Diet: A Case Study from Lesotho, Tanzania'. *Ecology of Food and Nutrition* 8, 87-93.

Flight, C., 1976b, 'The Kintampo Culture and its Place in the Economic Prehistory of West Africa', in J.R. Harlan, J.M.J. de Wet, and A.B.L., Stenmler, eds., *Origins of African Plant Domestication*. The Hague, Mouton, 211-221.

Fouraste, F., 1984, *La fonction sociale du guérisseur, in: Revue de psychologie médicale*, T. 8, p. 77-81.

Fouraste, F., 1982, *Quelques remarques sur la dynamique de la pratique du guérisseur et sur les rapports à la médecine scientifique*, Brazzaville, 5ème colloque du CAMES, Septembre.

Fouraste, Raymond, François, 1988, «Pour une essai de définition des médecines de tradition en Afrique de l'ouest», in: *Bulletin de liaison médecine traditionnelle et pharmacopée*, Vol. 2, No. 1, pp. 67-71.

Francis-Boeuf, C., 1937, «L'industrie autochtone du fer en AOF», *Bulletin du Comité d'Etudes Historiques et Scientifiques de l'AOF*, T. XXI, No. 3, 403-464.

Fredoux, A. and J. P. Tastet, 1976, «Apport de la palinologue à la connaissance paléogéographique du littoral ivoirien entre 8000 et 12000 ans», *Seventh African Micropaleontological Colloquium*, Ile Ife, Nigeria.

Freyre, G., 1974, *Maîtres et esclaves, la formation de la société brésilienne*, Paris, Gallimard, 2è édit. (1ère édit. 1952), 551p.

Froelich, J.C., 1968, «Sorciers et magiciens question de mots», in: *L'Afrique et l'Asie*, No. 83-84, 3ème-4ème trimestre, pp. 74-79.

Fuglestad, F., 1977, «Quelques réflexions sur l'histoire des institutions de l'ancien royaume du Dahomey et de ses voisins», in: *Bulletin de l'IFABN*, Tome 39, série B, No. 3, p. 493-517.

Gaillet, L., 1917, *Coulibaly: Les Sénégalais sur la terre de France, portraits, anecdotes, souvenirs*, Paris, Jouve et Cie, 153p.

Gaillet, L., 1976, «Coulibaly: Histoire du Sodabi», in *La croix du Bénin*, No. 401, janvier-février, p. 3.

Gallais, A., 1967, *La delta intérieur du Niger*, (2 vols.) Mémoire No. 79, Dakar, Institut Fondamental de l'Afrique Noire.

Gallay, A., 1966, «Quelques gisements néolithiques du Sahara malien», *J. Soc. Africanistes*, 36, 167-208.

Ganlson, Robert, G., 1990, 'Book Review', in: *African Studies Review*, Vol. 33, No. 1, April, pp. 164-165.

Garcia, L.M., 1976, «Archives et traditions orales: A propos d'une enquête sur la politique du royaume du Danhomé à la fin du 19ème siècle», in: *Cahiers d'Etudes Africaines*, No. 61-62, p. 189-206.

Gbenonvi, R. et Vgnonde, J.N., 1983, «Nyo nu xà, nyo nu len dó gbè towe mè...», *Binndi e Jannde, Bulletin pour la promotion des langues africaines*, 9-10, pp. 115-121, Paris.

Gelb, I.J., 1973, «Pour une théorie de l'écriture», Paris, Flammarion, *Idées et Recherches*, 304p.

Genest, Serge, 1980, «Phytothérapie et Médecine africaine: quelques réflexions d'un anthropologue en marge d'une réunion d'experts», in: *Revue canadienne des études africaines*, Vol 13, No. 3, pp. 497-499.

Gibbal Jean-Marie, 1984, «Le signe des génies», in: *Cahiers d'études Africaines*, T. XXIV-2, No. 94, pp. 193-203.

Gille, B., 1968, *Histoire de la métallurgie*, «Que sais-je?» No. 96, PUF, 127p.

Girard, René, 1972, *La violence et le sacré*, Paris, Grasset, 451p.

Githens, T. S., 1949, *Drug Plants of Africa*. University of Pennsylvania Press, 125pp.

Glaze, Anita, J., 1981, *Art and Death in a Senufo Village*. Bloomington, Indiana University Press.

Glélé, A.M., 1974, *Le Danxome (Dahomey): du pouvoir Adja à la nation Fon*, Paris, Hubia, 286p.

Gluckman, M., 1955, *Custom and Conflict in Africa*. New York, Barnes and Noble.

Gluckman, Max, 1967, «Crise morale et solution magique», in: *Cahiers de l'ISEA*, série V - 10, No. 2, février, pp. 5-48.

Gnanvo Cyprien, 1986, «L'enseignement des mathématiques dans les langues africaines (problèmes théoriques et linguistiques): le cas du Bénin», *Actes du colloque international sur Langues Africaines et philosophie*, pp. 230-233.

Godonou, A., 1985, *L'artisanat traditionnel du fer à Porto-Novo (de la fin du XVIIe siècle à nos jours)*, Flash, UNB, 73p.

Good, Charles, M., 1987, *Ethnomedical Systems in Africa: Patterns of Traditionnal Medicine in Rural and Urban Kenya*, New York, the Guilford Press, 354p.

Goodman, L S. and A Gilman, 1980, *The Pharmacological Basis of Therapeutics*. Macmillan, New York, Baillière and Tindall, London, 6th ed.

Goody, J. and Watt, I., 1963, «The Consequences of Literacy», *Comparative Studies in Society and History*, 5, 304-45, (reprinted in J Goody (ed.), *Literacy in Traditional Societies*. Cambridge University Press, 1968).

Goody, J., 1971, 'The Impact of Islamic Writing on the Oral Cultures of West Africa', in: *Cahiers d'Etudes Africaines*, No. 43, pp. 455-466.

Goody, J., 1977, «La raison graphique», *Les Editions de Minuit*, Paris.

Goody, J., 1979, «La raison graphique: la domestication de la pensée sauvage», Paris, *les Editions de Minuit*, «Le sens commun», 275 p.

Goody, J., 1986, *La logique de l'écriture: aux origines des sociétés humaines*, Paris, Armand Colin, 198p.

Goucher, C.L., 1981, 'Iron is Iron Till it is Rust: Trade and Ecology in the Decline of West African Iron Smelting', *Journal of African History*, 22, 179-189.

Goucher, C.L., 1984, *The Iron Industry of Bassar, Togo: An Interdisciplinary Investigation of African Technological History*, PhD. Thesis, University of California at Los Angeles.

Gouegan Dominique, 1984, *Enseignement et mathématique*, Paris, ACCT.

Gravrand, R.P., 1966, «Le Lup serer. Phénomène de l'emprise des Pangol et Psychothérapie des possédés», in: *Psychopathologie africaine*, Vol II, No. 2, pp. 195-226.

Gravrand, R.P. Henri, 1975, «Noq et Sorcellerie dans les çonceptions serer», in: *Psychologie africaine*, No. 2, Vol XI, pp. 179-216.

Gréaule, M., Dieterten, G., 1951, «Signes graphiques soudanais», Paris, Herman et compagnie, 88p., in: *Actualité scientifique et industriels USB*, l'Homme, Cahiers d'ethnologie de géographie et de linguistique.

Greene, D. L., 1966, *Dentition and the Biological Relationships of Some Meroitic, X-Group and Christian Populations from Wadi Halfa*, Sudan, *Kush* 14, 285-88.

Grégoire, J., 1953, «Contribution à l'étude du kinkeliba» (Combretum micranthem Don.) Thèse de Doctorat en Pharmacie, Université de Marseille.

Griaule, M., Dieterlen,G., 1935, «Calebasses dahoméennes», in: *journal de la société des africanistes*, Tome V, fasc. 2, pp. 203-246.

Griaule, M., 1937, *Notes sur la divination par le Chaval*, in: Null. Com. et Hist. et Scienct. AOF, T. 20, pp. 113-141.

Guarisma, G., Whlhelm, J.G. Möhlig, 1986, *La méthode diatectométrique appliquée aux langues africaines*, Berlin, Dietrich Reiner, Verlag, 425p.

Haaland, R., 1989, 'Man's Role in the Changing Habitat of Mema during the Old Kingdom of Ghana', *Norwegian Archaelogical Review*, 13 (1): 31-46.

Hadfield, R.P., 1949, 'Traits of Divine Kingship in Africa', London, Watts and Co, 134p.

Hagedorn, H., 1980, 'Fluvial Processes in the Sahara', *Palaeoecology of Africa*: 12, 115-23.

Hagege, C.l., 1978, *La phonologie panchronique: Comment les sens changent dans les langues?*, Paris, PUF, 223p.

Hagege, C.I., 1985, *L'homme de paroles*, Fayard, Paris.

Hagege, Claude, 1986, *La structure des langues*, Paris, PUF, 125 p.

Haillot, Jean, 1936, «Sur la géomancie et ses aspects africains», in: *Bulletin, Com. His. et Scientif. AOF*, T. 19, pp 91-139.

Hallen, Barry, 1976, «Phenomenology and the Exposition of African Traditional Thought», *Second Order*, 5 1976, 45-65.

Hallen, Barry and J.O. Sodipo, 1986, *Knowledge, Belief and Witchcraft: Analytic Experiments in african Philosophy*. London, Ethnographica.

Hamilton, A., 1972, 'The Significance of Patterns of Distribution shown by Forest Plants and Animals in Tropical Africa from the Reconstruction of Upper Pleistocene Paleoenvironments: A Review', *Palaeoecology of Africa* 9, 63-67.

Harborne, J. B., T. J., Mabry and H. Mabry, 1975, *The Flavonoids*, Part 2, Chapman and Hall, I vol., 1204pp.

Harlan, J. R., J. M. J. de Wet, and A. B. L. Stemler, 1976, (eds.) *Origins of African Plant Domestication*. The Hague, Mouton.

Harris, D. R., 1972, 'The Origins of Agriculture in the Tropics, *American Scientist* 60, 180-93.

Harris, D. R., 1976, 'Traditional Systems of Plant Food Production and the Origins of Agriculture in West Africa, in Harlan, de Wet & Stemler (eds.), 311-356.

Hau, Kathleen, 1959, 'Evidence of the Use of the Pre-portuguese Written Characters by the Bini', in: *Bulletin de l'IFAN*, série B, Tome XXI, No. 12, pp. 109-154.

Heckel, Edouard, 1884, *Des kolas africaines au point de vue botanique, chimique et thérapeutique*, Paris, Flammarion, 85p.

Hegba, M., 1979, *Sorcellerie, réalité ou chimère dangereuse?* Abidjan, Inades.

Hegba, Meinrad, P., 1985, *Sorcellerie et prière de délivrance: réflexion sur une expérience*, Abidjan, INADES, 254p.

Henige, D. P., 1974, *The Chronology of Oral Tradition: Quest for a Chimera*, Oxford, Claren Don Press, 265p.

Henry, T. A., 1949, *The Plant Alkaloids*, 4th ed. Churchill: London, 803pp.

Herbert, W., 1984, *Red Gold of Africa Copper in Precolonial Eugenia, History and Culture*, University of Wisconsin Press, Madison & London, 433p.

Herskovits, M. J., 1938, *Dahomey: An Ancient African Kingdom*. 2 vols. New York, J J Augustin.

Heusch (de), Luc, 1985, *Sacrifice in Africa*. Trans. L. O'Brien and A. Morton, Bloomington, Indiana University Press.

Hiernaux, J., 1968, *La diversité Humaine en Afrique sub-Saharienne*, Brussels.

Higgs, E. S., and M. R. Jarman, 1972, 'The Origins of Plant and Animal Husbandry', in E S Higgs, eds., *Papers in Economic Prehistory*, Cambridge, Cambridge University Press, 3-13.

Higounet, C., 1976, *L'écriture*, 5è éd., Paris, PUF, «Que sais-je?», 128p.

Hillaire-Marcel, C., 1979, Les Teneurs en isotopes stables des faunes pléistocènes en milieu continental pour les reconstitutions paléoclimatiques. Premiers commentaires après une étude préliminaire de faunes à *Cerastoderma glaucum* et à *Melania tuberculota* du Wadi Shad (Libye). *Bulletin de l'Association sénégalaise pour l'étude du Quaternaire de l'Ouest africain*, 56, 79-85.

Houis, M., 1980, «Oralité et Scipturalité», in: *Eléments de recherche sur les langues africaines*, AGECOOP.

Houis, Maurice, 1981, «La relation de détermination en syntagmes et composés nominaux», *Afrique et Langage*, No. 16, p. 5, Paris.

Hounkpatin Capo et Zinzindohoué, Noélie, 1975, *Akanta wowo glo nu yé à* (vocabulaire théorique de mathématique en wacigbè en gengbè), Cnl, Porto-Novo.

Hountondji, P.J., 1970, *L'idée de science dans les Prolégomènes et la première recherche logique de Husserl*, thèses pour le doctorat de 3è cycle, Paris (inédit).

Hountondji, P.J., 1973, «La philosophie et ses révolutions», in *Les Cahiers philosophiques africains*, Nos. 3 et 4, Lubumbashi, Zaïre.

Hountondji, Paulin, 1987a, *Address Delivered to Seminar on Endogenous Knowledge*, National University of Benin, Cotonou, 10 December.

Hountondji, Paulin, 1987b, 'Le particulier et l'universel', *Bulletin de la société française de philosophie*, No. 4, October-December.

Hounwanou, R.T., 1984, *Le FA, une géomancie divinatoire du golfe du Bénin*, Ed. Les NEA

Hows, Maurice, 1971, *Anthropologie Linguistique de l'Afrique noire*, Paris, PUF, 232p.

Hurard, Paul, 1960, «Contribution à l'étude du cheval du fer, et du chameau au Sahara oriental» (I - le Fer), in: *Bulletin de l'IFAN*, Tome XXII, série B, No. 1-2, p. 134-178.

Hurard, P., 1964, «Nouvelle contribution à l'étude du fer au Sahara et au Tchad», in: *Bulletin de l'IFAN*, série B, Tome XXVI, No. 3-4, juillet-octobre, pp. 257-396.

Hutchinson, J. and J. M. Dalziel, 1954-1972, *Flora of West Tropical Africa*. Crown Agents, Milbank, London, 2nd. ed., 3 vols., published in 5 parts.

Idemudia, O. G. and D. E. U., Ekong, 1968, Constituents of Some West African Members of the Genus *Terminalia. First Inter-African Symposium on Traditional Pharmacopoeias and African Medicinal Plants*. OUA/STRC, Dakar, Publ. No. 104.

Inikori, J.E., 1978, «La traite négrière et les économies atlantiques de 1451 à 1870», in: *La traite négrière du XVè au XIXè siècles: Histoire générale de l'Afrique, Etudes et documents 2*, Paris, UNESCO, pp. 58-91.

Iroko, Abiola, Félix, 1982, «Le rôle des termitières dans l'histoire des peuples de la République du Bénin des origines à nos jours», in: *Bulletin de l'IFAN*, T. 44, série B, No. 1-2, janv-avril, pp. 50-75.

Iroko, Abiola, Félix, 1984, «Le spectacle de la mort à Cotonou des origines à nos jours: un essai d'histoire des mentalités», in: *Le mois en Afrique*, No. 227-228, pp. 133-133.

Irvine, F. R., 1930, *Plants of the Gold Coast*. Oxford University Press, London, 868pp.

Irvine, F. R., 1961, *Woody Plants of Ghana*, 2nd ed., Oxford University Press, London, 868pp.

Iyasera, Soloman, O., 1975, 'Oral Tradition in the Criticism of African Literature', in: *The Journal of Modern African Studies*, Vol. 13, No. 1, pp. 107-119.

Izard, M., 1985, «Les peuples et les royaumes de la boucle du Niger et du bassin des volta du XIIe au XVè siècles», in: *Histoire générale de l'Afrique*, T. IC, l'Afrique du XIIe au XVIè siècles, ch. IX, UNESCO/NEA, Paris, 237-263.

Jackson, Michael, 1978, 'An Approach to Kuranko Divination', *Human Relations* 31 (2) 117-38.

Jacob, Alain, 1974, *Armes blanches de l'Afrique Noire*, Paris, Rou-Radesley, 83p.

Jacob, André, 1982, «Comptes rendus» (P. Bordier, Ce que parler veut dire. L'économie des échanges klinguistiques, ed. Fauard, 1986, 244 p.), in: *L'homme et la Société*, No. 65-66, juillet-déc., pp. 197-198.
Jacob, André, 1982, «Le langage et à la révolution», in: *L'Homme et la Société*, No. 63-64, janvier-juin, pp. 3-6
Jacquemain, H., 1970, Recherches sur les anthocyanes foliaires de trois arbres tropicaux: *Mangifera indica L., Theobroma cacao L., Lophira alata* Banks ex Gaertn. Thèse Paris, 1970, *Plantes Médicinales et Phytothérapie*, 4, 230-50, 306-41; (1971) 5, 45-94.
Jahoda, Gustav, 1971, *The Psychology of Superstition*. New York, Penguin.
Jaulin, Robert, 1961, *La géomancie: Analyse formelle*, Paris, Mouton, 199p.
Jaynes, Julian, 1976, *The Origins of Consciousness in the Breakdown of the Bicameral Mind*. Boston, Houghton-Mifflin.
Johnson, Gabriel Kuaovi, 1952, «Le cauri chez les Gen Mina du bas Togo», in: *Notes Africaines*, No. 53, janvier, pp. 20-21.
Johnson, Gabriel Kwakovi, 1965, *Numérotation en langue Gen ou Gegbe - mina - popo du bas Togo*, essai d'un nouveau mode de comptage, Lomé, Institut Togolais de Sciences Humaines, 16p.
Jousse, Marcelle, 1978, *L'Anthropologie du geste: le parlant, la parole et le souffle*, Paris, Gallimard, 329p.
Jousse, M., 1981, *Le style oral*, Fondation Marcel Jous, Paris (1ère édition).
Jules-Rosette, Benneta, 1978, 'The Veil of Objectivity: Prophecy, Divination', *American Anthropologist* 80(3), 549-70.
Julliot, C.I., 1919, *L'éducation de la mémoire*, Paris.
Junod, H.A., 1932, «Le sacrifice de l'ancestrolatrie Sud-Africaine», in: *Archives de psychologie*, T. XXIII, No. 32, juillet, pp. 305-335.
Kallaway, A., 1984, *Guirault, Guérisseurs, itinéraires des Andes, recherche sur les pratiques médicales et magiques*, Paris, ORSTOM, 668p.
Karl, E., 1968, *Traditions historiques orales au Dahomey et dans le Golfe du Bénin*, SL, UNESCO, 421p.
Karl, E., 1974, *Traditions orales au Dahomey, Bénin, Niamey, Centre Régional de Documentation pour la tradition orale*, 420p.
Karp, Ivan, 1960, Introduction to *Explorations in African Systems of Thought*, ed. Ivan Karp and Charles S. Bird, Bloomington: Indiana University Press, 1-10.
Keeley, L. H., 1980, *Experimental Determination of Stone Tool Uses*, Chicago.
Kerharo, J. and A. Bouquet, 1950, *Plantes Médicinales de la Côte d'Ivoire et Haute Volta* Vigot, Paris, 297pp.
Kerharo, J., 1968, «Les plantes magiques dans la pharmacopée traditionnelle (sénégalaise)», in: *Ethnoatria*, Vol. II, No. 11, Anno., pp. 3-6.

Kerharo, J., 1969, «La noix de cola, origine et histoire, emploi, chimie et parmacologie», in: *Médecine d'Afrique noire*, No. 6, Juin, 5p.

Kerharo, J., 1969, «Le facteur magico-religieux dans l'exercice de la médecine traditionnelle en milieu sénégalais», in: *Médecine d'Afrique Noire*, Tome XVI, No. 8-9, avril-septembre, p. 651-655.

Kerharo, J., 1974, *La pharmacopée sénégalaise traditionnelle, plantes médicinales et toniques* (avec la collaboration pour la partie botanique de G. Adam, Paris, Vigot Frères, 54p.

Khan, M. R., G. Ndaalio, M. H. H., Nkunya, H. Wevers and A. N. Sawhney, 1980b, 'Studies on African Medicinal Plants. Preliminary Screening of Medicinal Plants for Antibacterial Activity', *Planta Medica*, Suppl., 91-7.

Ki-Zerbo, J., 1969, «La tradition orale en tant que source pour l'his africaine», in: *Diogène*, septembre.

Ki-Zerbo, J., 1972, *Histoire de l'Afrique noire, d'hier à demain*, Hatier, Paris, 702p.

Kiethega, J.B., 1981, «La carte du fer en Haute-Volta», in: *Recherche, Pédagogie et Culture*, No. 55, sept-Déc: 83-86 + cartes.

Kiethega, J.B., 1988, «Etat des recherches sur la production traditionnelle du fer au Burkina Faso», Communication au *Séminaire sur l'Histoire*, Novembre, UNB, Abomey-Calavi, 30p.

Kikassa Lukala M., Kibwenge, E., 1986, «Le N'Kier, Un rituel de guérison chez les Yansi», in: *Le mois en Afrique*, No. 243-244, avril-mai, pp. 115-128.

Kirwen, Michael C., 1987, *The Missionary and the Diviner*. Mary Knoll, N.Y., Orbis Books.

Klaus, D., 1980, 'Climatological Aspects of the Spatial and Temporal Variations of the Southern Saharan Margin', *Palaoecology of Africa* 12, 315-31.

Kokwaro, O., 1976, *Medicinal Plants of East Africa*. East African Literature Bureau, Nairobi, Dar-es-Salaam.

Koly, Dominique, 1985, «Rcherche linguistique théorique et appliqué», in: *La définition d'une stratégie relative à la promotion des langues africaines*, UNESCO, CLT/85/WS/72, p. 229-226., Document de la réunion d'experts Conakry, Guinée du 21 au 25 septembre.

Kossou, B., 1988, «Cultures africaines. Comment survivre?», in: *Entente africaine*, revue trimestrielle, No. 74, septembre, p. 57 à 63.

Krzyzaniak, L., 1978, 'New Light on Early Food-production in the Central Sudan', *Journal of African History*, 19, 159-72.

Kuukure, Edward, 1985, *The Destiny of Man: Dagaare Beliefs in Dialogue with Christian Eschatology*. Frankfurt am Main: Peter Laing.

Labouret, H., 1922, «La divination en afrique Noire», *L'Anthropologie*, 31, 334-60.

Labouret, H., 1934, «Divination par les cauris à la Côte d'Ivoire», in: *Bulletin du musée de l'ethnographie du Trocadéro*, No. 6, juillet-décembre, pp. 4-11.
Lallo, J. W., G. J. Armelagos and R. P. Mensforth, 1977, 'The Role of Diet, Disease, and Physiology in the Origin of Porotic Hyperostosis', *Human Biology* 49(3), 471-83.
Lambo, T. A., 1961, 'A Form of Social Psychiatry in Africa', *World Mental Health*, 13(4), 190-203.
Lambo, T. A., 1968, 'Schizophrenia: Its Features and Prognosis in the African', in: *Deuxième Colloque Africain de Psychiatrie* (Dakar, Senegal, 5-9 mars) *Compte rendu*. Paris, Audecam.
Lambrecht, F. L., 1964, 'Aspects of the Evolution and Ecology of Tsetse Flies and Trypanosomiasis in the Prehistoric African Environment', *Journal of African History* 5(1), 1-24.
Langley, Ph., Ngom, M., 1979, *Technologies villageoises en Afrique de l'ouest et du centre Dakar*, ENDA-UNICEF, 412p.
Lapassade, Georges, 1982, «Les thérapies de la transe», in: *L'Homme et la société* No. 65-66, juillet-décembre, pp 77-106.
Laplatine, F.R., 1976, *Maladies mentales et thérapies traditionnelles en Afrique*, Paris, Delange, 156p.
Larelle, Louis, 1947, *La parole et l'écriture*, Paris, L'artisan du livre, 251p.
Lavondés, H., 1963, «Magie et langage», in: *L'homme*, Paris, Mouton, T. 3, No. 3, sept-décembre, pp. 109-117.
Laya, Diouldé, 1978, *La tradition orale, problèmatique et méthodologie des sources de l'histoire africaine*, Niamey, CRDTO, 18p.
Le Golf, Jacques, et Nora, P., 1974 (sous la direction de), *Faire de l'histoire*, 3 volumes, Editions Gallimard, Paris, pp. 230, 352 et 281.
Lebat, Serge, 1969, «Les gisements de minerai de fer d'Afrique noire occidentale» (Libéria, Sierra Léone, Guinée), in: *Cahiers d'Outre-Mer*, No. 85, janvier-mars, pp. 75-87.
Lebeuf, J. P., 1958, «Santé mentale et possession», in: *Désordres mentaux et santé mentale en Afrique au sud du sahara/Mental Disorders and Mental Health in Africa South of the Sahara* (CCTA/SCA-WFMH-WHO Meeting of Specialists on Mental Heath, Bukavu) (SDcientific Council for Africa South of the Sahara, publ. No. 35), London Commission for Technical Co-operation in Africa South of the Sahara, pp. 164-67.
Lebiche, A., n.d., «Notes pour servir à l'histoire Maure (notes sur les forgerons, les Kunta, et les maures du Hod)», in: *Bulletin de l'IFAN*, No. 2, pp. 737-750.
Lechat, P. F., 1978, Bisseliches, F Bournerias, H Dechy, Y Juillet, G. Lagier, C Merynignac, B Rouveix, P Sterin, A Warnet and S Weber, *Pharmacologie Médicale*, 3rd edn., Masson, Paris, 677pp.

Leger, J.M., 1982, «Incidences de certaines croyances popu-populaires (sorcellerie) sur la pratique médicale courante», in: *Revue Médicale Suisse Romande* 102p., pp. 629-639.

Lehman, J. P. & Memel Foté, H., 1967, «Le cercle du prophète et du sorcier», *Psychopathologie Africaine*, 3(1), 81-119.

Lepreux, Marc, 1954, *Médecine, magie, sorcellerie*, Paris, PUF, 287p.

Leroi-Gouchan, A., 1950, *Evolution et Techniques - Milieu et Techniques*, Paris, Albin Michel, 512p.

Leroi-Gourhan, André, 1974, «Les voies de l'histoire avant l'écriture» (Ways and Byways of History Before Writing), in: *Le Golf, Jacques and Nore, Pierre*, (eds.) Faire de l'histoire (Making History), Gallimard, Paris.

Levi Makarius, Laura, 1974, *Le sacré et la violence des intérêts*, Paris, Payot, 379p.

Levi-Strauss, C., 1974, *Anthropologie structurale*, éd. Plon, Paris.

Levi-Strauss, C.I., 1955, *Tristes tropiques*, Gallimard, Paris.

Lévy-Bruhl, Lucien, 1966, *Primitive Mentality* (1923), Boston, Beacon Press.

Lévy-Strauss, Claude, 1966,. *The Savage Mind*. Chicago University of Chicago Press.

Lewis Hall, L., 1988, *Hausa Medecine: Illness and Well Being in a West African Culture*, Durham (North Cardinal), Duke University Press, 369p.

Lhote, H., 1952, «La connaissance du fer en Afrique Occidentale», Encyclopédie mensuelle d'Outre-Mer, 25 septembre, 262-272.

Lhote, H., 1977, «Technique des potiers de la région de Tessaoua (Niger)», in: *Notes Africaines*, No. 53, janvier, pp 12-18.

Lienhardt, Godrey, 1970, *Divinity and Experience: The Religion of the Dinka*, Oxford Clarendon Press.

Lo, Modou, 1984, *Pharmacopée sénégalaise pratique*, Dakar, (thèse), pharmacie, 164p.

Loewe, Michael and Carmen Blacker, eds., 1981, *Oracles and Divination*, Boulder, Colorado Shambhala.

Lombard, J, 1967, «Les cultes de possession en Afrique noire et le Bore Hausa», *Psychopathologie Africaine*, 3 (3), 419-39.

Lombard, J., 1987, «Contribution à l'histoire d'une ancienne société politique du Dahomey: la royauté d'Allada», in: *Bulletin de l'IFAN*, Tome XXXIX série B, No. 1-2, p. 40-66.

MacArthur, R. H., 1972, *Geographical Ecology*, New York, Harper and Row.

MacGaffey, Wyatt, 1981, 'African Ideology and Belief: A Survey', *African Studies Review* 24(2-3), 227-74.

Mair, Lucy, 1969, *Witchcraft*, London, Weidenfeld and Nicolson.

Makinde, M. Akim, 1988, *African Philosophy, Culture and Traditional Medicine* (Monographs, International Studies Africa Series No. 53). Ohio, Ohio University Press, 154p.

Makki, A., 1989, «Vers une communauté de recherche pour le développement endogène» (congrès du CRDE, Bamako, Mali 30/1 au 4/2 1989), in: *Génève-Afrique*, Vol.XXVII, No. 1, pp. 123-126.

Maldiney, Henri, 1982, «Langue et révolution», in: *L'homme et la société*, No. 63-64, janvier-juin, pp. 117-150.

Maley, J., 1972, «La sédimentation pollinique actuelle dans la zone du lac Tchad» (Afrique Centrale), *Pollen et Spores* 3, 253-307.

Maret (de), P., 1981, «L'évolution monétaire du Shaba central entre le 7è et le 18è siècle», *African Economic History*, 10.

Martinet, A., 1970, *Eléments de linguistique générale*, Paris Armand Colin.

Martinet, André, 1975, *Exploitation des langues et reconstruction*, Paris, PUF, 261p.

Marwick, M. G., 1973, 'How Real is the Charmed Circle in african and Western Thought?' *Africa* 43(1), 59-70.

Mary, André, 1963, «L'alternative de la vision et de la possession dans les sociétés religieuses et thérapeutiques du Gabon», in: *Cahiers d'Etudes Africaines*, Vol. XXII - 3, No. 91, pp. 281-310.

Masson, G., 1939, «Médecins et sorciers en pays bamiléké», in: *L'Anthropologie* T. 49, No. 3-4, juillet, p. 313-332.

Mauny, R., 1952, «Essai sur l'histoire des métaux en Afrique occidentale», in: *Bulletin de l'IFAN*, T. XIV, No. 2, Avril 1952, pp. 545-595.

Mauny, R., 1970, *Les siècles obscurs de l'Afrique noire - Histoire et archéologie*, Paris, Fayard, 314 pages.

Mauny, R., 1973, «Datation au carbone 14 d'amas de coquillages des lagunes de Basse Côte d'Ivoire», *West African Journal of Archaeology*, 3, 207-14.

Maupoil, B., 1943, *Contribution à l'étude de l'origine musulmane de la géomancie au bas Dahomey*, Paris, Université de Paris, 95p.

Maupoil, B., 1961, *La géomancie à l'ancienne Côte des Esclaves* (Travaux et Mémoires de l'Institut d'Ethnographie, No. 42), Paris, Institut d'Ethnographie XLII, 688p. (nouv. édit., 1981).

Maurice, Albert, 1958, «Vestige du néolithique et croyances au nord Dahomey», in *Notes Africaines* No. 79, juillet, pp. 67-172.

Mc Master, Mary, A., 1985, 'Advances in the Study of African Iron Technology', in: *Canadian Journal of African Studies*, Vol 19, No. 2, pp. 449-451, (Compte rendu de: Kense 1983 (Français), Traditional African Iron Working, Galgary Alberta, Department of Archaelogy, University of Calgary, 206p.

McMaster, D.N., n.d., 'Speculations on the Coming of the Banana to Uganda', *Journal of Tropical Geography* 16, 57-69.

Medeiros (de), F., 1989, «Premières fouilles archéologiques et alli, au Togo, à Notse», *Education béninoise*, No. 3-4: 128-132.

Medeiros (de), F., 1989, «Africanisme et historiographie africaine», communication au colloque du cinquantenaire de l'Institut Fondamental d'Afrique noire, Dakar (Sénégal) février-mars.

Megaw, J. V. S., 1977, *Hunters, Gatherers and First Farmers Beyond Europe*, Leicester,.

Memel Foté, H., 1962, «Rapport sur la civilisation animiste», in: *Colloque sur les religions*, Paris, Présence Africaine, pp. 31-58.

Michelet, Julet, 1966, *La sorcière*, Paris, Flammarion, 314p.

Middleton, John, 1955, 'The Concept of Bewitching in Lugbara', in: *Africa*, T. 25, No. 3, juillet, pp. 252-260.

Mokhtar, G (ed.), 1981, UNESCO *General History of Africa*-11, London.

Monfouga-Nicolas, J., 1972, *Ambivalence et culte de possession*, Paris, Anthropos.

Monteil, C., 1931, «La divination chez les Noires de l'Afrique occidentale française», *Bulletin du Comité d'Etudes Historiques et Scientifiques de l'Afrique Occidentale française*, 14(1-2), 72-136.

Montserrat, Palau Marti, 1958, «Croyances africaines», in: *Notes Africaines*, No. 80, oct., pp. 106-107.

Moore, Omar Khayyam, 1979, 'Divination - A New Perspective', in *Reader in Comparative Religion*, 4th ed., William A. Lessa and Evon Z. Vogt, 376-79, New York, Harper and Row.

Morat, Paul, 1965, «Sur le Dahomey Méridional» (compte rendu de «les pays du bas oumé» par Paul Pélissier), in: *Revue de Géographie de l'Afrique occidentale*, No. 1-2, pp. 191-196.

Mortabau Degbe, Faustin, 1991, *Contribution à l'étude de la pharmacopée traditionnelle au bénin*, Dakar thèse pharmacie, 138p.

Mounim, Georges, 1974, *Histoire de la Linguistique des origines au 20ème siècle*, Pathé Diagne, Dakar, 54p.

Mulonda, K., Bakodianjila, T., Tshimanga, M. et Matuhu, M., 1986, «Le Nupongo», in: *Le mois en Afrique*, No. 239-240, pp. 106-114 (1ère partie).

Mulonda, K., Bakodianjila, T., Tshimanga, M. et Matuhu, M., 1986, «Le Mupongo», in: *Le mois en Afrique* No. 241-242, février-mars, pp. 108-120 (2ème partie).

Munson, P. J., 1976, 'Archaelogical Data on the Origins of Cultivation in the Southwestern Sahara and their Implications for West Africa', in *Harlan et al.*, 187-210.

Murdoch, G. P., 1959, *Africa in Peoples and their Culture History*, New York, McGraw-Hill.

Ndiaye, Moctar, Justin, 1977, *Contribution à l'étude de la pharmacopée traditionnelle au Sénégal oriental*, Dakar, Université, 85p.

Needham, Rodney, 1972, *Belief, Language, and Experience*, Oxford, Blackwell.

Needham, Joseph, 1986, 'Science and Civilization in China', Vol. 6, 1, *Botany*, Cambridge, Cambridge University Press.

Nehaer, N., 1979, 'Awka Who Travel: Itinerant Metal Metalsmith of Southern Nigeria', *Africa*, 49 (4): 352-355.

Nescott, Roger, W., 1967, *African Languages and African Prehistory*, Boston University Press, 10p.

Ngoma, F., 1963, *L'initiation Ba-Kongo et sa signification*, Paris Centre d'étude des problèmes sociaux indigènes, Collection de mémoires.

Ngubane, Harriet, 1977, *Body and Mind in Zulu Medicine*, London, Academic Press.

Nguyen Ba Tuoc, 1963, *Recherches botaniques, chimiques et pharmacodynamiques sur quelques drogues vermifuges d'Indochine*, Thèse de Pharmacie, Paris, 120pp.

Niane, D.T., 1985, «Le Mali et la deuxième expansion manden», in: *Histoire général de l'Afrique*, vol. IV. L'Afrique du XIIè au XVIè siècles, Paris, UNESCO/NEA, ch. VI: 141-196.

Obichama, E.N., 1967, 'Transition from Oral Tradition Toliterary Tradition', in: *Présence Africaine*, No. 63, 3e trismestre, pp. 14O-161.

Odutola, F. A. and D. E. U. Ekong, 1968, 'The Chemistry of some Traditional Antitussive Drugs of Nigeria, Communication, *Interafrican Symposium of Traditional Pharmacopoeias and African Medicinal Plants*, Dakar.

Ojha, D., S. N. Tripathi and G. Sing, 1966, 'Role of an Indigenous Drug (*Achyranthes aspera*) in the Management of Reaction of Leprosy', Preliminary observations, *Leprosy Review*. 37, 115.

Okou, Gani, 1965, «Superstitions Nord-dahoméennes», in: *Notes Africaines*, No. 65, janvier, pp. 16-20.

Oliver, B., 1960, *Medicinal Plants in Nigeria*, Private ed., Nigerian College of Arts, Science and Technology, 138pp.

Ortigues, M. C. & Ortigues, E., 1973, *Oedipe africain* (rev. ed.), Paris, Union Générale d'Editions, (1ère éd. 1966).

Palou, J., 1980, *La sorcellerie*, Paris, PUF, 128p.

Pareinder, Geoffrey, 1986, *Esprits et sorciers d'Afrique Noire*, Paris, Laffont, 143p.

Parin, Paul, 1976, «Anthropologie et psychiatrie», in: *Psychopathologie africaine*, Vol. XII, No. 1, pp. 91-107.

Paris, R. R. and H. Moyse, 1963, *Abrégé de matière médicale, matières premières d'origine végétale*, I vol., Vigot, Paris.

Paris, R. R. and H. Moyse, 1965, *Précis de matière médicale*, I vol., Masson et Cie, Paris.

Paris, R. R. and H. Moyse, 1967, *Précis de matière médicale*, Vol. II, Masson et Cie, Paris.

Paris, R. R. and H. Moyse, 1971, *Précis de matière médicale*, Vol. III, Masson et Cie, Paris.
Park, G. K., 1963, 'Divination and its Social Contexts', *J. Royal Anthropological Inst.*, 93(2), 195-209.
Parkington, J. E., 1972, 'Seasonal Mobility in the Later Stone Age', *African Studies*, 31, 223-43.
Parrinder, Geoffrey, 1963, *Witchcraft: European and African*, London, Faber and Faber, 215p.
Parrinder, Geoffrey, 1986, *Esprits et sorciers d'Afrique noire*, Paris, Laffont, 143p.
Paulme, D., 1965, «Oracles grecs et devins africains», *Revue d'Histoire des Religions*, 159, 145-157.
Pauwels, R.P., 1949, 'The Masaka a Cylinder: An Interpretation of its Use', by M. Requaert, (with on appendix dealing with divination by means of fat), in: *The Uganda*, Vol. XIII, No. 1, pp. 23-27.
Pauwels, R.P., 1953, «La magie du Rwanda», in: *Annalilateranensi*, vol 17, pp. 83-115.
Pauwels, R.P., 1954, «La divination au Rwanda», in: *Kango overzee*, T.XX, No. 4-5, pp. 293-368.
Peake, H. J. E., 1927, 'The Beginnings and the Early Spread of Agriculture', *Nature* 119, 894-96.
Peake, H. J. E., 1928, *The Origins of Agriculture*, London, Ernest Benn.
Peek, Philip, M., 1981, 'The Power of Words in African Verbal Arts', *Journal of American Folklore*, 94(371), 19-43.
Peek, Philip, M., 1982, 'The Divining Chain in Southern Nigeria', in *African Religious Groups and Beliefs*, ed. S. Ottenberg, Meerut, India, Folklore Institute, 187-205.
Peek, Philip, M., 1985, 'Ovia Idah and Eture Egbedi: Traditional Nigerian Artists', *African Arts* 18(2), 54-59, 10.
Pelt, J. M., 1959, *Contribution à l'étude des huiles de chaulmoogra africaines*, Thèse de Doctorat en Pharmacie, Université de Nancy.
Pelton, Robert, D., 1980, *The Trickster in West Africa*, Berkeley, University of California Press.
Penel, Jean-Dominique, 1986, «Langues africaines et philosophie des sciences», actes du colloque international sur Langues africaines et philosophie, Cotonou, 10 décembre, pp. 79-100.
Petrequin, P., 1984, *Habitat lacustre du Bénin: une approche ethno archéologique*, Paris, Recherche sur les civilisations, 214p.
Phillipson, D. W., 1975, 'The Chronology of the Iron Age in Bantu Africa', *Journal of African History* 16, 321-42.

Phillipson, D. W., 1985, *African Archeology*, Cambridge, Cambridge University Press.

Pianka, E. R., 1974, *Evolutionary Ecology*, New York, Harper and Row.

Podlewski, André Michel, 1971, «La dynamique des principales populations du nord Cameroun», in: *Cahiers de l'ORSTOM*, série sciences humaines, Vol. VII, No. spécial, pp. 29-34.

Pole, L.M., 1975, 'Iron Working Apparatus Techniques: Upper Region of Ghana', *West African Journal of Archaelogy*, 5: 11-39.

Porteres, R., 1938, «A propos de l'industrie du fer en Afrique occidentale dans la zone forestière», *Bulletin du Comité d'études Historiques et Scientifiques de l'AOF*, t. XXI, No. 3, 463-466.

Portères, R., 1950, «Vieilles agricultures de l'Afrique intertropicale», *Agronomie tropicale* 5, 489-507.

Portères, Roland, 1960, «La monnaie de fer dans l'ouest africain au XXè siècle», in: *Journal d'Agriculture Tropicale et de Botanique Appliquée*, Vol VII, No. 1-2-3, pp. 97-109.

Portères, R., 1962, «Berceaux agricoles primaires sur le continent africain», *Journal of African History* 3, 195-210.

Portères, R., 1976, 'African Cereals: Eleusine, Fonio, Black Fonio, Teff, *Brachiaria, paspalum, Pennisetum*, and African Rice', in J.R. Harlan, J.R.J. de Wet and A.B.L., Stemler, eds., Origins of African Plant Domestication, The Hague, Mouton, 409-52.

Posnasky, M., 1973, 'Aspects of Early West African Trade', *World Archaeology*, 5, 149-62.

Posnasky, M. and McIntash, R., 1976, 'New Radiocarbon Dates for Northern and Western Africa', *Journal of African History*, 17, 161-95.

Posnasky, M., 1976, 'Archaelogy and the Origins of the Akan Society in Ghana', in: *Sieveking et al.*, 49-59.

Poynter, F. N. L., 1971, «Médecine africaine», in: *Médecines traditionnelles et art d'Afrique noire*, ed. J. Sonolet, Paris, Expansion Scientifique Française, pp. 5-9 (Introduction).

Preneuf, Chantal, 1969, «L'homme qui fait planter les arbres», in: *Psychopathologie africaine*, Vol. 5, No. 3, pp. 395-460.

Quenum, Faustin, 1965, «Athiémé, divination chez les Adjas», in: *Traits d'Union*, No. 6, janvier-février, pp. 9-11.

Quine, W. V. O., 1975, 'Mind and Verbal Dispositions', in *Mind and Language*, Oxford University Press.

Rabeding, J. F., 1976, *Pratique de divination à Madagascar, technique de Sikily en pays Sakalava*, Paris, ORSTOM, 234p. (mémoire).

Radji, A., 1987, «Médecine et pharmacopée traditionnelles en République Populaire du Bénin», in: *Bulletin de liaison ACCT*, Vol. 1,.

Ramat, Paolo, 1985, *Typologie linguistique*, Paris, PUF, 139p.

Rattray, R. S., 1923, *Ashanti*, London, Oxford University Press.

Rattray, R. S., 1916, 'The Iron Workers of Akpafu', *Journal of Royal Anthropological Institute*, vol. XLVI: 431-435.

Ravise, A., 1970, «Industrie néolithique en os de la région de St. Louis, Sénégal», *Notes Africaines*, 128, 97-102.

Ray, Benjamin, 1976, *African Religions: Symbols, Ritual and Community*, Englewood Cliffs, N.J., Prentice-Hall.

Rebout, Georges, 1948, «Un axiome universel», in: *La revue scientifique*, No. 3288, janvier, pp. 21-26.

Retel-Laurentin, A., 1969, *Oracles et ordalies chez les Nzakara*, Paris, Mouton.

Rigby, Peter, 1975, 'Prophets, Diviners, and Prophetism: The Recent History of Kiganda Religion', *Journal of Anthropological Research*, 31(2), 116-48.

Rivallain, J. et Iroko, A.F., Paléomonnaies africaines, les cauris, 25-40, Les collections monétaires. Administration des monnaies et médailles, Paris, 1986.

Rivallain, J., and Iroko, A. F,.1986, «Paleomonnaies africaines, les cauris», 25-40, *Les collections monétaires, administration des monnaies et médailles*, Paris.

Rivière, Claude, 1983, «Bibliographie», in: *Le Mois en Afrique*, No. 227-227, décembre 1984-Jjnvier 1985, pp 169-170 - de: Auge, Marc, Herzlich, Claudine, Le sens du Mal-Anthropologie, Histoire, Sociologie, de la Maladie, Paris, 280p.

Rivière, Claude, 1984, «La grossesse chez les Evé du Togo», in: *Le Mois en Afrique*, No. 227-228, pp. 120-132.

Rognon, P., 1976, *Le massif de l'Atakora et ses bordures: études géomorphologique*, Paris, CNRS.

Sadji, M., 1974, «Le mythe et la sorcellerie», in: *Notes Africaines*, No. 41, janvier, pp 16-20.

Sahlins, M. D., and E. R. Service, (eds.), 1960, *Evolution and Culture*, Ann Arbor, University of Michigan Press.

Sangmuah, E., 1968, 'The Healing (Spiritual) Therapy in Ghana, Ankaful Hospital, Ghana', in: *Deuxième Colloque Africain de psychiatrie* (Dakar, Sénégal, 5-9 mars), Compte rendu, Paris, Audecam, pp. 104-111.

Sarnthein, M., 1978 'Sand Deserts during Glacial Maximum and Climatic Optimum, *Nature* 272, 43-46.

Sauer, C. O., 1952, *Agricultural Origins and Disperals*, New York, American Geographic Society.

Sauer, M., 1969, *Seeds, Spades, Hearths and Herds*. (Reprint of 1952 ed.) Cambridge, Mass, MIT Press.

Saussure de, F., 1969, *Cours de linguistique générale*, Payot, Paris.

Schneider, J. L., 1967, «Evolution du dernier lacustre AND peuplements préhistoriques au Pays-Bas du Tchad», *Bulletin de l'Association sénégalaise pour l'étude du Quaternaire de l'Ouest africain* 14-15, 19-23.

Sene, P. M., 1985, «La parole pensée», in *Notre Librairie*, No. 81 octobre-décembre.

Servant, M. and S. Servant-Vildary, 1970, «Les formations lacustres et les diatomés du Quaternaire récent du fond de la cuvette tchadienne», *Revue de géographie physique et de géologie dynamique* 12(1), 63-76.

Shaw, B. D., 1976, 'Climate Environment and Prehistory in the Sahara', *World Archaelogy* 8(2), 133-149.

Shaw, T., 1981, 'The Late Stone Age in West Africa and the Beginnings of African Food Production', in *Roubet et al.*, 213-35.

Silla, Ousmane, 1968, «Religion traditionnelle et technique thérapeutiques des lébu du Sénégal», in: *Bull. de l'IFAN*, tome XXX, série B, No. 4, octobre, pp. 1566-1580.

Smith, A. B., 1974, 'Preliminary Report of Excavation at Karkarichinkat Nord and Sud, Tilemsi Valley, Mali, Spring 1972', *West African Journal of Archaelogy*, 4, 33-55.

Smith, A. B., 1979, 'Biogeographical Considerations of Colonization of the Lower Tilemsi Valley in the Second Millennrum B.C.', *Journal of Arid Environments* 2, 355-361.

Soglo, G., 1987, «Gù, dieu des forges: culte et rites», in: *Cahiers des Archives du sol*, I:81-98.

Soule de Laffont, D., 1958, *Rapport complémentaire sur le gisement de fer de la rive sénégalaise du bassin de la Falémé (Sénégal)*, Dakar, Haut. Comm. de la Rép. en Afrique occidentale française, service de Géologie et de Prospection Minière, 44p.

Souroy, J. Ch., 1952, *Sorciers noirs et sorciers blancs, la magie, la sorcellerie et ses drames en Afrique*, Bruxelles, Librairie encyclopédique, 264p.

Souza (de), S., 1987, *Flore du Bénin, catalogue des plantes du Bénin, Tome 1*, publié par la Mission Française de Coopération et d'Action culturelle de Cotonou, Bénin.

Souza (de), S., 1988, *Flore du Bénin*, noms des plantes dans les langues nationales béninoises, Tome 3, publié par la mission française de coopération et d'action culturelle de Cotonou, Bénin.

Sow, I., 1977, *Psychiatrie dynamique africaine* (Bibliothèque scientifique), Paris, Payot.

Spooner, B. J., 1973, *The Cultural Ecology of Pastoral Nomads*, Modules in Anthropology No. 45, Reading, Mass, Addison-Wesley.

Stanton, W. R., 1962, 'The Analysis of the Present Distribution of Varietal Variation in Maize, Sorghum, and Cowpea in Nigeria as an Aid to the Study of Tribal Movements', *Journal of African History* 3, 251-61.

Steveking, G. de G. *et al.*, 1976, *Problems in Economic and Social Archaeology*, London.

Stoller, Paul, and C. Olkes, 1987, *In Sorcery's Shadow: A Memoir of Apprenticeship among the Songhay of Niger*, Chicago, University of Chicago Press.

Summers, R., 1969, *Ancient Mining in Rhodesia*, Salisbury.

Suret-Canale, J., 1973, *3ème édition Afrique Noire: géographie civilisations, histoire*, Paris, Editions Sociales, 395p.

Surgy (de) Albert, 1982, *La géomancie et le culte d'AFA chez les EVHE du littoral*, Paris, publications orientalistes de France, 44p.

Surgy (de) Albert, 1987, *La divination chez les Mwaba-Gurma (Nord Togo): L'initiation du devin et la pratique divinatoire*, Paris, L'Harmattan, Vol. 2, 319p.

Sutton, J.E.J., 1982, 'Archaelogy in West Africa: A Review of Recent Work and a Further List or Radiocarbon Dates', *Journal of African History*, 23,3: 291-313.

Sylla, Yéro, 1985, *Manuel de linguistique africaine. L'argumentation en syntaxe*, Dakar, UNESCO, 22p.

Tchitchi, Y. Tousaint, 1984, *Systématique de l'àjagbè, thèse pour le Doctorat de 3ème cycle*, Université Sorbonne Nouvelle, Paris III.

Tchitchi, Y. Toussaint, 1986, «Langues africaines et problèmes de terminologies», Actes du colloque international sur le thème *Langues africaines et philosophie*, pp. 1-23.

Tchitchi, Y. Toussaint, 1987, «Typologie de l'énoncé nominal dans quatre parlers gbè», *Cahiers d'études linguistique* No. 2, Abomey-Calavi.

Terell, J., 1977, 'Biology, Biogeography of Man', *World Archaelogy* 8(3), 237-48.

Thomas, Jacqueline, M.C., 1980, *La linguistique africaniste française: en France et en Afrique: le point sur la question*, Paris, SELAF, 114p.

Thomas, L. V., 1977, *Les sages dépossédés: univers magiques d'Afrique noire*, Paris, René Laffont, 306p.

Thompson, Judith, Susan, M. Perry, Gérald, J., 1991, 'Juju-soup: The Witch Herbalist's Solution for Infertility', in *African Studies Review*, Vol. 33, No. 1, avril, Georgia, Emory University, pp. 55-64.

Tiando, E., 1978, «Les techniques du fer en milieu Waaba, Tangamba, Daataba» annexe VI, in: *Perspctive historique des populations de l'Atakora, l'exemple des Waaba-Tangamba-Daataba*, mémoire de maîtrise, UNB Abomey-Calavi, 182-192.

Tidjani, Abdou Serpos, 1943, «Un procédé de divination au Dahomey, la gourde-pendule», in: *Bulletin de l'IFAN*, Vol. V, No. 1-4.

Tixier, J., 1963, *Typologie de l'Epipaléolithique du Maghreb*, Mémoires du CRAPE 2, Paris, Arts et Métiers Graphiques.

Tohoun Benjamin, 1979, «La numération décimale: le cas aja», Communication No. 2, *Actes du Séminaire National de Formation Linguistique*, Lokossa, 3-12 avril, Cnl pp. 164-178.

Toure, R.G., Demonbynes, P, 1958, *Outils traditionnels de l'Afrique Occidentale*, Bambey, CRA, 35p.

Traoré, Dominique, 1965, *Comment le noir se soigne-t-il, ou Médecine et magie africaines*, Paris, Présence Africaine, 647p.

Trautmann, René, 1940, *La divination à la Côte des Esclavages et à Madagascar: Le Vôdoû Fa-Le Sikidy*, Dakar, Institut Français d'Afrique Noir.

Tubiana, Joseph, 1980, «Les langues et l'Etat: Autonomies, indépendances», in: *Revue d'Etudes Politiques et Economiques Africaines*, No. 180-181, p. 143-148.

Turnbull, C. M., 1961, *The Forest People*, New York.

Turner, V. W., 1968, *The Drums of Affliction: A Study of Religious Processes among the Ndembu of Zambia*, Oxford Clarendon Press and the International African Institut.

Turner, Victor, 1967, *The Forest of Symbols*, Cornell University Press.

Tylecote, R. P., 1975, 'The Origin of Iron Smilting in Africa', *West African Journal of Archaeology*, 5, 1-19.

Ucko, P. J. and Dimbleby, G. W., 1969, *The Domestication and Exploitation of Plants and Animals*, London.

Uiso, F. W., 1979, *Traditional Medicine Research Unit, Annual Report*, Muhimbili Medical Center, University of Dar-es-Salaam, Tanzania.

Vansina, J., 1961, *De la tradition orale. Essai de méthode historique*, Tervuren, Musée royal d'Afrique centrale.

Vavilow, N. I., 1926, *Studies on the Origin of Cultivated Plants*, (Russian and English), Leningrad, Institute of Applied Botanical Plan Breeding.

Vendreyes, J., 1968, *Le langage: introduction linguistique à l'histoire*, Paris, Albin Michel, 444p.

Verger, Pierre, 1957, *Notes sur le culte des oracles et vodun à Bahia? La Baie de tous les Saints au Brésil et à l'ancienne côte des esclaves en Afrique*, Dakar, IFAN; No. 4, 609p.

Vernant, J-P, 1975, *Les origines de la pensée grecque*, Paris, PUF, 135p.

Vincke, J.L., n.d., «Linguistique Africaine: De la science exacte à la science morale», in: *Canadian Journal of African Studies*, Vol. 22, No. 2, pp. 310-316.

Wai-Ogusu, B., 1973, 'Was there a Sangoan Industry in West Africa?' *West African Journal of Archeology*, 3, 191-6.

Wantchecon, M. A., 1983, *Contribution à l'histoire des technologies anciennes du Bas-Bénin: l'exemple du travail du fer à Allada, des origines du royaume à la conquête aboméenne en 1724*, TER. Ecole Normale Supérieure, UNB, 47 p. + annexes.

Wantchecon, M. A, 1987, «Notes sur l'histoire de la métallurgie du fer dans l'ancien royaume d'Allada», in *Cahiers des Archives du sol*, No. 1, 73-81.

Waterlot, E. G., 1926, *Les bas-reliefs des bâtiments royaux d'Abomey* (Dahomey), Paris, Institut d'Ethnologie, Mémoire de l'Institut d'Ethnologie de Paris.

Watt J. M. and M. G. Breyer-Brandwijk, 1962, *The Medicinal and Poisonous plants of Southern and Eastern Africa*. Livingstone, Edimburgh and London, I vol., 1057pp.

Watt, J. M., 1967, 'African Plants Potentially Useful in Mental Health', *Lloydia*, 30, 1-22.

Weisrock, A. and P. Rognon, 1977, «Evolution morphologiqsue des basses vallées de l'atlas atlantique marocain», *Géologie méditerranéenne*, 4, 313-34.

Westerlund, David, 1985, *African Religion in African Scholarship*, Monograph No. 7, Studies Published by the Institut of Comparative Religion at the University of Stockholm, Almquist and Wiksell International.

Westerman, D. Bryan, M.A., 1970, *The languages of West Africa*, London, International African Institute, 277p.

White, L. A., 1959, *The Evolution of Culture*, New York, McGraw-Hill.

Willet, F., 1962, 'The Microlithic Industry from Old Oyo, Western Nigeria', *Actes du quatrième congrès panafricain de préhistoire et de l'étude du Quaternaire*, 261-71.

Williams, M. A. J., and Faure, H. (eds.), 1980, *The Sahara and the Nile*, Rotterdam, Balkema.

Wing J. Van, 1921, *Etudes Bakongo: sociologie-religion et magie* (2nd ed.), Bruges, Desclée de Brouwer (1ère éd.).

Winkelman, Michel, 1982, 'Magic : A Theoretical Reassessment', *Current Anthropology* 23(1), 37-66.

Xaio, P., 1983, 'Recent Developments on Medicinal Plants in China', *Journal of Ethnopharmacology*, 7, 95-109.

Yai, J. Olobiyi, 1968, «Remarques sur lEtat actuel des recherches linguistiques au Dahomey», in: *Présence Africaine*, No. 68, 4ème trismestre, pp. 153-163.

Yangni, Angaté, 1980, «La Médecine traditionnelle», *Bull. Ac. Nat. Médecin*, No. 5, 164p., 428-435.

Zahan, D., 1960, *Sociétés d'initiation bambara: le N'domo, le Korè*, Paris, Mouton.

Zahan, D., 1979, *The religion, Spiritually and Thought of Traditional Africa*, Chicago University of Chicago Press.

Zempleni, A., 1968, *L'interprétation de la thérapie traditionnelle du désordre mental chez les Wolof et les lébous* (Sénégal), Thèse de 3è cycle en psychologie, Paris, 543p.

Zempleni, A., 1969, «La thérapie traditionnelle des troubles mentaux chez les Wolof et les Lébou (Sénégal): principes», *Social Science and Medicine*, 3, 191-205.

Zohoun, Th, Dramane, K., 1988, «La perception du concept de la médecine préventive dans la société traditionnelle africaine: A propos de l'expérience de la République Populaire du Bénin», in: *Bulletin médical pharm*, Vol. 2, No. 1, pp. 57-65.

Zuesse, Evan, M., 1979, *Ritual Cosmos: The Sanctification of Life in african Religions*, Athen, Ohio University Press.

www.ingramcontent.com/pod-product-compliance
Lightning Source LLC
Chambersburg PA
CBHW071414230926
51846CB00001B/83
* 9 7 8 2 8 6 9 7 8 0 4 0 8 *